Readers tell us that EATER'S CHOICE really works . . .

"Using the 10% saturated fat diet in your book I lowered my lipids from 347 mg/dL to 204 mg/dL. . . . The magnitude of the results was both rewarding and surprising."

Joe D. Burek, D.V.M., Doylestown, Pennsylvania

"I started on the 3% saturated fat regime and lowered my cholesterol from 249 to 145 without exercise and lost the 20 pounds I wanted to lose in the process. . . . Thank you for writing such a simple, easy-to-understand book."

Cary Lichtenstein, Chicago, Illinois

"Thank you for your wonderful book. . . . I have had a cholesterol problem for 3 years and have been unable to decrease it. After only 2 weeks on your food plan, my cholesterol dove from 220 to 199."

Mildred Kani, Kenner, Louisiana

"Thought you'd like to know that between your great recipes and sat-fat/cholesterol information and my husband's will power, he went from 340 to 220 in 4 months. We couldn't have done it without you!"

Adrienne Breen, Chicago, Illinois

and gives them the facts they need . . .

"Bravo! Your book provides everything one should know in order to outwit the heart attacker."

Mundy Torok, Dover, New Jersey

"Your book is a revelation — what I've been looking for for years. Now for the first time I have facts and figures, and it's simple for me to stay within our fat budget. It's very exciting to know what to do."

Bernadette Stubbs, San Jose, California

"I am proud to say that after 3 weeks and 5 days my total cholesterol went from 301 to 209. Thank you for your book, which made counting the sat-fats easy and fun."

Gary Crouch, San Antonio, Texas

EATER'S CHOICE is recommended by experts . . .

"I've recommended your book to all my patients needing cholesterol-control diets. I've given it numerous times as a gift — even since Christmas."

Mary H. Belenky, R.D., Arnold, Maryland

"Among all the cholesterol books from the technical/professional point of view, yours is the best."

Richard N. Podell, M.D., M.P.H., New Providence, New Jersey

"I loved your book! I am a nurse and work for a cardiologist. We have recommended your book to many of our patients."

Debbie Ouillette, Pinconning, Michigan

"I am the Health Educator for our Health Department. I have found your book to be an excellent, clear, and *practical* resource."

Eric Triffin, West Haven, Connecticut

and provides delicious eating!

"My compliments to the chef!"

Marcia Dunn, Pittsburgh, Pennsylvania

"A whole new way of living with food."

Carol Beatty, Montpelier, Vermont

"One of our patients came in for a check-up — cholesterol 301. I suggested *Eater's Choice*. Last week his cholesterol was 171. . . . He and his wife feel like they are eating gourmet meals all the time."

Naomi Shaiken, New York, New York

"The recipes are fantastic! No boredom here. I have not tried one that we haven't liked. Yours is the first book I turn to when trying to decide what to cook for company."

Debbie Bailey, Pittsburgh, Pennsylvania

"My husband had a 410 cholesterol count, and the diet sheets his doctor gave him totally confused me. I got *Eater's Choice*, and at the end of 6 weeks his chol was 198! . . . As an Iowa farm girl I learned to cook using all the 'good' things — lots of butter, eggs, cream, and meat. This gives you an idea of what a total change it has been for me. . . . Best of all, my husband tells anyone who listens how well he eats, how good the meals are, and how pleased he is."

Jean M. Gray, Scottsdale, Arizona

EATER'S CHOICE

A FOOD LOVER'S GUIDE TO LOWER CHOLESTEROL

Dr. Ron Goor and
Nancy Goor

Illustrations by Nancy Goor

For Dennis, Alicia, Michael & Angie, Best wishes! Ron & Nancy Goor

Third Edition

HOUGHTON MIFFLIN COMPANY
Boston New York

Copyright © 1987, 1989, 1992 by Ronald S. Goor
and Nancy Goor

For information about permission to reproduce
selections from this book, write to Permissions,
Houghton Mifflin Company, 215 Park Avenue
South, New York, New York 10003.

Library of Congress Cataloging-in-Publication Data
Goor, Ron.
  Eater's choice : a food lover's guide to lower
  cholesterol / Ron Goor and Nancy Goor ;
illustrations by Nancy Goor. — 3rd ed.
      p.   cm.
  Includes bibliographical references and index.
  ISBN 0-395-60572-5
  1. Low-cholesterol diet.   2. Low-cholesterol
diet — Recipes.   I. Goor, Nancy.   II. Title.
RM237.75.G66   1992   91-34002
613.2'6 — dc20   CIP

Printed in the United States of America

BTA 10 9 8 7 6 5

Book design by Joyce C. Weston

To the staff and participants of the
Coronary Primary Prevention Trial, whose
dedication and perseverance helped prove
that lowering blood cholesterol reduces
the risk of heart attack.

And to Charles Suther,
whose encouragement helped make
this book possible.

Acknowledgments

The authors wish to thank the many people who have contributed to the development of this book: Annette Arbel, Mary Evelyn Bedenbaugh, Robert Betting, Buffie Brownstein, Judy Chiostri, Karen Feinstein, Leslie Goodman-Malamuth, Charles and Jeanette Goor, Alex and Dan Goor, Ilene Gutman, Nancy Hallsted, Anita Hamel, Mary Hanke, Barbara Hilberg, Arlene Howard, Dr. Donald Hunninghake, Grace Hyslop, Eleanor Iverson, Sally and Carl Jones, Ann Jons, Esther Krashes, Dr. John LaRosa, Suzanne Lieblich, Bonnie Liebman, Morton Liftin, Eva MacLowry, Berengere and Jean-François Maquet, Sherri McKissick, Joy Mara, Alyssa Mezebish, Martin and Helen Miller, Linda Nelson, Nancy Ocshner, Dr. James and Ruth Phang, Muriel Rabin, Helen Rosenfeld, Isabelle Schoenfeld, Dr. Helmut Schrott, Judith Sheard, Lian Tsao, Philip Wagenaar, and Linda York.

CONTENTS

A NOTE ON THE THIRD EDITION

IN THE TWO YEARS since the first revision of *Eater's Choice* was published, interest in cholesterol has continued to grow. The National Institutes of Health (NIH) have announced cholesterol guidelines for children and adolescents. Recently published scientific evidence has shown that lowering blood cholesterol can cause regression of plaque blocking the coronary arteries. New cholesterol-lowering drugs have been introduced. Health fads, such as oat bran and fish oil tablets, have come and gone. Tropical oils are fast disappearing from our food supply. An explosion of new food products, claims, and marketing has capitalized on the public's desire to reduce cholesterol levels. Nonfat food substitutes have entered the market, and "Lite," "Lean," "Lower-in-fat," and "97% fat-free" products dominate grocery shelves. Even fast-food restaurants have jumped on the "low-fat" bandwagon.

To keep *Eater's Choice* current and responsive to your needs, we have made numerous changes and additions. You will be happy to know that we have reorganized the Food Tables and added new foods (including Chinese restaurant food and a multitude of commercial foods). At the suggestion of a reader, Robert R. Betting, we have inserted the very useful Food Tables Index to help you find specific foods in the Food Tables. We have also added a chapter to introduce and clarify the recommendations of the "National Cholesterol Education Program Report of the Expert Panel on Blood Cholesterol Levels in Children and Adolescents." We have expanded our discussion of lipoproteins to include lipoprotein ratios. To help you cope with high-fat commercial foods, we examine actual food labels and provide specific instructions on how to order out in restaurants. We have included step-by-step directions on how to keep a food record — the most effective tool for changing from a heart-risky, high-sat-fat diet to a heart-healthy diet that is low in saturated fat. And we discuss new information on exercise, olive oil, hydrogenated vegetable oils, and the importance of diet on the effectiveness of cholesterol-lowering drugs.

We have added 49 new, easy, and scrumptious low-sat-fat recipes to the 230 in the first revision. Try Blueberry Soup, Turkey with Capers, Chicken Fajitas, Cumin Wheat Bread, and Meringue Shells with Fresh Strawberries and Warm Raspberry Sauce for starters. If you own the original *Eater's Choice*, that means that you now have 80 new recipes (including 30 new recipes from the first revised edition). Writing *The Choose to Lose Diet* made us extremely aware of total fat as well as saturated fat. As a result, we have reduced the total fat calories of many of the *Eater's Choice* recipes. To help those following Choose to Lose, a list of the total fat calories of all the recipes in this edition begins on page 535.

We would like to thank you for your wonderful letters. When you write that you have lowered your cholesterol from 280 to 190, or that your friends adore Apricot Chicken Divine, or that your doctor recommended the book to you or you recommended *Eater's Choice* to your doctor (!), or that your whole family is eating more healthfully, we feel very, very good.

Our goals for this edition remain unchanged: we want you to understand how foods affect blood cholesterol and the risk of heart disease and, more specifically, how to evaluate your own diet and learn how to make heart-healthy food choices. High cholesterol is one of the few medical conditions that **you** can control simply and without sacrifice. Having a sat-fat budget allows you to fit in your high-sat-fat favorites as well as judge the sat-fat "cost" of all foods. The nearly 300 recipes in *Eater's Choice* allow you to experience the true pleasure of eating delicious food while lowering your cholesterol. Good luck!

— Dr. Ron Goor and
Nancy Goor

FOREWORD

MODERN MEDICINE deserves much credit for improving the health and longevity of Americans by reducing the incidence of many infectious diseases and other causes of death of the past. However, as Americans live longer, diseases of a somewhat different nature — chronic diseases — are taking a relatively larger toll. Just when many people reach the peaks of their careers or a much deserved retirement, their lives may be devastated by heart disease or cancer. Heart disease alone accounts for 50 percent of the deaths in the United States. It is a major cause of disability and a major drain on our emotional and financial resources, both national and personal.

Heart disease is the result of multiple risk factors associated with our high living standard: rich foods, smoking, lack of exercise. In other words, the American way of life may be dangerous to our health. But I am convinced that lifestyles can be changed; in fact, they are changing. Scientific evidence has proven that quitting smoking reduces the incidence of lung cancer and heart disease. Lowering blood pressure reduces the incidence of stroke and heart disease. It is gratifying to see the decline of these diseases in the segments of the population that have made changes. As a consequence, mortality from heart disease has declined by 30 percent and that from stroke by 45 percent in the past twenty years.

While an individual cannot be given a guarantee, these trends show that the adoption of a sensible lifestyle can prevent the development of diseases that threaten both the length and quality of life.

Now a major national public health campaign is being launched against a third, equally potent risk factor for heart disease: high blood cholesterol. Recent evidence has shown that lowering high levels of blood cholesterol will indeed reduce the risk of heart disease. Blood cholesterol levels can be lowered by eating less saturated fat and cholesterol.

The first step is consciousness raising. We need to become aware of the hazards of elevated blood cholesterol levels. To discover if you are at increased risk for heart disease, know your blood cholesterol number. High blood cholesterol is a silent killer. There are no symptoms to warn you until the disease is fully developed, and by then it is often too late. Sudden death can be the first symptom.

If your blood cholesterol is too high, take steps to lower it with the help of your physician. It is up to you, however, to take control over this risk factor. Learn what can be done about it, make the necessary changes, and stick to them.

One of the changes to lower blood cholesterol recommended by the American Heart Association is to reduce total fat intake to 30 percent of daily caloric intake, saturated fat intake to 10 percent, and cholesterol intake to no more than 300 mg per day. Many people find this advice hard to apply. What does it mean in practical terms? How much of which foods should you eat to consume 10 percent of calories from saturated fat?

I have found that *Eater's Choice* addresses these questions in an easy, effective way. *Eater's Choice* discusses the saturated fat content of foods along with a comprehensive discussion of various risk factors of heart disease. Armed with this knowledge, you can figure out exactly what you should be eating to follow the American Heart Association guidelines. The *Eater's Choice* approach to lowering blood cholesterol works because *you* choose the foods you eat.

Eater's Choice is a valuable tool for physicians and other health professionals. Because it uses a quantitative assessment, both you and your physician know exactly what changes you must make in your eating pattern to achieve a healthy blood cholesterol level. Most important, *Eater's Choice* gives those at risk the facts and skills they need to modify their own diet in order to lower their cholesterol. I have found that people who assume responsibility for their own problems are more likely to devise solutions they can live with and thus achieve results that will be lasting.

Eater's Choice will help you discover that a healthy way of eating can also be delicious and satisfying. Far from being a sacrifice, eating heart-healthy foods makes the good life worth living. This book should become a handbook for the making of a modern public health campaign designed to improve the quality of life for all Americans.

— *Julius Richmond, M.D.*
Former Surgeon General of the United States and Assistant Secretary of Health,
Department of Health and Human Services

Professor of Health Policy Research and Education, Harvard University

INTRODUCTION

LIKE MILLIONS of other Americans, I come from a family with a history of heart disease. My father had his first of three heart attacks when he was only thirty-one. I was three years old at the time. I grew up with heart disease. It was there, but I didn't take it too seriously.

When I was thirty-one, my blood cholesterol level was measured for the first time. It was 311 mg/dL, the doctor told me — an abnormally high level that put me at very high risk for heart disease, especially with my family history. He sent me to the National Institutes of Health (NIH) to be screened for participation in a clinical trial. The trial was designed to test the effect of lowering blood cholesterol on the risk of heart disease.

At NIH, physicians explained the degree of risk associated with my blood cholesterol level and the nature of the experiment. The experiment included coronary angiography. This test involves inserting a tube through a leg artery up to the heart. A dye is injected so that the amount of blockage of the coronary arteries can be visualized. The mortality rate for the test was only 1 in 100, I was assured.

Learning about the risks of the experiment as well as the risk associated with my elevated blood cholesterol level scared the hell out of me. Although I was excluded from participating in the study (my blood cholesterol level dropped below the cut-off point for entry into the study when I went on the mild study diet), this experience may well have saved my life.

For the first time, I began to realize the seriousness of high blood cholesterol. I was a heart attack just waiting to happen. But equally important, I got a taste of what it is like to be a patient, to have tests done on me and to think of myself as sick. This was hard to take. After all, I was a young man of thirty-one, and I felt great.

This experience taught me two lifesaving lessons. First, although I felt fit and vigorous, I was actually at high risk for heart disease because of my high blood cholesterol level. And with my family history, it could not be ignored. Second, I could lower my blood cholesterol level simply by changing what I ate.

It was too bad it took me all those years to realize the wisdom of my parents' advice about the foods I ate. They were always recommending a low-cholesterol, low-fat diet. I resented their insistence when there seemed to be little relevance to my health. My father was the one who was sick, not I.

How foolish I was. Coronary heart disease is a slow, insidious disease that begins in childhood and develops without symptoms over decades. Then, all of a sudden, boom — a heart attack that may be fatal and, if not, will certainly change your life.

My NIH experience changed my life. I wanted to do something professionally about cholesterol and heart disease. I took my wife and young sons to Boston and added a master of public health degree to my Ph.D. in biochemistry. I then returned to Bethesda, where I got a job as the National Coordinator of the Coronary Primary Prevention Trial at the National Heart, Lung, and Blood Institute of the National Institutes of Health. As I will explain later, this trial was developed to test the hypothesis that lowering your blood cholesterol really does lower your risk of heart disease.

I was involved with this trial for seven years, from its beginning to its end. After it was successfully completed, I took a new job in the Heart Institute as Coordinator of the National Cholesterol Education Program. I wanted to get the word out to the public, physicians, and dietitians about blood cholesterol, diet, and heart disease.

After a year and a half, I became convinced that the way to reach the public was for my wife and me to write a book — this book, which is filled with the information I have gained as a professional in this field. This is not just an academic subject for me. I have lowered my blood cholesterol from 311 mg/dL to 200 mg/dL merely by changing the foods I eat. My two young sons consider heart-healthy eating the natural way to eat. They are not even aware that they are reducing their risk of coronary heart disease and developing healthy habits for the future; they just enjoy eating good food.

Changing my eating habits has been an easy, inexpensive, and pleasant way for me to lower my risk of heart disease. That is what this book is all about. I want to tell *you* how to do it.

— *Dr. Ron Goor*

ONE

EATER'S CHOICE

FOR YOU   1

THIS BOOK was written for you, whether you are an average, healthy American, a recipient of a triple coronary artery bypass or an angioplast, or a survivor of four heart attacks. If you are in good health, it will give you the knowledge and skills to help you stay healthy and improve your chances of avoiding heart disease and possibly some common forms of cancer. And if you already have heart disease, this book will give you the tools to help you slow down further progression of your condition or even reverse it.

THE INSIDIOUS DISEASE

It may be difficult for you to worry about heart disease if you are healthy, active, and in the prime of life. But here are some alarming statistics that should jar you out of your complacency.

- Fifty percent of Americans die of heart disease.
- Heart disease is the leading cause of death in the United States, outnumbering deaths from cancer and accidents combined.
- Three Americans suffer heart attacks every minute.
- One American dies from a heart attack every minute.
- The first symptom for half the victims of heart disease is death.
- More than 500,000 Americans die from heart attacks each year.
- More than 650,000 Americans are hospitalized for heart attacks each year.
- More than 5 million Americans have angina or other symptoms of heart disease. Many of these people lead highly restricted, painful, and fearful lives.

Choose Not to Be a Part of These Grim Statistics. These statistics are a national shame. They need not be true. Heart disease is not a natural consequence of aging. The epidemic of heart disease is a product of the way we live. By changing our lifestyles, we can make an impact on our health.

In fact, it is already happening. Coronary heart disease has declined by 30 percent in the past twenty years and stroke has decreased even more. Many experts believe that the lifestyle changes Americans are making are reducing the incidence of heart disease. Americans are consuming less cholesterol and saturated fat and have lower blood cholesterol levels. They are smoking fewer cigarettes. They have lowered their blood pressure. They are exercising more.

The lifestyle changes you and your family make can also make a difference. You can increase the chances that you and your family will escape coronary heart disease by the way you choose to live.

But you must act now. The first symptom of half of those who die of heart attacks is death itself. All the improvements in emergency coronary care are of no help in such cases. This high rate of sudden death places an important premium on *prevention*. No one but you can make the necessary decisions that affect your heart disease risk.

Three Major Risks

How do you know if you are at increased risk for coronary heart disease? You are at increased risk if you

- smoke,
- have high blood pressure (over 140/90),
- have elevated blood cholesterol (over 200 mg/dL).*

These are the three major risk factors for coronary heart disease that you can control.

One Plus One Equals Four. The presence of any one of the risk factors (high blood cholesterol, cigarette smoking, or high blood pressure) *doubles* your risk of coronary heart disease. Having two of these risk factors *quadruples* the risk. Thus, if you smoke and have high blood pressure, your risk is enhanced fourfold. And if you smoke, have high blood cholesterol, and have high blood pressure, your risk increases *eightfold* (see Figure 1). It certainly makes you think. We hope it will make you stop smoking, seek advice on con-

---

*Milligrams of cholesterol per deciliter of blood

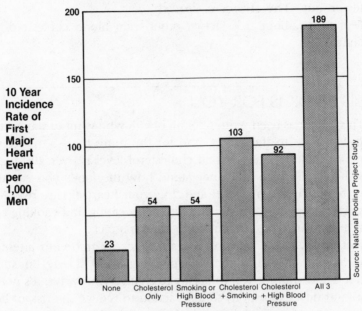

Risk of Coronary Heart Disease Increases with Additional Risk Factors

10 Year Incidence Rate of First Major Heart Event per 1,000 Men

Source: National Pooling Project Study

Risk Factor Status at Entry

Figure 1: Risk Factors for Coronary Heart Disease *The three major risk factors — blood cholesterol, blood pressure, and smoking — have additive effects on the incidence rate of coronary heart disease.*

Adapted with permission from the Journal of Chronic Diseases, *vol. 31, Pooling Project Research Group, "Relationship of Blood Pressure, Serum Cholesterol, Smoking Habit, Relative Weight, and ECG Abnormalities to Incidence of Major Coronary Events: Final Report of the Pooling Project." Copyright 1978, Pergamon Press, Ltd., and with permission of the American Heart Association, Inc.*

trolling your high blood pressure, and continue reading this book to find out how to lower your blood cholesterol.

What do all these risks mean and how do they apply to you and your life decisions? Perhaps this analogy will help you understand: Suppose that life is like playing Russian roulette. In this game of Russian roulette, you have a partially loaded gun pointed at your head. Obviously, the more chambers that contain bullets, the higher the chance that you will die.

Think of risk factors as the bullets in the chamber of the gun. The more risk factors for coronary heart disease you have, the greater are the chances you will have a heart attack and, perhaps, die. The question is: Do you want to play with one chamber loaded or two or three or four? **The choice is yours!**

(For more about risk factors other than blood cholesterol, see Chapter 9.)

THIS BOOK IS FOR YOU

This book has been written for all of you who want to stay healthy and enjoy life to the fullest, and for the more than 50 percent of American adults whose blood cholesterol level is over 200 mg/dL. This book will help you understand how the foods you eat affect your blood cholesterol level and thus your heart disease risk. Most important, it will teach you the necessary eating and cooking skills to reduce your chance of suffering a heart attack.

Act Now. Don't wait for a heart attack to grab your attention. The clogging of your arteries is happening NOW, slowly, but surely, and it won't wait for you to decide to change your ways. It's not too late (and never too soon) to take action to reduce the risk of heart disease for yourself, your spouse, and your children.

A Special Note to Those Who Already Have Heart Disease

Especially if you already have angina or have had a coronary by-pass operation or a heart attack, you can benefit from this book. As we will explain in Chapter 3, you can slow or stop the progression of the life-threatening blockage of the coronary arteries and, in some cases, even reverse it.

A Special Note to the Total Population

This book is for everyone. The *Eater's Choice* low-fat eating plan and recipes are not just for people who are worried about coronary heart disease. The National Cancer Institute recommends a diet low in fat and high in fiber to help prevent some common cancers, such as colon and breast cancers. A similar low-fat diet is also recommended for diabetics. For those concerned with their looks as well as their health, eating foods low in fat is one of the best ways to lose weight and stay trim. You'll feel better, too. As Dr. Richmond points out in the Foreword, "Far from being a sacrifice, eating heart-healthy foods makes the good life worth living." So, no matter who you are, take this book to heart.

Remember:

1. Heart disease is the leading cause of death in the United States.
2. Three major risk factors for coronary heart disease are high blood cholesterol, high blood pressure, and cigarette smoking.
3. *You* can control the three major risk factors of heart disease.

2 IT'S YOUR HEART — KEEP IT TICKING

YOU GO to the doctor for a physical. You're feeling great. You're not *too* heavy — well, just a few pounds; a bit soft and blubbery around the middle. But, you've never felt better. You get a little breathless walking up steps, but other than that, you feel like a twenty-year-old. Your doctor sits you down. His expression is serious. "You are in good physical condition," he tells you, "but your blood cholesterol is 245." "So?" you ask. "So," he answers, "you're a good candidate for a heart attack. The higher your blood cholesterol, the higher your risk of heart disease."

You feel a queasy sensation in your stomach. Your head begins to spin. "What is blood cholesterol?" you ask. "How does it affect my heart?" You've read about cholesterol in the newspapers. You remember something about HDL, or good cholesterol, and triglycerides, but it never really sank in. Now you're ready to listen. You *need* to understand it. It's *your* heart. It's *your* life.

THE HEART AND HEART DISEASE

The heart is a muscle that pumps blood throughout the body to deliver nutrients to all the body's cells and to remove waste materials. Just how much work the heart does is mind-boggling. Even while you rest or sleep, the heart beats between 70 and 80 times each minute and pumps nearly 5 quarts of blood. That adds up to about 100,000 beats and about 1800 gallons of blood pumped each day.

During vigorous exercise, the heart can increase its output nearly fivefold. Blood is kept moving through the extensive network of arteries, capillaries, and veins by the pumping heart at such a rate that

Figure 2: The Heart and Coronary Arteries *The coronary arteries and the network of vessels branching off from them come down over the top of the heart like a crown (corona) and supply the heart muscle with oxygenated blood. Drawing by Judy Beavers.*

blood can make the trip from the heart to the big toe and back in less than one minute.

In order to do all this work, the heart muscle needs a constant supply of nutrient-rich, oxygenated blood. This is supplied by the coronary arteries that branch off from the aorta (see Figure 2).

What Is Atherosclerosis? The underlying cause of coronary heart disease is a process called atherosclerosis. Atherosclerosis is the clogging of the coronary arteries with fatty, fibrous, cholesterol-laden deposits (called atheromata or plaques). These deposits thicken the artery wall, thus narrowing the channel through which the blood flows. Plaques are caused by an excess of cholesterol in the blood (see Figure 3).

When Does Atherosclerosis Begin? In countries where people eat foods high in saturated fat, plaques begin to develop in childhood. Plaque formation progresses at different rates in different people, depending on their ability to metabolize fat. (Both high blood pressure and smoking speed up the rate of atherosclerosis.) Over the course of the first three to four decades of life, plaque deposits gradually increase and the openings of the coronary arteries gradually narrow (see Figure 4).

Figure 3: Plaque Removed from a Coronary Artery *This plaque acquired the shape of the coronary artery that it completely blocked. Photo by Maggie Moore, laboratory of Dr. William C. Roberts, NHLBI.*

Figure 4: Progression of Blocking of a Coronary Artery *The progressive blocking of a coronary artery by the accumulation of plaque is shown in these three cross-sections.*

During this time there are usually no symptoms. You feel good. You are active, in your prime, enjoying the good life. Then suddenly, or so it seems, the inevitable occurs. An artery that feeds blood to the heart muscle becomes 75 percent or more blocked with plaque.

What Is Angina? If you are lucky, the first symptom of coronary heart disease may be angina pectoris. This mildest and earliest symptom is brief chest pain, usually experienced upon exertion. Angina occurs because not enough blood can get through the blocked arteries to supply oxygen to the heart muscle cells. Cells deprived of oxygen for only a few minutes can recover if you rest, thereby reducing

Figure 5: Damage to the Heart Muscle After a Heart Attack *The shaded area shows the extent of dead heart muscle resulting from the blockage of a coronary artery. Drawing by Judy Beavers.*

the demand on the heart. If the oxygen supply is cut off for longer periods, permanent damage to the heart may result.

The First Symptom May Be Your Last. If you are not so lucky, a small blood clot may become lodged in the narrowed artery and completely block the flow of blood to part of the heart. This part of the heart muscle dies. Result: **heart attack or sudden death** (see Figure 5).

WHAT IS CHOLESTEROL AND WHY DO WE HAVE IT?

Let's backtrack. The doctor says your blood cholesterol is too high. What does heart disease have to do with cholesterol?

Cholesterol is an odorless, white, powdery substance (see Figure 6). It is like a fat in that it does not mix with water. We are concerned with cholesterol because in excess it forms plaque, which clogs the coronary arteries and causes heart disease.

Cholesterol also has many beneficial and vital functions. It is a necessary ingredient of the cell walls of *all* animals, including humans. Cholesterol in the cell wall helps make your skin waterproof and also slows down water loss by evaporation from the body. Cho-

Cholesterol

Figure 6: Chemical Structure of Cholesterol *Cholesterol is a fatlike substance with a sterol ring structure. It is found in foods and in the VLDL, LDL, and HDL lipoproteins in the blood.*

lesterol is also used in the formation of the steroid and sex hormones. Cholesterol acts as an insulator in the myelin sheath that surrounds nerves and allows normal transmission of nerve impulses.

Cholesterol is transported in the blood stream together with fats. It is in this capacity that cholesterol becomes implicated in heart disease.

FAT FACTS

In your blood right now are various kinds of particles carrying fat around to do useful work or get stored for later use. Everyone has his or her own balance of the various kinds of particles, depending on diet, heredity, and physical activity. Because we now know one kind of particle is good and another bad, it is worth knowing which is which.

Lipoproteins

Fats* in your body (and in foods) generally occur as *triglycerides.* They are transported in blood, which consists mainly of water. They are broken down and their energy released by enzymes,** which function in a water medium. However, fats do not mix with water. So fats are packaged into particles to keep them from separating out

---

*Fats are one of the five major classes of nutrients; the other four are proteins, carbohydrates, minerals, and vitamins.

**Enzymes are proteins that speed up chemical reactions without themselves being changed.

from the water in the blood. These particles, which also contain proteins and cholesterol, are called *lipoproteins* (*lipo* means fat). Four of the major types of lipoproteins are very low density lipoproteins (VLDL), low density lipoproteins (LDL), high density lipoproteins (HDL), and chylomicrons.

VLDL Lipoproteins. The liver uses excess carbohydrates and fats from the foods you eat to make triglycerides (fats). These triglycerides are packaged into VLDL (very low density lipoprotein) particles for distribution from the liver to the rest of the body. VLDL particles contain large amounts of triglycerides and lesser amounts of cholesterol, protein, and other fats. VLDL particles are produced and released into the blood stream in large quantities after meals.

LDL Lipoproteins: The Bad Cholesterol. As the VLDL particles circulate through the blood stream, triglycerides are removed from the particles and enter cells, where they are used as a source of energy. The fat-depleted VLDL particles are called LDL (low density lipoprotein) particles. The cholesterol and protein that remain constitute a large part of the LDL particles.

LDL particles remain in the blood stream for different periods of time in different people. The longer the LDL particles remain in the blood stream, the greater the chance they will become oxidized and taken up by cells called monocytes. Monocytes that have become engorged with LDL-cholesterol lodge in the coronary artery wall. As more and more LDL is oxidized, taken up by monocytes, and lodged in the artery walls, the artery channel becomes more and more narrow. You know the result. When blood can no longer flow through a coronary artery, the part of the heart supplied by that artery dies. Result: heart attack.

Thus, the higher the LDL level in the blood, the more cholesterol is available to clog the coronary arteries and the higher is the risk of developing atherosclerosis and coronary heart disease. The cholesterol in LDL deserves its name of "bad cholesterol."

In some people, LDL particles are quickly removed from the blood stream by special LDL receptors on cell surfaces. Once inside the cells, cholesterol from the LDL particles is broken down. When these fortunate people with a normal or high number of LDL receptors have their blood cholesterol measured, their LDL is very low.

Other people have reduced numbers of fully functioning LDL receptors (the genetic constitution and diet of the individual determines the number and activity of the LDL receptors). In these people, LDL particles remain in the blood stream longer, producing a higher LDL level in the blood. Since LDL particles are so rich in cholesterol, a high LDL level results in a high blood cholesterol level.

HDL Lipoproteins: The Good Cholesterol. HDL (high density lipoprotein) particles are the smallest of the lipoprotein particles. HDL removes cholesterol from LDL particles and cells and transports it to the liver. Here most of the cholesterol is broken down into bile acids and excreted into the small intestine. Some of the cholesterol is reprocessed into new VLDL particles.

By removing cholesterol from LDL, HDL prevents cholesterol from accumulating in the coronary arteries and thus protects against the development of heart disease. The higher the HDL level, the more cholesterol is removed from the blood stream and the lower is the risk of heart attack. The lower the HDL level, the less cholesterol is removed from the blood stream, and the greater is the risk of heart disease.

Cholesterol. While cholesterol is not a lipoprotein, it is contained in all the lipoproteins. It is of particular interest because it is a major culprit in the formation of plaque.

Cholesterol in the blood is derived partly from cholesterol in the foods you eat and partly from cholesterol made in the liver and the intestine. Because cholesterol is so vital to the normal functioning of the body, all of the body's cholesterol needs can be met by cholesterol made in the liver. In addition, each cell in the body can make cholesterol. Even if you consumed no cholesterol at all (i.e., if you were a strict vegetarian), your body would manufacture enough cholesterol for proper growth and development. However, consumption of too much cholesterol can overload your system and end up as plaque in your coronary arteries.

Note: Cholesterol in foods is not the only, or even the most important, nutrient that affects your blood cholesterol level. The amount of saturated fat in foods is a more important factor in raising blood cholesterol levels, as we will see in Chapter 5.

What *Your* Cholesterol and Lipoprotein Values Mean

All this talk about lipoproteins and cholesterol is very abstract. You want to know about *your* lipoproteins and *your* cholesterol. What do the numbers that you receive from your doctor or from a blood cholesterol screening mean? Do your levels put you at increased risk for heart disease?

First, the total blood cholesterol reading is the sum of the cholesterol in your VLDL, LDL, and HDL particles. Thus, if your total blood cholesterol level is 250, the breakdown may look like this:

$$\begin{array}{r} 45 \text{ mg/dL of HDL-cholesterol} \\ + \quad 20 \text{ mg/dL of VLDL-cholesterol} \\ + \; 185 \text{ mg/dL of LDL-cholesterol} \\ \hline 250 \text{ mg/dL of total cholesterol} \end{array}$$

HDL. Average HDL-cholesterol levels for adult males are about 45 mg/dL and about 55 mg/dL for adult females. Levels lower than average place you at increased risk. The lower they are, the greater your risk. Levels below 35 mg/dL should be a cause for concern. Levels above the average decrease your risk. The higher they are, the lower your risk.

If your HDL is low, you can raise it, but only within narrow limits. Regular aerobic exercise and losing weight if you are overweight will increase your HDL levels. On average, nonsmokers have higher HDL levels than smokers.

A low HDL-cholesterol level coupled with other heart disease risk factors, such as high blood pressure, smoking, or a family history of heart disease, significantly increases risk. You should see your physician and take vigorous steps to reduce these risk factors. You should lower your blood pressure, stop smoking, exercise regularly, and lose weight if you are overweight.

If your HDL-cholesterol is low, you should make a determined effort to lower your LDL-cholesterol. Give your HDL a break. If you eat too much saturated fat, you have an abundance of LDL particles circulating in your blood. To remove the cholesterol from the LDL in your blood, you need a lot of HDL particles. But you don't have a lot of HDL particles. So, the cholesterol in the LDL that the HDL cannot handle remains in the blood and is eventually deposited in your artery walls. However, if you eat less saturated fat, fewer LDL particles circulate in your blood. This gives your HDL a fighting chance. Your HDL particles, although limited in number, are able to remove cholesterol from the smaller amount of LDL particles in your blood so the LDL-cholesterol won't end up clogging your arteries.

Because of their sex hormones, most premenopausal women have higher levels of HDL than do men of the same age. During the thirty or so years that women are protected from developing atherosclerosis by high levels of HDL, many men are accumulating plaque at a fast rate. As a result, many men begin to experience heart disease at early ages (as early as their forties). This is not to imply that women are immune to heart disease. Once women reach menopause and lose their protective hormones, they too begin to develop plaque at a fast rate. Women's risk may rise as much as a thousandfold after menopause. In fact, heart disease is the leading cause of death in women, occurring fifteen to twenty years later than in men.

VLDL and Triglycerides. VLDL is not measured directly. It is calculated from your triglyceride level as follows:

$$VLDL = triglycerides \div 5.$$

Triglycerides can be measured only after a twelve-hour fast.

Average values of triglycerides are about 140–150 mg/dL for men and about 100–120 mg/dL for women. Triglycerides are considered a risk factor for heart disease at levels above 150 mg/dL, especially when coupled with an HDL level below 40 mg/dL. If your triglycerides are too high, restrict your intake of simple sugars (sweets) and alcohol (an important factor in raising triglycerides), exercise regularly, and lose weight if you are overweight. Eating less simple sugar, less saturated fat, and more complex carbohydrates (grains, vegetables, and fruits) will help you lose weight and thus lower your triglycerides.

LDL. Average levels of LDL-cholesterol are about 135–145 mg/dL for men and about 120–135 mg/dL for women. About half of American adults have levels higher than these. Such levels are too high for long-term health and are the major reason heart disease is the leading cause of death in this country.

You can lower your LDL-cholesterol levels by changing the foods you eat and by losing weight. Specifically, eating foods low in saturated fats and cholesterol lowers your LDL. Eating less saturated fat increases the number of LDL receptors, thus allowing for increased removal of LDL (bad) cholesterol from the blood. Eating less cholesterol reduces the amount of cholesterol available to be made into lipoproteins in the liver and released into the blood.

The majority of total blood cholesterol is carried in the LDL. Since the total blood cholesterol level is a reflection of the LDL level, it is usually sufficient to monitor only total blood cholesterol. In the rest of this book, we will refer only to total blood cholesterol. But you should know that when you reduce your total blood cholesterol by changing the foods you eat, you are primarily lowering your LDL level and thus your risk of heart disease.

LIPOPROTEINS AND YOUR RISK OF HEART DISEASE

LIPOPROTEIN	RISK INCREASES IF:	TO REDUCE YOUR RISK:
HDL	Low	Exercise regularly Stop smoking Lose weight if overweight
VLDL (Triglycerides)	High	Restrict alcohol Exercise regularly Lose weight if overweight Eat less simple sugar (sweets) Eat less saturated fat
LDL	High	Eat less saturated fat Eat less cholesterol Lose weight if overweight

Lipoprotein Ratios

Your doctor, health professional, or lab report may have expressed your cholesterol numbers in the form of a ratio. The ratio of total cholesterol to HDL-cholesterol, or the ratio of LDL-cholesterol to HDL-cholesterol, is a shorthand measure of heart disease risk which has been reduced to one number. Ratios take into account the fact that total cholesterol by itself does not tell the full story of your risk. Remember, the higher your LDL level, the higher your risk of coronary heart disease. The higher your HDL level, the lower your risk.

The following example shows how completely different lipoprotein ratios may produce the same total cholesterol level.

	Fred	*Ted*
LDL-cholesterol	120 mg/dL	165 mg/dL
HDL-cholesterol	65 mg/dL	30 mg/dL
VLDL-cholesterol	35 mg/dL	25 mg/dL
Total cholesterol	220 mg/dL	220 mg/dL
Total/HDL ratio	3.4	7.3
LDL/HDL ratio	1.8	5.5

In this example, Fred is at much lower risk than Ted despite the fact that both have the same total cholesterol level.

The Two Ratios. Two different ratios are commonly used. Be sure you know which is being used to describe your risk because the actual numerical values of the ratios are quite different.

1. **Total cholesterol/HDL-cholesterol ratio:** you are considered to be at lower risk if your ratio is below 5.0. Dr. William Castelli of the Framingham Study (see page 21) feels the ideal ratio is under 3.5.
2. **LDL-cholesterol/HDL-cholesterol ratio:** you are considered to be at lower risk if your ratio is below 3.0.

Ratios as Predictors. With total cholesterol levels between 200 and 240 mg/dL, the ratios are better predictors of your risk than either LDL or total cholesterol alone. However, if your total cholesterol is over 240 mg/dL, LDL alone is the best predictor of risk. Even if your HDL is high, making your ratio look good, it can never be high enough to protect you from such high LDL levels.

Likewise, if your total cholesterol level is very low, your ratio will not be a useful predictor of risk. Persons with very low total cholesterol levels, and thus low LDL levels, do not need high HDL levels to protect them. For example, HDL levels are low among rural Japanese, but so are LDL levels. Despite the resulting ratio, heart disease is rare in these people.

YOU CAN CHOOSE TO LOWER YOUR RISKS

Chylomicrons: Yet Another Lipoprotein

If you are sitting there chuckling because you gobble up Quarter Pounders and stuff Wendy's cheese potatoes down your gullet with abandon and still maintain a low total and LDL-cholesterol level, wipe the smile from your lips. New scientific studies show that even with low LDL-cholesterol levels, eating a diet high in fat and saturated fat puts you at risk for heart disease. Eating a low-fat, low-sat-fat diet is still the healthiest route for everyone.

Here's why. In addition to getting fat from the liver, cells get fat directly from the fat in the foods you eat. The fat that you eat is transported from the intestine to the rest of the body in chylomicron particles produced in the intestine. As the chylomicrons circulate through the blood stream, fat is removed and almost all — 97 percent — goes directly into your fat stores, those plump places around your waist, hips, and thighs. The fat-depleted chylomicrons become chylomicron remnants. Under normal conditions, chylomicron remnants are rapidly removed from the blood stream and broken down in the liver (good news). However, studies have shown that animals fed diets high in fat and saturated fat accumulate large amounts of chylomicron remnants in their blood. Because there are too many remnants for the body to dispose of quickly, they remain circulating in the blood for a period of time. Eventually they are oxidized and taken up by cells called monocytes which lodge in the artery wall, causing atherosclerosis, or narrowing of the coronary arteries (bad news). So even if your total or LDL-cholesterol levels always read low, eating a diet high in fat and saturated fat can clog your arteries and put you at high risk for heart disease.

The bottom line is that a diet low in fat and saturated fat is heart-healthy, no matter if your cholesterol is sky-high or 170 mg/dL. And that's what this book is all about. *Eater's Choice* gives you the most effective, inexpensive, safe, and palatable way to lower your risk: **change the foods you eat.** YOU can stop clogging your arteries simply by eating a low-fat and low-sat-fat diet. YOU can make a difference in your heart's destiny.

By the time you finish Chapter 10, you should be convinced that it really does matter what foods you pour into your body. If you bought a new car and wanted to keep it in tiptop operating condition, you would never fill it with dirty gas oozing big globs of grease that could collect in the pipelines and clog the fuel line. You would make sure you fed it the best gas available. Why not treat yourself as well as you treat your car?

Remember:

1. The heart is a living pump that must be constantly supplied with oxygen and nutrients via the coronary arteries.
2. Atherosclerosis is the process by which the coronary arteries are progressively blocked by cholesterol-rich deposits.
3. Heart attacks occur when a coronary artery becomes 75 percent or more blocked. A heart attack involves death of the part of

the heart muscle normally supplied by the blocked coronary artery.

4. Cholesterol in the blood is found in the lipoprotein particles involved in fat transport: VLDL, LDL, and HDL. Total blood cholesterol is the sum of the cholesterol in VLDL + LDL + HDL.

5. High levels of HDL cholesterol ("good" cholesterol) lower the risk of heart disease. You can raise your HDL by exercising regularly, losing weight if you are overweight, and stopping smoking.

6. High levels of LDL cholesterol ("bad" cholesterol) raise the risk of heart disease. You can lower your LDL and your risk of coronary heart disease by eating less saturated fat and cholesterol.

THE EVIDENCE 3

A T THE END of the last chapter, we categorically stated that you could lower your blood cholesterol and thus stop clogging your arteries by changing your eating habits. Before you consider a major revamping of your old eating style, you may want proof that the change will indeed lower your blood cholesterol level and that lowering your blood cholesterol will reduce your risk of coronary heart disease.

Without drowning you in a sea of scientific data, we will merely touch on a few of the more important studies that show that:

1. elevated blood cholesterol is a risk factor for coronary heart disease;
2. blood cholesterol levels can be raised or lowered by the foods you eat;
3. lowering blood cholesterol reduces the risk of coronary heart disease.

EVIDENCE PART I: ELEVATED BLOOD CHOLESTEROL IS A RISK FACTOR FOR CORONARY HEART DISEASE

The Framingham Study

For almost forty years, investigators have been studying the health of the population of Framingham, Massachusetts, paying particular attention to risk factors for heart disease. Blood cholesterol levels have been measured and remeasured, heart attacks have been recorded. Even today, data on the original participants and their chil-

Risk of Coronary Heart Attack Rises as Blood Cholesterol Increases

Average Annual Incidence Rate of Heart Attack per 10,000 Men

Blood Cholesterol (mg/dL)

Source: Framingham Study

Figure 7: Coronary Heart Disease Risk and Blood Cholesterol Risk of coronary heart disease rises with increasing blood cholesterol levels. Risk increases rapidly as blood cholesterol levels rise above 200 mg/dL.

dren are being collected and analyzed. The results of this long-term population study are conclusive: **blood cholesterol levels predict the future incidence of heart attacks.**

The relationship between blood cholesterol levels and heart attacks is shown in a curve popularly known as the "Framingham risk curve" (see Figure 7). This curve is smooth and continuous. As blood cholesterol levels go up, risk of heart attack rises. At blood cholesterol levels above 200 mg/dL, risk rises rapidly. The risk is four times greater at a blood cholesterol level of 300 mg/dL than at a blood cholesterol level of about 200 mg/dL. (The Framingham risk curve could just as accurately be expressed in terms of LDL-cholesterol level instead of total blood cholesterol.) Although even the lowest blood cholesterol levels carry some risk of coronary heart disease, Dr. William Castelli, director of the Framingham Study, has stated that no one with a blood cholesterol level below 150 mg/dL has ever had a heart attack in Framingham.

EVIDENCE PART II: BLOOD CHOLESTEROL LEVELS CAN BE LOWERED (OR RAISED) BY DIET

Blood cholesterol levels are not set in concrete. They can be changed. To a large extent YOU can lower (or raise) your blood cholesterol level by what you eat. Here's the evidence to prove it.

International Comparisons

Comparing diets of countries with low and high coronary heart disease rates reveals a direct correlation between the amount of saturated fat in the diet and the blood cholesterol level and incidence of heart disease among the different populations.

The rates of coronary heart disease among countries varies almost tenfold from a low of 100 per 100,000 in Japan to a high of 900 per 100,000 in Finland. The Japanese eat little beef (a food high in saturated fat) and much fish (a food low in saturated fat and rich in polyunsaturated fat). The Finns, on the other hand, eat large amounts of cheese and whole milk products — foods high in saturated fat.

Countries with high average blood cholesterol levels and high rates of coronary heart disease have diets in which saturated fat accounts for over 15 percent of total calories. This includes the United States, Scotland, England, Finland, and Holland. Countries with very low blood cholesterol levels and very low coronary heart disease rates have diets in which saturated fats contribute less than 10 percent of total calories. Such countries include Japan and Greece.

Is the Evidence Valid? How can we be sure that these differences in coronary heart disease rates among countries are really due to dietary differences and not to genetic differences?

Japan to Hawaii: Changing Dietary Habits. An interesting study of Japanese migrants to Hawaii and San Francisco sheds light on this question. Japanese in Japan have one of the lowest rates of coronary heart disease. They have low blood cholesterol levels (the average blood cholesterol level was found to be less than 170 mg/dL) and eat a diet in which fat contributes only about 10 percent of total calories and saturated fat only about 3 percent. By Western standards, this is a very low fat diet.

The Japanese who have migrated to Hawaii have adopted some Western dietary habits. They eat a diet higher in fat and saturated fat than the typical Japanese diet but not as high as a typical American diet. The Japanese in Hawaii have higher blood cholesterol levels and higher rates of coronary heart disease than those in Japan but not as high as those in San Francisco.

Japan to Hawaii to San Francisco: Accumulating Bad Dietary Habits and Plaques. The Japanese who have migrated to San Francisco have gone even further in adopting American dietary habits, have blood cholesterol levels similar to native Americans, and, alas, have rates of coronary heart disease similar to Americans. Clearly, it is diet, and not genetics, that is raising the blood cholesterol levels and consequently the coronary heart disease rates of the migrants.

Japan Revisited: A Postscript. Alas. In the last few years, American fast food has been introduced to Japan and has become extremely popular. As you would expect, Japanese blood cholesterol levels are rising and the incidence of acute myocardial infarctions (heart attacks) has increased fivefold.

Vegetarians Provide Evidence. Most Seventh-Day Adventists are ovo-lacto vegetarians and thus eat some eggs and dairy products. Some, however, are strict vegetarians and eat no animal products at all. Others eat meat.

In general, those who are strict vegetarians have the lowest blood cholesterol levels. Ovo-lacto vegetarians (the majority of Adventists) have slightly higher blood cholesterol levels. Those who eat meat have the highest levels. *The vegetarian Adventists (including ovo-lacto vegetarians) have significantly lower heart disease rates than other Americans of the same age and sex.* It should be kept in mind that Adventists also do not drink coffee or alcohol or smoke tobacco.

Dietary Studies in Normal Volunteers. The strongest and most direct evidence that diet affects blood cholesterol levels comes from studies of normal volunteers whose intakes of saturated, polyunsaturated, and monounsaturated fats and cholesterol are varied under tightly controlled conditions on special hospital wards. These studies show that LDL cholesterol levels decrease when dietary saturated fat and cholesterol are decreased and when dietary polyunsaturated fat is increased. Removing saturated fat from the diet has two times the blood cholesterol–lowering impact as does adding an equal amount of polyunsaturated fat. Note: The best strategy for lowering cholesterol is to reduce saturated fat in your diet. The benefits can be tremendous — up to a 33 percent lowering of total blood cholesterol levels. For the relative merits of saturated versus poly-unsaturated fats, see the discussion on page 39.

How Your Heredity Fits In

At this point a question always seems to pop up. If blood choles-terol levels are affected by diet, why do people who eat exactly the same diet have different blood cholesterol levels?

Your blood cholesterol level is determined by how your genetic constitution affects the metabolism of the fats and cholesterol you eat. In other words, blood cholesterol level depends on an interac-tion between genetics and diet — that is, how sensitive you are to the amounts of saturated fats and cholesterol you eat.

We are a population with a great range of genetic constitutions affecting the control of blood cholesterol levels. Upon exposure to the typical high-fat, high-cholesterol American diet, these different genetic constitutions are expressed as widely divergent blood cho-lesterol levels. Thus, some people can eat large amounts of saturated fat and cholesterol and maintain a blood cholesterol level of 150 mg/ dL. Other people on the same fatty diet maintain a blood cholesterol level of 350 mg/dL.

The Japanese in Japan show much less variability in blood cho-lesterol levels. However, the fact that there is much genetic variabil-ity in the Japanese population is revealed when they are exposed to a typical American diet of high saturated fat and cholesterol. Thus, one person with a blood cholesterol of 170 mg/dL in Japan may find it rise to 230 mg/dL on a San Francisco diet, while another may find it rise to 280 mg/dL, while yet another may find it rise only to 180 mg/dL.

EVIDENCE PART III: LOWERING BLOOD CHOLESTEROL REDUCES YOUR RISK OF CORONARY HEART DISEASE

The big question that remains is: Does lowering elevated blood cholesterol levels in humans reduce the risk of coronary heart dis-ease? The answer is a resounding and definite YES.

The Coronary Primary Prevention Trial Gets Results

In 1973, the National Heart, Lung, and Blood Institute (one of the National Institutes of Health) began a ten-year study, the Coronary Primary Prevention Trial (CPPT), to test the lipid hypothesis: lowering blood cholesterol levels reduces the incidence of coronary heart disease.

The basic plan of the study was as follows. To test the lipid hypothesis, two groups of men with identical risks of coronary heart disease were selected. At the outset, both groups had identical average blood cholesterol levels of almost 300 mg/dL. Both groups followed a mild cholesterol-lowering diet. In addition, one group received a drug (cholestyramine) that lowered their blood cholesterol levels while the other group received a placebo that looked and tasted like the real drug but had no blood cholesterol–lowering effect. During the study, the only risk factor difference between the two groups was the lower blood cholesterol level of the drug-treated group.

CPPT Results: Lowering Blood Cholesterol Cuts Risk. At the end of the ten years, there was a definite difference in the incidence of coronary heart disease between the two groups. The group treated with the active drug had a lower average blood cholesterol level and a lower incidence of fatal and nonfatal heart attacks than the group that was not drug-treated.

Blood cholesterol levels in the drug-treated group were, on average, 9 percent lower than those in the placebo group. The incidence of fatal and nonfatal heart attacks in the treated group was 19 percent lower than in the placebo group. (There were reductions of a similar magnitude in new cases of angina, coronary bypass surgery, and electrocardiographic abnormalities in the treated group.)

This figures out to a fantastic ratio: for every 1 percent reduction in blood cholesterol, there was a 2 percent reduction in risk. Thus, participants who achieved a 25 percent reduction in blood cholesterol reduced their risk of heart attack by 50 percent.

These results may be applicable to you. For every 1 percent you reduce your blood cholesterol, your risk may be reduced by as much as 2 percent. Pretty good odds.

Another NIH Study Confirms CPPT Results. Another NIH study, which was conducted at the same time, also tested the lipid hypothesis. It produced results that could actually be seen in the coronary arteries. In this study, men and women were chosen with elevated blood cholesterol levels and atherosclerotic narrowing of their coronary arteries. They were randomly divided into two groups. Both groups followed a mild cholesterol-lowering diet. One treatment group received a blood cholesterol–lowering drug (cholestyramine) and the other a placebo.

At the beginning of the study, both groups underwent coronary angiography to evaluate the extent of atherosclerosis or narrowing of their coronary arteries. (Coronary angiography is a technique that uses an iodine-containing dye and x-ray pictures to allow visualization of the coronary arteries.) At the end of the study, five years later, the severity of atherosclerosis of the coronary arteries of both groups was once more assessed by coronary angiography.

The results were dramatic. Investigators could actually *see* that lowering LDL-cholesterol levels in the drug treatment group prevented the further narrowing of the coronary arteries.

In 1987 these results were confirmed. The Cholesterol-Lowering Atherosclerosis Study (CLAS) was an angiographic study of middle-aged men who had undergone coronary bypass surgery. Those men who were treated with a combination of drugs (colestipol and niacin) and diet had lower LDL levels, higher HDL levels, and, as a result of these changes, significantly less accumulation of atherosclerotic plaque than those not treated with a combination of drugs and diet. More exciting, 16.2 percent of the drug-and-diet-treated group experienced regression of atherosclerotic plaque.

Diet Versus Drug. You may wonder how we can assume that lowering blood cholesterol levels by diet is effective in reducing risk of coronary heart disease when the CPPT and the NIH and CLAS studies were drug studies.

Participants in the placebo group in the CPPT showed a range of reduction of LDL-cholesterol levels. These reductions were achieved by diet alone since these men received no active drug. Just as in the drug group, the greater the reduction in LDL-cholesterol by diet, the greater was the reduction in the incidence of coronary heart disease.

A follow-up study of the participants in the CLAS study who did not receive drugs showed the effect of diet on the development of new plaque-containing lesions in their coronary arteries. During the study, those whose fat intake averaged 27.5 percent of total calories developed **no new** plaque-containing lesions. But, those whose fat intake averaged 34 percent of total calories did develop new lesions. Those participants who reduced their LDL-cholesterol by an average of 7 percent developed *no new* lesions, while those who reduced their LDL levels by only 0.6 percent did develop new lesions.

Proof in the Pudding: Low-Fat Diet Causes Reversal. The most dramatic demonstration to date that a diet low in fat and saturated fat can actually reverse the narrowing of the coronary arteries comes from the Lifestyle Heart Trial. The trial consisted of 41 patients with angiographic evidence of coronary heart disease. The 22 participants in the experimental group consumed a very low fat diet (less than 10 percent of total calories), exercised regularly, and participated in a stress management program. Their total blood cholesterol levels were reduced by 24 percent and LDL levels by 37 percent. The 19 control subjects who followed no particular diet or exercise or stress program got no significant cholesterol reduction.

Angiographic analysis of the coronary arteries of the experimental group showed the following dramatic results: At the beginning of the study, the plaque in the coronary arteries was so thick it narrowed the openings to 60 percent of the original diameter. After only one year, plaque was reduced (regressed) so that the diameter opened up to 62.2 percent. In the control group, just the reverse was true. The plaque accumulated (progressed), closing the diameter even further, from 57.3 percent to 53.9 percent.

The results were even more dramatic when lesions that reduced the artery diameter by more than 50 percent were considered. After a year, plaque in the experimental group's arteries *regressed* so that the average diameter enlarged from 38.9 percent to 44.2 percent of the original opening and *progressed* in the control group, narrowing the opening from 38.3 percent to 35.6 percent of the original.

You may look at these results and think, 2.2 percent regression and 3.4 percent progression, or even 5.3 percent regression and 2.7 percent progression — what's the big deal? But you must remember that this study measured regression or progression after only *one* year. These percentages will be more impressive to you when you realize that reducing the diameter of your arteries 3.4 percent year after year will eventually narrow them to 25 percent or less of the original diameter. When the openings of coronary arteries are reduced this much, small blood clots floating through the blood stream can get caught in the narrowed artery and block the flow of nutrient-rich blood to the heart muscle. You know the result: heart attack.

On the other hand, just think how clear your arteries can become if the plaque that clogs them is reduced 2.2 percent or 5.3 percent, year after year.

These results are inspiring. But before you restrict yourself to a diet limited to 10 percent of total fat, be advised that it is unclear whether such a restrictive diet — mainly fruits, vegetables, greens, soybean products, egg white, and nonfat milk — is truly necessary to achieve regression. Regression was achieved in the CLAS study with a much less stringent diet.

The Benefits. In conclusion, definite regression can be expected in 16 to 47 percent of people, provided they lower their LDL level by 34 to 48 percent for 3 to 5 years. As proved in these studies, the main benefit of a diet low in saturated fat is that progression (continued narrowing of the coronary arteries) can be slowed, stopped, and in some cases reversed. Not a bad reward for just eating a lot of delicious low-fat food!

Remember:

1. The higher the blood cholesterol, the greater is the risk of developing coronary heart disease.
2. Blood cholesterol levels are determined in part by genetic factors and in part by the foods you eat.
3. Reductions of up to 33 percent in blood cholesterol level can be achieved by diet alone.
4. Reducing blood cholesterol levels lowers risk of fatal and nonfatal heart attack.

4 IS YOUR BLOOD CHOLESTEROL TOO HIGH?

T HE CORONARY Primary Prevention Trial (CPPT) results were positive. **Lowering blood cholesterol (and LDL) prevented heart attacks.** The lipid hypothesis was proven.

What do these results mean to you personally? How high is *your* risk? How much do *you* have to lower your blood cholesterol to reduce your risk?

NATIONAL INSTITUTES OF HEALTH RECOMMENDATIONS

To provide guidelines to physicians and the public, the National Cholesterol Education Program of the National Institutes of Health (NIH) convened an Adult Treatment Panel. This distinguished panel of scientists and physicians reviewed all of the available scientific and medical data and, on October 5, 1987, made the following recommendations (see Appendices for a more complete summary of the Adult Treatment Guidelines):

• Know your blood cholesterol number.

NATIONAL INSTITUTES OF HEALTH RECOMMENDATIONS

BLOOD CHOLESTEROL LEVELS, MG/DL

AGE	RECOMMENDED	BORDERLINE-HIGH RISK	HIGH RISK
20 +	under 200	200–239	240 +

- Keep your blood cholesterol below 200 mg/dL by diet (and drugs, if necessary).
- Diet is the first line of treatment to reduce blood cholesterol below 200 mg/dL and should be given a fair and rigorous trial for at least 6 months before even considering drugs. In fact, most adults can expect to lower their blood cholesterol below 200 mg/dL by diet alone.
- The presence of coronary heart disease or other risk factors for heart disease, such as male sex, family history of premature heart attack (before age 55), cigarette smoking, high blood pressure, low HDL (below 35 mg/dL), diabetes, cerebrovascular or peripheral vascular disease, and severe obesity (30 percent or more overweight) indicate the need for more vigorous therapy.

What Is Normal Blood Cholesterol?

The NIH recommendations are very definite: keep your blood cholesterol level below 200 mg/dL. However, you may be (or may already have been) told by health professionals that a blood cholesterol much higher than 200 mg/dL is *normal*. These advisers are not trying to dig you an early grave. They are just confusing the two meanings of normal — normal in a statistical sense and normal meaning disease-free.

But you must understand what normal means in reference to your blood cholesterol so you will not be lulled into a false sense of security about your blood cholesterol level. Ask for numbers. Blindly accepting your blood cholesterol level as "normal" may be injurious to your long-term health.

"Normal" Statistically Speaking. Here's what "normal" means in a statistical sense. You begin with a curve (see Figure 8) which plots the percentages of Americans with different blood cholesterol levels. This curve looks like many other curves, for example, curves that plot the distributions of weights, heights, or blood pressures in a population. In all such curves, persons with normal values in a statistical sense are found in the middle 95 percent of the curve. In Figure 8, normal blood cholesterol would include values that range from about 150 mg/dL to about 300 mg/dL.

Normal Is Not Necessarily Healthy. Just because values occur *often* in a population, this does not make them normal in the healthy

Current American Population Distribution

Figure 8: Current U.S. Distribution of Blood Cholesterol   *The average blood cholesterol level for adult Americans is about 215–220 mg/dL. Over 50 percent of American
adults have blood cholesterol levels above 200 mg/dL.*

sense. Blood cholesterol levels in the statistically normal range of
200 to 300 mg/dL are too high for long-term health. That is why
there is an epidemic of heart disease in this country, why 550,000
people die of heart disease each year — one each minute — and why
5.4 million people have been diagnosed as having coronary heart
disease.

As one physician so wisely explained, "We confuse normal with
optimal. Normal in America is to have a heart attack in middle age,
and we don't think that is good. We need new optimal levels. Somewhere around 180 to 200."

A Truly Normal Distribution. If the current distribution of
blood cholesterol levels in the United States is not normal, what
would a distribution of truly normal blood cholesterol levels (i.e.,
levels not associated with disease) look like? In Figure 9, an "ideal"
distribution of normal blood cholesterol levels (i.e., levels associated

**Comparison of Ideal and Current
American Population Distributions**

*Figure 9: Comparison of Current U.S. Blood Cholesterol Distribution with an
Ideal Distribution* The ideal distribution of blood cholesterol levels exhibits lower
levels than the current U.S. distribution and has an average of about 150 mg/dL. Only
a small percentage of the ideal population has blood cholesterol levels above 200 mg/dL.

with little or no heart disease) is shown together with the distribution of current levels in the United States.

You can see that the entire ideal curve of normal blood cholesterol
levels is shifted to lower levels. It has an average level of 150 mg/dL
instead of 215–220 mg/dL. Only a small percentage of the ideal population has blood cholesterol levels above 200 mg/dL. In this ideal-
ized population, a blood cholesterol level of 230 mg/dL is highly elevated rather than normal. Where does your blood cholesterol fit on
this curve?

Relating Risk to Blood Cholesterol Levels
in Different Populations

In Figure 10, shading indicates cholesterol levels (above 200 mg/
dL) associated with increased risk of heart attack. You can see several
interesting facts.

Average is *Not* "Normal"

*Figure 10: Average is **NOT** Normal*   *The shading indicates blood cholesterol levels associated with increased risk of heart attack.*

First, very few people in the ideal population are at increased risk of heart attack due to elevated blood cholesterol levels. Heart disease would be relatively rare in this population. Those few people at highest risk have cholesterol levels slightly above 200 mg/dL, levels currently considered normal in the United States. A real-life example proves the point. The distribution of blood cholesterol levels among rural Japanese farmers and fishermen is essentially identical to the ideal distribution. Heart disease in Japan is indeed rare: one-tenth the rate in the United States.*

Second, a study of these curves makes it clear that a large percentage of the current population of the United States is at increased risk of heart disease due to elevated blood cholesterol levels. Alas, heart disease is not at all rare in the United States. Over 50 percent

---

*As the Japanese diet becomes more Americanized, so will Japanese heart-health statistics. "Rare" will no longer describe the heart disease rate in Japan.

BYPASS PATIENTS — TAKE HEED

Bypass operations may eliminate the symptoms of heart disease, such as angina; but they do not cure the underlying atherosclerotic process, which goes on depositing fat in your coronary arteries. Bypass artery grafts have been found to accumulate plaque at a faster rate than the original arteries they replaced. They accumulate plaque at a faster rate the higher your blood cholesterol level. It is common for such grafts to close completely within three to five years. *This need not happen.* You can slow or even reverse the clogging of your bypass artery graft by changing what you eat and thereby lowering your blood cholesterol level.

---

of the population has blood cholesterol levels above 200 mg/dL, a level at which the risk curve begins to rise steeply. It is no coincidence that the NIH Adult Treatment Panel recommends that people with elevated blood cholesterol levels take action to reduce them to below 200 mg/dL.

While those people with very high blood cholesterol levels (say, above 280 mg/dL) are clearly at very high risk, they account for only a small percentage of the total population and thus for only a small percentage of the number of heart attacks. There are many more people with "normal" levels of about 225–235 mg/dL and they account for the great bulk of heart disease.

Now you can see why we recommend that you should insist on knowing your blood cholesterol level. Know your numbers. Don't settle for a statement that your cholesterol is normal.

AVERAGE BLOOD CHOLESTEROL OF HEART ATTACK PATIENTS

In fact, the average blood cholesterol level of patients admitted to coronary care units with heart attacks is about 225–235 mg/dL. The average blood cholesterol level of persons receiving coronary artery bypass grafts is also about 225–235 mg/dL. These levels are mistakenly considered normal by many health professionals. Pretty scary news, yes?

Because many of these patients do not have high blood pressure, do not smoke, and have no family history of premature heart disease, until recently they were considered to have no risk factors for heart disease. But today their blood cholesterol of, say, 225–235 mg/dL is understood to be a prime factor in the development of their disease.

AN ACTION PLAN FOR ALL AMERICANS: EAT LESS FAT

No matter whether you have been told that your blood cholesterol level is normal or that you are at borderline-high or high risk, if you want to reduce your risk of coronary heart disease you must get your blood cholesterol level down to below 200 mg/dL. The recommended method is to change the foods you eat.

The National Institutes of Health (NIH) and the American Heart Association (AHA) recommend that all Americans over the age of two years adopt a diet that reduces total dietary fat intake. (See Chapter 12 for a discussion of cholesterol and children. For more information about dietary fats and their effects on blood cholesterol levels, see the next chapter.) Total fat should be reduced to no more than 30 percent of total calories. The fat calories should be evenly distributed among the three types of fat as follows:

	FATS (% OF TOTAL CALORIES)				CHOLESTEROL (MG PER DAY)
	TOTAL	SAT.	MONO.	POLY.	
AHA and NIH recommend no more than	30	10	10	10	200–300
Current U.S. intake	40	17	16	7	470

In addition, intake of total calories should be reduced, if necessary, to correct obesity and to maintain desired body weight.

You may find these recommendations complicated and difficult to follow. That is why we developed *Eater's Choice*. As we explain in the next chapter, *Eater's Choice* not only simplifies the AHA recommendations by focusing only on reducing saturated fat intake, but also provides a method for translating the abstract guidelines into actual food choices.

Eat Right and Your Blood Cholesterol Will Show It

Do not be discouraged if your blood cholesterol level is too high. The picture is not bleak. Most people can lower their blood cholesterol simply by changing the foods they eat. In fact, it takes only about three weeks to see a change in your blood cholesterol level. Of course, you must make enough changes in the foods you eat and stick with them for your blood cholesterol level to fall below the danger zone and stay there.

You may expect to achieve dramatic reductions of your blood cholesterol — reductions up to 30 percent, depending on your responsiveness to diet and how much you change the foods you eat. Reductions of 10 to 15 percent are common. Thus, if your starting blood cholesterol level is 270 mg/dL, you might be able to lower it by about 80 mg/dL (about a 30 percent decrease) to 190 mg/dL. If your starting blood cholesterol level is 240 mg/dL, you might be able to lower it by about 70 mg/dL (about a 30 percent decrease) to 170 mg/dL.

How much you can lower your blood cholesterol by changes in the foods you eat depends on the following factors:

- your original eating pattern;
- your heredity, which determines how responsive your blood cholesterol is to changes in your diet;
- how much you change the foods you eat.

The higher the amount of saturated fat and cholesterol in your original eating pattern and the higher your resulting blood cholesterol, the greater will be the fall in your blood cholesterol with a decreased intake of saturated fat and cholesterol.

Those Who Need It the Most Benefit the Most. As you can see from the above, although the percentage decrease is the same for both, the person with the higher blood cholesterol level achieved a greater reduction (80 mg/dL decrease) in response to a blood cholesterol–lowering eating plan than did the person with a lower starting level (70 mg/dL decrease). Both will benefit from changes in what they eat, but persons with the highest risk can expect a larger absolute reduction. This should motivate those most in need of reducing their coronary heart disease risk.

Your Own Private Statistics. Enough of official edicts. You are already on your way to eradicating heart disease — even if it's only your own. The next chapters will help you apply all you have learned about blood cholesterol, foods, and heart disease to your own life. You will set personal blood cholesterol–lowering goals and learn how to meet those goals.

Remember:

1. A blood cholesterol level considered to be "normal" in the United States may be too high for long-term health. Over 50 percent of the adult American population has blood cholesterol levels above 200 mg/dL, the point at which risk begins to rise sharply.
2. All adults are advised to reduce their blood cholesterol below 200 mg/dL by adopting a diet that reduces total dietary fat intake.

EATER'S CHOICE: EATING FOR LIFE

YOU HAVE BEEN inundated with statistics, biochemical explanations, and evidence. Enough! Let's get started with practical advice to improve and lengthen your life. Let's get started with the *Eater's Choice* plan for lowering your blood cholesterol level.

Eater's Choice is the name given to this plan because it is an eating plan with choice — your choice. *Eater's Choice* gives you the knowledge to decide your own personal blood cholesterol goals and tailor your food choices to meet these goals.

Eater's Choice focuses on the saturated fat content of foods as the basis for making food choices. You determine the amount of saturated fat you should eat to lower your blood cholesterol and you keep track of how much saturated fat you are eating.

FATS

Total fat in a food is the sum of three kinds of fat: saturated fat, monounsaturated fat, and polyunsaturated fat. Each has a different effect on the blood cholesterol level. Foods contain mixtures of these different types of fat in different proportions (see Figure 11). No food contains pure saturated, monounsaturated, or polyunsaturated fat.

Saturated Fat. Saturated fat is called saturated because all the carbon atoms in the long fat molecule carry the maximum possible number of hydrogen atoms; that is, the carbon atoms are *saturated* with hydrogen atoms (see Figure 12). Saturated fat is generally solid at room temperature. Foods high in saturated fats are beef, lamb, veal, pork, and whole milk dairy products, including butter and cheese. Five kinds of vegetable fats are saturated: coconut oil, palm oil, palm kernel oil, cocoa butter (in chocolate), and hydrogenated

COMPOSITION OF FATS

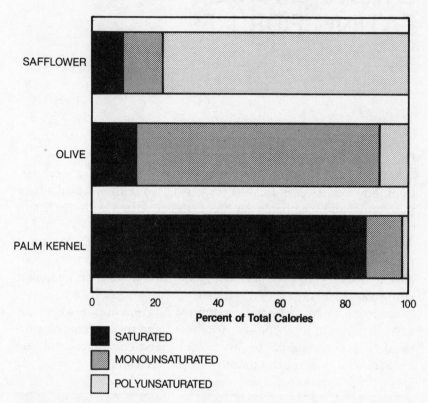

Figure 11: Composition of Fats   *Total fat in a food is the sum of three kinds of fat: saturated fat, monounsaturated fat, and polyunsaturated fat. This graph shows that all fats are mixtures of the three types of fats. Safflower oil is called a polyunsaturated fat because it contains more polyunsaturated fat than either mono or saturated fat. Olive oil is called a monounsaturated fat because it contains mainly, but not exclusively, monounsaturated fat. Palm kernel oil is called a saturated fat because it contains predominantly saturated fat. Look closely to see that palm kernel oil contains a tiny amount of polyunsaturated fat.*

vegetable oil. In general, animal fats are high in saturated fats and plant fats are low. **Saturated fat raises LDL-cholesterol and total blood cholesterol levels.**

Monounsaturated Fat. Monounsaturated fat has one point of unsaturation; that is, there are two fewer hydrogen atoms than in a

Triglyceride

Glycerol **Fatty Acids**

Figure 12: Chemical Structures of the Fats *Triglycerides are composed of three fatty acids attached to a glycerol molecule: In saturated fats all the carbon atoms (C) in the molecule carry the maximum possible number of hydrogen atoms (H). Monounsaturated fat has one point of unsaturation and thus can absorb two additional hydrogen atoms. Polyunsaturated fat has two or more points of unsaturation and thus can absorb four or more additional hydrogen atoms.*

fully saturated fat (see Figure 12). The richest source of mono-unsaturated fat is olive oil. Recent scientific evidence indicates that monounsaturated fat lowers total blood cholesterol by lowering LDL-cholesterol without lowering HDL-cholesterol. In addition, new studies show that olive oil prevents the oxidation of LDL par-ticles. The oxidation of LDL particles promotes their uptake by monocytes. LDL-filled monocytes are deposited in coronary artery walls, causing the narrowing (atherosclerosis) that may eventually block blood from flowing to the heart muscle. By preventing the oxidation of LDL particles, olive oil helps retard the atherosclerotic process.

Polyunsaturated Fat. Polyunsaturated fat has two or more points of unsaturation; that is, there are four or more fewer hydro-gen atoms than in a fully saturated fat (see Figure 12). Polyunsatu-rated fats are generally liquid at room temperature. In general, vegetable oils, except coconut, palm, palm kernel, and cocoa butter, are high in polyunsaturated fat. Polyunsaturated fat lowers blood LDL-cholesterol levels and, to a much lesser extent, HDL-cholesterol levels.

Because consumption of large quantities of polyunsaturated fats lowers HDL-cholesterol and has been implicated in the development of certain cancers in animals, we recommend limiting intake of poly-

CHOLESTEROL CONTENTS
OF SELECTED FOODS*

(The American Heart Association recommends that your intake
of cholesterol should not exceed 200–300 mg each day.)

FOOD	PORTION	CHOLESTEROL, MG
Dairy		
Butter, regular	1 pat	11
Cheeses		
cottage, creamed	1 cup	31
2%	1 cup	19
low-fat	1 cup	10
natural and processed	1 oz	16–35
Egg yolk	1 large	213**
Milk		
whole	1 cup	33
2%	1 cup	18
skim	1 cup	5
Yogurt		
low-fat	8 oz	10–14
nonfat	8 oz	0–1
Meat, Fish, Poultry		
Cooked beef, veal, pork, chicken, turkey, fish	1 oz	18–25
Crab, cooked	1 oz	28
Kidney, beef, cooked	1 oz	200
Liver		
beef, cooked	1 oz	126
chicken, simmered	1 oz	180
Scallops, cooked	1 oz	15
Shrimp, cooked	1 oz	43
Plant Products		
Fruits		0
Grains		0
Vegetables		0
Vegetable oils		0

*Adapted from *Composition of Foods*, Handbook No. 8, U.S. Department of Agriculture.
**In previous editions of *Eater's Choice*, we reported the cholesterol content of an egg
yolk as 274 mg. Based on updated lab measurements, the Egg Board has revised the
cholesterol content of egg yolks to an average of 213 mg per yolk (range: 180–230 mg).

unsaturated fat to about 5–7 percent of total calories and when possible, choosing olive oil instead. (See the discussion of trans fats on page 80.)

Dietary Cholesterol. Dietary cholesterol raises LDL-cholesterol. Cholesterol is found *only* in animal products, such as beef, pork, poultry, fish, cheese and other whole milk dairy products, and eggs. Especially rich sources of cholesterol are egg yolks and organ meats, such as liver, pancreas, and brain. Cholesterol is *not* found in foods made from plants, such as vegetables, fruits, nuts, or seeds.

FOCUS ON SATURATED FAT, NOT CHOLESTEROL

Eater's Choice focuses on the saturated fat content of foods because, of the four dietary constituents that influence blood cholesterol levels (saturated fat, monounsaturated fat, polyunsaturated fat, and cholesterol), saturated fat is the most potent determinant of blood cholesterol levels. The more saturated fat you remove from your daily consumption, the more your LDL-cholesterol level will fall.

Monounsaturated fats, olive oil in particular, have a positive effect on heart disease by preventing the oxidation of LDL particles and thus limiting their uptake by monocytes and deposition in the artery walls. However, the consumption of too much fat of any variety is not healthy. Fats have more calories per unit weight than either proteins or carbohydrates. Fat contains 9 calories per gram while proteins and carbohydrates each have only 4 calories per gram. **Fats make you fat.** In addition, fats have been implicated as a risk factor for some common cancers, such as breast, colon, and prostate. (If you are interested in learning more about how fat affects your health and/or you are interested in reducing the fat from your body, read our book *The Choose to Lose Diet*, Houghton Mifflin, 1990.)

Eater's Choice focuses on the saturated fat and *not the cholesterol content of the foods you eat* for the following reasons. First, with only a few easy to remember exceptions, saturated fat and cholesterol occur in the same foods; they are fellow travelers. So, by avoiding foods high in saturated fat, you are also avoiding foods high in cholesterol. The exceptions are: egg yolks and organ meats (brain, pancreas, liver, kidneys), which are high in cholesterol but have only moderate amounts of saturated fat. On the other hand, coconut oil, palm oil, palm kernel oil, hydrogenated vegetable oil, and cocoa butter (in chocolate) are very high in saturated fat but have no cholesterol.

Second, the cholesterol you eat has much less effect on raising blood cholesterol levels than does saturated fat. Many people assume that all you have to do to lower your blood cholesterol level is to eat less cholesterol. Eggs are loaded with cholesterol. Eat fewer eggs and your blood cholesterol problem is licked, so the argument goes. However, contrary to popular belief, the amount of fats, especially *saturated fats,* that you eat has a much greater effect on your blood cholesterol level than does the amount of cholesterol you consume.

Of course, this does not mean that you should eat unlimited numbers of eggs or other high-cholesterol foods. Remember that the American Heart Association and the Adult Treatment Panel recommend a daily cholesterol intake of no more than 200–300 mg (one large egg yolk contains 213 mg). Avoid foods high in cholesterol. Think before you eat.

Third, keeping track of only saturated fat makes *Eater's Choice* a simple yet effective plan to follow. The simpler a plan is to follow, the more likely you are to follow it and the more likely you are to succeed in lowering your blood cholesterol level.

HOW TO REDUCE YOUR SATURATED FAT INTAKE

You can reduce your saturated fat intake in two ways:

1. Reduce the amount of fat you eat by substituting foods high in complex carbohydrates (starches) and fiber (such as rice, whole-grain pastas, breads, and cereals, vegetables, and fruits) for foods high in saturated fat. And replace high-fat foods with low-fat or nonfat foods, such as sour cream with low-fat yogurt. (See the food tables at the end of the book for the saturated fat contents of common foods.)
2. Substitute foods high in unsaturated fat (such as olive oil or margarine) for foods high in saturated fat (such as butter, lard, and beef tallow). Go light on margarine (see the discussion of trans fats on page 80).

The Total Diet Counts

As you establish your new eating plan, you must remember that to lower your blood cholesterol you will have to make changes in what you eat. **You will have to make enough changes to make a difference.** What is important are the amounts and types of fats you eat and not the actual foods that supply them. Individual foods either raise or lower your blood cholesterol level by the way they contribute to the daily total of total fat, saturated fat, polyunsaturated fat, and cholesterol.

But how many changes do you have to make to make a difference? How much is enough? *Eater's Choice* is a plan that allows you to determine how much is enough by keeping track of your saturated fat intake. How you set your daily saturated fat budget will depend on how much you want to reduce your blood cholesterol level. Periodic monitoring of your blood cholesterol level will tell you if your change in food choices has made a sufficient difference in lowering it or if you must make more changes in your eating pattern.

You need not wait months to see if your heart-smart eating behavior has lowered your blood cholesterol level. It takes only about three weeks to achieve up to 30 percent lowering of your blood cholesterol if you have made the right food choices.

While the types and amounts of fats and not the foods that contain them are important to the health of your body, which foods contain the fats you eat are of utmost importance to you. Thus, 30 calories of saturated fat from bacon or from cheesecake may have identical effects on your blood cholesterol level but undoubtedly quite different effects on your palate and psyche. And that is why *Eater's Choice* is useful for you. You tailor your food choices to fit your saturated fat budget *and* your taste buds.

Cold Turkey: A Dish for Some. Before we delve into *Eater's Choice* we realize some of you may not want to take the trouble to monitor your sat-fat (saturated fat) intake. You may wish to restrict your diet totally to foods low in saturated fat: fish, white meat turkey or chicken without skin, loads of vegetables and fruits, bread (made without hydrogenated oils), oatmeal, rice, pasta, skim milk, low-fat yogurt and cottage cheese, tub margarine and olive, safflower, sunflower, or corn oil, etc.

Going cold turkey means completely eliminating all foods high in saturated fat. This includes red meats, such as beef, veal, lamb, pork, ham, and cold cuts, as well as whole milk dairy products, such as cheese, sour cream, cream, whole milk, 2% milk, butter, and ice cream, in addition to most commercial snacks and baked goods and other products made with palm oil, palm kernel oil, coconut oil, hydrogenated vegetable oil, cocoa butter, or lard.

If you want to try this approach, all the recipes in this cookbook are dishes you can eat with complete freedom. They are designed to be low in saturated fat *and* delicious.

Take It Easy: A Strategy for Others. If you feel there are too many foods that you cannot give up without sinking into a deep depression, that life would not be worth living without brie and crackers, *Eater's Choice* gives *you* control over your choices of food and still allows you to lower your blood cholesterol level.

Of course, you will not be able to eat *everything* you want in the amounts and as often as you want, but you will be able to eat that brie if you make enough low-fat choices in your diet to compensate for the added saturated fat. This is a flexible plan that you will change and modify until you reach your target low blood cholesterol level.

A STEP-BY-STEP GUIDE TO *EATER'S CHOICE*

First, if you have not already done so, have your physician measure your total blood cholesterol. (New technology is now available to measure blood cholesterol in mere minutes from a drop of blood taken from your finger. This revolutionary advance in blood analysis will make it possible to have your blood cholesterol measured at your work place, health clinic, even shopping malls, as well as at your physician's office.) If your total blood cholesterol level is elevated, you should also know your levels of HDL, triglycerides, and LDL. (Remember: a twelve-hour fast is required before your blood is drawn to measure triglycerides and LDL.) See Chapter 2 for a discussion of all the lipoproteins in the blood.

Ask for numerical values. Make sure you know both your HDL and your LDL levels in addition to your total blood cholesterol. Remember, the lower your HDL level, the higher your risk and the greater the incentive to lower your LDL level.

NOTE: Cholesterol levels measured within three months after a heart attack, surgery, or other physical trauma may be abnormally low.

Set Your Blood Cholesterol Target

Set your own personal blood cholesterol goals. You know what your blood cholesterol level is. You know that you want it to be below 200 mg/dL. Recall from the Framingham risk curve (Chapter 3) that the lower your blood cholesterol level, the lower your risk of coronary heart disease.

Perhaps you want to lower your blood cholesterol level in stages. Perhaps it is now 260 mg/dL and you want to take it down to 230 mg/dL as the first step. Fine. You just have to tailor your eating to meet this goal. After a month, have your blood cholesterol level measured again. When you have achieved your goal of 230 mg/dL and feel comfortable with your new eating pattern, you are ready to make additional diet changes to lower your blood cholesterol to 200 mg/dL.

Know Your Desirable Body Weight

Because the amount of saturated fat allowed on the *Eater's Choice* plan is based on the number of calories you eat each day, you need to know how many calories you consume or should consume. If you are overweight, you should choose your desirable weight as a goal. You may already know your desirable weight. If not, Table 1 on page 48 lists desirable weights for men and women of different heights and body frame sizes.

To help keep your weight down, you should also exercise. (Be sure to consult your doctor about what exercises you can do safely.) Even just walking for twenty minutes or more each day will help you lose weight. (And you'll feel better too!) Losing weight if you are overweight will contribute to reducing your blood cholesterol

---

ON EXERCISE AND LOSING WEIGHT

Contrary to popular opinion, the main value of exercise is not burning calories, but building and preserving muscle. By exercising, you force your body to burn fat from the fat stores rather than protein from the muscle tissue. By engaging in regular aerobic exercise and eating a low-fat diet, you maximize depletion of your fat stores and thus ensure permanent weight loss.

Table 1: Desirable Weights for Adults Age 25 and Over*
(weight in pounds without clothing)

HEIGHT WITHOUT SHOES		FRAME		
(FEET)	(INCHES)	SMALL	MEDIUM	LARGE
Men				
5	1	112–120	118–129	126–141
5	2	115–123	121–133	129–144
5	3	118–126	124–136	132–148
5	4	121–129	127–139	135–152
5	5	124–133	130–143	138–156
5	6	128–137	134–147	142–161
5	7	132–141	138–152	147–166
5	8	136–145	142–156	151–170
5	9	140–150	146–160	155–174
5	10	144–154	150–165	159–179
5	11	148–158	154–170	164–184
6	0	152–162	158–175	168–189
6	1	156–167	162–180	173–194
6	2	160–171	167–185	178–199
6	3	164–175	172–190	182–204
Women				
4	8	92–98	96–107	104–119
4	9	94–101	98–110	106–122
4	10	96–104	101–113	109–125
4	11	99–107	104–116	112–128
5	0	102–110	107–119	115–131
5	1	105–113	110–122	118–134
5	2	108–116	113–126	121–138
5	3	111–119	116–130	125–142
5	4	114–123	120–135	129–146
5	5	118–127	124–139	133–150
5	6	122–131	128–143	137–154
5	7	126–135	132–147	141–158
5	8	130–140	136–151	145–163
5	9	134–144	140–155	149–168
5	10	138–148	144–159	153–173

*Courtesy of Metropolitan Life Insurance Company, New York, N.Y., 1959
For persons between 18 and 25 years of age, subtract 1 pound for each year under 25.

and LDL levels (and blood pressure), raising your HDL level, and reducing your risk of coronary heart disease morbidity and mortality. For more information about weight loss and exercise and a budget plan to lose weight, read *The Choose to Lose Diet: A Food Lover's Guide to Permanent Weight Loss,* by Dr. Ron Goor and Nancy Goor and Katherine Boyd (Houghton Mifflin, 1990).

Determine Your Frame

In order to use the table of desirable weights (Table 1) you need to know if your body frame is small, medium, or large. You can determine this by placing your left thumb and middle finger around your right wrist. Squeeze your fingers as tightly as possible. If the thumb and finger overlap, you have a small frame. If they just touch, your frame size is medium. If they do not touch, then you have a large frame. This method is a bit crude, but accurate enough for our purpose. Find your desirable weight by sex, height, and frame size on the chart.

Know Your Ideal Daily Caloric Intake

In order to determine your daily caloric intake, you must know your approximate daily level of activity (daily energy expenditure) in addition to your desirable weight. To determine your level of activity, try to identify which of the following five descriptions most accurately describes your level of activity during the preceding week. Choose a lower level of activity if you are not sure which of two levels best describes your activity.

Activity Levels*

Very Sedentary. Limited activity, confined to a few rooms or a house. Slow walking, no running. Most major activities involve sitting.

Sedentary. Activities involve mostly walking or some sporadic slow running at a jogging speed of approximately ten minutes per mile. Recreational activities include bowling, fishing, target shooting, horseback riding, motorboating, snowmobiling, or other similar activities. Less than ten minutes of continuous running (faster than a jog) per week.

---

*From *The DINE System* by Dr. Darwin Dennison

Moderately Active. Activities include golf (eighteen holes), doubles tennis, sailing, pleasure swimming or skating, aerobic dancing, Jazzercise, downhill skiing, or other similar activities. Between ten and twenty minutes of continuous running at least three times per week.

Active. More than twenty minutes of sustained activity, such as jogging, swimming, competitive tennis, or cross-country skiing, more than three times per week or more than forty-five minutes of recreational tennis, paddle ball, or other activities at least three times per week.

Super Active. At least one and a half hours of vigorous activity (training for competitive athletics, full-court basketball, mountain climbing, weight training, football, wrestling, or other similar activity) four days per week or more than two and a half hours of recreational activity four or more times per week.

Your Daily Caloric Needs

Use Table 2 to determine the number of calories you should consume each day. First, locate your desirable weight along the left-hand column. Making sure you use the correct row for your sex, find the number of calories under the column for your activity level.

This is the calorie level that will maintain your desirable weight based on your activity level. If your activity level changes, as it might with changes in season, you should determine your level of caloric intake anew. If you want to lose weight and you are not doing so after two or three weeks, determine your caloric intake using a lower activity level.

The following example will help you understand how to determine your desirable caloric level.

George is 5 feet 9 inches tall. He determines by the wrist test that he is of medium frame. To find how much he should weigh, he locates his height in the left-hand column of Table 1. Looking across the row for 5 feet 9 inches, he finds his weight range under the frame column labeled Medium. His weight range is 146–160. George actually weighs 160 pounds but wants to lose 10 pounds and weigh 150 pounds.

George jogs for thirty minutes five times a week. After reading the descriptions of various activity levels above, he determines that his activity level is Active. He finds his desirable weight (150) in the left-

Table 2: Ideal Caloric Level Based on Goal Weight, Activity Level, and Sex

DESIRABLE WEIGHT	SEX	ACTIVITY LEVEL				
		VERY SEDENTARY	SEDENTARY	MODERATELY ACTIVE	ACTIVE	SUPER ACTIVE
90	M	1170	1260	1350	1440	1530
	F	1053	1134	1215	1296	1377
95	M	1235	1330	1425	1520	1615
	F	1111	1197	1282	1368	1453
100	M	1300	1400	1500	1600	1700
	F	1170	1260	1350	1440	1530
105	M	1365	1470	1575	1680	1785
	F	1228	1323	1417	1512	1606
110	M	1430	1540	1650	1760	1870
	F	1287	1386	1485	1584	1683
115	M	1495	1610	1725	1840	1955
	F	1345	1449	1552	1656	1759
120	M	1560	1680	1800	1920	2040
	F	1404	1512	1620	1728	1836
125	M	1625	1750	1875	2000	2125
	F	1462	1575	1687	1800	1912
130	M	1690	1820	1950	2080	2210
	F	1521	1638	1755	1872	1989
135	M	1755	1890	2025	2160	2295
	F	1579	1701	1822	1944	2065
140	M	1820	1960	2100	2240	2380
	F	1638	1764	1890	2016	2142
145	M	1885	2030	2175	2320	2465
	F	1696	1827	1957	2088	2218
150	M	1950	2100	2250	2400	2550
	F	1755	1890	2025	2160	2295
155	M	2015	2170	2325	2480	2635
	F	1813	1953	2092	2232	2371
160	M	2080	2240	2400	2560	2720
	F	1872	2016	2160	2304	2448
165	M	2145	2310	2475	2640	2805
	F	1930	2079	2227	2376	2524
170	M	2210	2380	2550	2720	2890
	F	1989	2142	2295	2448	2601
175	M	2275	2450	2625	2800	2975
	F	2047	2205	2362	2520	2677
180	M	2340	2520	2700	2880	3060
	F	2106	2268	2430	2592	2754
185	M	2405	2590	2775	2960	3145
	F	2164	2331	2497	2664	2830

| | | ACTIVITY LEVEL | | | | |
DESIRABLE WEIGHT	SEX	VERY SEDENTARY	SEDENTARY	MODERATELY ACTIVE	ACTIVE	SUPER ACTIVE
190	M	2470	2660	2850	3040	3230
	F	2223	2394	2565	2736	2907
195	M	2535	2730	2925	3120	3315
	F	2281	2457	2632	2808	2983
200	M	2600	2800	3000	3200	3400
	F	2340	2520	2700	2880	3060
205	M	2665	2870	3075	3280	3485
	F	2398	2583	2767	2952	3136
210	M	2730	2940	3150	3360	3570
	F	2457	2646	2835	3024	3213
215	M	2795	3010	3225	3440	3655
	F	2515	2709	2905	3096	3289
220	M	2860	3080	3300	3520	3740
	F	2574	2772	2970	3168	3366

hand column of Table 2. Looking across the row for 150 for males (M), he finds his ideal caloric intake level under the Active column. George's ideal daily caloric intake is 2400 calories.

Reduce Saturated Fat to 10 Percent of Total Calories or Less

Now that you have determined *your* calorie level, you can figure out how much saturated fat you should eat each day. Your daily allotment of saturated fat will ultimately depend on the initial level of your blood cholesterol and how much your blood cholesterol drops in response to a lower saturated fat intake.

The first step for everyone, no matter how high your initial blood cholesterol level, is to reduce your saturated fat intake to no more than 10 percent of your total calories. We call this the *Eater's Choice* 10 Percent Plan. (Those with high-risk blood cholesterol levels — see National Institutes of Health recommendations in Chapter 4 — should consider starting directly with the *Eater's Choice* 6 Percent Plan discussed on page 53.)

In practical terms, what does that mean? Here is George again. George should consume 2400 calories a day to maintain his desirable weight. His blood cholesterol level is 250 mg/dL. To lower his blood cholesterol below 200 mg/dL, he must reduce his saturated fat intake to 10 percent or less of his daily calories. Ten percent of 2400 calories is 240 calories of saturated fat. George should eat no more than 240 calories of saturated fat each day.

To help you visualize what 240 calories of saturated fat means in terms of foods, there are:

- 45 calories of saturated fat in 1 cup of whole milk;
- 100 calories of saturated fat in 4 ounces of lean, broiled ground beef;
- 12 calories of saturated fat in 4 ounces of roasted chicken breast without skin;
- 117 calories of saturated fat in a Burger King Double Cheeseburger.

You can use the blank worksheet on page 55 to determine *your* daily sat-fat budget. Use George's worksheet as a guide.

Once you go on the *Eater's Choice* plan, you will want to monitor your blood cholesterol levels periodically to see how you are doing. Remember, it only takes two to three weeks for blood cholesterol levels to respond to changes in eating patterns. At first you should check at more frequent intervals — six weeks, six weeks, three months, six months — until your blood cholesterol stabilizes at its new lower level. Then have it checked every twelve months. Do not get upset if your blood cholesterol level fluctuates slightly — this is normal.

To prevent your blood cholesterol from rising, you must continue to follow the *Eater's Choice* plan, to keep your sat-fat intake at 10 percent or less of your calories. Your blood cholesterol level is affected by what you eat and will jump right back to its previously high level if you return to your old eating habits.

Eater's Choice 6 Percent Plan

If after about three months your blood cholesterol has not fallen below 200 mg/dL, you will need to switch to the *Eater's Choice* 6 Percent Plan. As you might guess, on the 6 Percent Plan you reduce your sat-fat intake to no more than 6 percent of your total calories. In George's case, he would eat no more than 144 (6 percent of 2400) calories of saturated fat a day on the *Eater's Choice* 6 Percent Plan.

Again, once you have brought your blood cholesterol below 200 mg/dL you must continue to follow the *Eater's Choice* 6 Percent Plan.

WORKSHEET TO DETERMINE
YOUR DAILY SAT-FAT BUDGET

Name ___GEORGE_____ Date __1/10/92__

STEP 1: DETERMINE YOUR DESIRABLE WEIGHT

    A. Sex: Male __X__   Female _____

    B. Height: __5__ feet __9__ inches

    C. Frame (wrist method):

    Small _____   Medium __X__ Large _____

    D. Weight Range (Table 1): __146 - 160__

    E. Desirable Weight: __150__

STEP 2: DETERMINE YOUR DAILY CALORIC INTAKE

    A. Activity Level Very Sedentary _____
       (see text):

       Sedentary _____

       Moderately Active _____

       Active __X_____

       Super Active _____

    B. Daily caloric intake (use Table 2): __2400__

STEP 3: DETERMINE YOUR DAILY SAT-FAT BUDGET

DAILY SAT-FAT BUDGET:

    __10__ % of daily caloric intake = __240__

WORKSHEET TO DETERMINE YOUR DAILY SAT-FAT BUDGET

Name _____ Date _____

STEP 1: DETERMINE YOUR DESIRABLE WEIGHT

    A. Sex: Male _____ Female _____

    B. Height: _____ feet _____ inches

    C. Frame (wrist method):

       Small _____ Medium _____ Large _____

    D. Weight Range (Table 1): _____

    E. Desirable Weight: _____

STEP 2: DETERMINE YOUR DAILY CALORIC INTAKE

    A. Activity Level Very Sedentary _____
       (see text):

                  Sedentary _____

                  Moderately Active _____

                  Active _____

                  Super Active _____

    B. Daily caloric intake (use Table 2): _____

STEP 3: DETERMINE YOUR DAILY SAT-FAT BUDGET

DAILY SAT-FAT BUDGET:

    _____% of daily caloric intake = _____

As described above, monitor your blood cholesterol periodically — six weeks, six weeks, three months, six months — and then once a year after you are sure your blood cholesterol has stabilized below 200 mg/dL.

For some, moving to a 4 percent plan may be necessary if strict adherence to a 6 percent plan has failed to reduce their blood cholesterol to below 200 mg/dL.

The Appeal of *Eater's Choice*

The main goal of *Eater's Choice* is to help you lower your risk of heart disease. What you may find just as important is that it allows enough personal choice to keep both your psyche and taste buds happy. You will still be able to eat the fatty foods you love, but perhaps less often or in smaller quantities.

The menu plans in Part II will give you some idea of how well you can eat on an *Eater's Choice* 10 Percent or 6 Percent (or even 4 Percent) Plan. The recipes at the end of the book will satisfy your palate without overloading your sat-fat budget and will give you tips on how to modify high-fat recipes from other cookbooks to create low-fat dishes.

A Balanced Diet

Eater's Choice emphasizes eating less saturated fat to lower your blood cholesterol level, but you must remember that your diet has to be balanced. In your zeal to reduce your intake of fats, you must not forget that you need vitamins, minerals, proteins, fiber, and bulk. (The meal plans in Chapter 13 will give you examples of balanced low-fat meals.)

As you remove saturated fat from your diet, you will have to replace it with something else. Most health experts today recommend replacing the saturated fat calories you eliminate with calories from complex carbohydrates. Complex carbohydrates are found in whole-grain breads and pastas, fruits, and vegetables. Enriching your diet with these foods has the additional advantages of increasing your intake of vitamins, minerals, and fiber.

Insoluble fiber, such as in whole wheat, may help prevent certain cancers, such as colon cancer. Soluble fiber, such as in oat bran products, has been found to lower blood cholesterol levels.

ADDED BENEFITS OF *EATER'S CHOICE*

Weight Loss

One of the loveliest benefits of *Eater's Choice* is a natural loss of weight. Many people report losing 10–15 pounds, and some as much as 40. You will be eating less fat and thus fewer calories without necessarily eating less food.

"But," you ask in disbelief, "if I replace saturated fat with complex carbohydrates, won't I turn into a tub? Everyone knows carbohydrates are fattening." If this is what you think, get this myth out of your head.

All fats — saturated, polyunsaturated, and monounsaturated — contain 9 calories per gram. Proteins and carbohydrates, on the other hand, contain only 4 calories per gram. Carbohydrates have less than half the calories per unit weight than fats (4 versus 9) and thus twice the bulk per calorie. Carbohydrates fill you up at half the caloric cost. Carbohydrate calories, even in excess, are not stored as fat tissue. Excess fat calories are stored as fat tissue. Fat makes fat!

Fat makes fat! is the theme of our new book, *The Choose to Lose Diet*. *Choose to Lose* specifically focuses on total fat for weight loss. It is true that by reducing saturated fat in their diet, many people lose weight. However, just reducing saturated fat is not always enough. There are foods such as olive oil and margarine that are very low in saturated fat but very high in total fat, and thus fattening. So to lose weight you have to target total fat. Learn what your fat budget is and how, by reducing fat in your diet, increasing your intake of complex carbohydrates, and exercising aerobically (walking) every day, you can become lean and stay that way forever.

It is not the potato that makes you fat, it is what you do to it. A medium baked potato has a trace amount of fat. You glob 3 tablespoons of sour cream (23 fat calories per tablespoon) on top, and the innocent potato now contains 69 fat calories. A piece of bread has 9 fat calories per slice. When you slather it with butter or margarine at 100 fat calories per tablespoon, it becomes 109 fat calories or more per slice. It is the huge amount of fat in the American diet that leads to overweight and obesity.

Dr. William Castelli, director of the Framingham Heart Study, aptly concurs:

> If you take the lowly potato, it's about 100 calories, let's say. If you chop it up and cook it in fat, you're up to 275 to 300 calories from that original hundred calories. If you slice it up real fine and make potato chips, you're up to 400 calories over that original potato. Now what's the difference? Just fat. What kind of fat? Well, frequently it's totally saturated fat. Why? Well, someone learned that if you cook potato chips in a totally saturated fat, they stay crispier longer. The shelf life, you know, of the potato chip goes on and on and on and on. The shelf life of the person who eats it doesn't. That's our problem.

The fat calories for *Eater's Choice* recipes are listed on pages 535–46.

Expanding Your Palette

A whole new world of foods will be open to you as you replace your saturated fats with complex carbohydrates. Both your food palette and taste palate will be expanded as you explore new recipes that fit into your sat-fat budget. For starters, try Indian Vegetables (page 286) or Indonesian Chicken with Green Beans (page 212) or Calzone (page 311).

Regularity

An added benefit of removing fat from your diet and increasing fiber, particularly whole grains, fruits, and vegetables, is the increased regularity of your excretory system.

LAST RESORT: DRUGS

If diet does not reduce your blood cholesterol adequately and *you are really following your eating plan to the letter,* you may need to take drugs prescribed by a physician. The preferred drugs are bile acid sequestrants — either cholestyramine (Questran)* or colestipol (Colestid) and nicotinic acid (niacin).

The bile acid sequestrants bind bile acids in the intestine and prevent their reabsorption and return to the liver. The bile acids are excreted in the feces. To compensate for the loss of bile acids, the liver removes large amounts of LDL-cholesterol from the blood. The cholesterol is converted into bile acids, which are then secreted into the intestine, where they help emulsify dietary fats.

Niacin lowers blood cholesterol levels by reducing the formation of VLDL, thereby blocking the formation of LDL. In small amounts (about 100 mg per day), niacin is a vitamin and has no effect on blood cholesterol. In doses large enough to lower blood cholesterol (1000–3000 mg per day), niacin is a potent drug with side effects (such as flushing, an itching rash, gastric upset, and/or blurred vision) and potential toxicities. It is recommended that people taking large doses should be under a physician's supervision and should have their liver function, blood glucose, and blood uric acid monitored periodically. Large amounts of niacin should not be taken by people with the following conditions: peptic ulcers, liver disease, gouty arthritis, or some types of heart rhythm disturbances.

Lovastatin is the first of a new class of potent blood cholesterol–lowering drugs: HMG CoA reductase inhibitors. These drugs work by blocking the synthesis of cholesterol in the liver. To compensate, the liver increases the amount of cholesterol, mainly LDL-cholesterol, that it removes from the blood. At this writing, lovastatin holds much promise but long-term safety has not yet been established.

If this discussion produces a vision of a banana split with four scoops of ice cream covered with chocolate sauce and whipped cream in one hand and a glass of bile acid sequestrant in the other, you will be sorely disappointed. All the drugs have side effects or toxicities and, with the exception of niacin, cost between $800 and $3000 a year, depending on drug and dose. In addition, drug therapy does not make up for eating a high-fat diet. Drugs complement a blood cholesterol–lowering diet. In fact, the more you lower your blood cholesterol by diet, the more effective will be your use of drugs. In a study showing the role of diet on effectiveness of drug therapy, 80 percent of people who ate a low-fat diet in com-

(*continued on next page*)

*Questran was the drug used in the Coronary Primary Prevention Trial to lower blood cholesterol levels and incidence of heart attacks.

LAST RESORT: DRUGS (continued)

bination with the cholesterol-lowering drug, lovastatin, lowered their LDL to the recommended level. In contrast, only 50 percent of those taking lovastatin while continuing to eat a high-fat diet were able to lower their LDL-cholesterol to the recommended level. The more you lower your blood cholesterol by diet, the more effective the drug will be. And remember, a low-fat, cholesterol-lowering diet has additional benefits that drugs do not have, such as weight control, reduced risk of some common cancers, regularity, low cost, no unpleasant side effects, and great taste.

Remember:

1. *Eater's Choice* is a simple method for lowering blood cholesterol by limiting the amount of saturated fat you eat while giving you control over your food choices.
2. Step-by-Step Guide to *Eater's Choice:*
   a. Have your total blood cholesterol measured; if it is above 200 mg/dL, have all your lipoproteins measured — total cholesterol, LDL, HDL, and triglycerides.
   b. Set your blood cholesterol goal (not to exceed 200 mg/dL).
   c. Determine how much you should weigh.
   d. Determine how many calories you must eat to maintain that weight. Calorie requirements depend on your sex, frame size, and activity level.
   e. Multiply your total daily calorie allotment by 10 percent (or 6 percent) to determine your maximum daily saturated fat budget; follow eating plan and monitor blood cholesterol levels in three months.
   f. If blood cholesterol is still above 200 mg/dL after three months, begin the 6 Percent (or 4 Percent) eating plan.

MAKING THE RIGHT CHOICES

6

Now that you or your physician have figured out how many calories of saturated fat you should eat each day, you are probably eager to put *Eater's Choice* into action.

Obviously, since you are setting limits on the saturated fats you consume, you will have to know the saturated fat contents of foods that you eat. The food tables at the end of the book list foods, their caloric value, and the number of calories of saturated fat they contain. After you determine the number of calories of saturated fat in a given portion of food, you can budget it into your daily food intake in one of two ways.

If planning is impractical or not in your nature, you can keep a running total of what you eat for the day. When you reach your daily allotment of saturated fat, that is it — no more saturated fat until tomorrow.

If you are a planner type, you can determine what your meals will be for the day or a week and add up the saturated fat calories in advance. You can make choices before you eat. "Hmmm," you think, "I'll spend ——— sat-fat calories on ——— and ——— sat-fat calories on ———." Planning ahead also makes you a more efficient grocery shopper.

If you plan ahead, you can save up sat-fat calories for a particular day or special occasion. Perhaps you are going out to dinner Saturday night and want to splurge on a big steak and a rich dessert. By not spending your total saturated fat budget each day, you may be able to save enough sat-fat calories to eat a 6-ounce lean and trimmed porterhouse steak (78 sat-fat calories), 2 tablespoons of sour cream (28 sat-fat calories) on your baked potato, and a piece of cheesecake (89 sat-fat calories).

Likewise, even if you have spent your sat-fat budget for the day and your Aunt May insists that you try the strawberry whipped cream cake she has made *just for you,* you may take a piece without dropping dead on the spot. Blood cholesterol levels do not respond to a single day's food intake; they reflect the sum of the fats you have eaten over the past several weeks. To make up for the splurge, eat fewer sat-fat calories than allowed on your budget for the next few days. But try to limit overdrawing your sat-fat budget in emergency situations or your arteries will pay the penalty.

Keeping Track

The only way to *really* know if you are eating within your sat-fat budget is to write everything down. It is not enough just to *think* you are eating a low-sat-fat diet. Suppose you ate a piece of chicken because you know that chicken is a low-fat food. Did you eat a KFC (Kentucky Fried Chicken) thigh at 69 sat-fat calories? Or two at 138? Or was it a batter-fried chicken breast with skin at 44 sat-fat calories? Or perhaps you grilled a breast with no skin at 4 sat-fat calories? It makes a big difference. To lower your cholesterol and keep it low, you have to know *exactly* what you are eating and the only way to know is to keep an honest and accurate food record.

Keeping a food record is THE SKILL that will give you insight into the reason your cholesterol is elevated and the mastery to control it. (See pages 523–531 for details on how to keep a food record.)

Recording the sat-fat calories of the foods you eat gives you power. You learn which foods are making your cholesterol high so you can make changes. You analyze your food record to discover which high-sat-fat foods you can't live without, which ones you can eat less of, and which ones you can eliminate altogether. You know how many sat-fat calories you have eaten so you can make room for splurges. You learn if your diet is balanced; if it is filled with enough fruits, vegetables, whole grains, and low- or nonfat dairy foods. How could you know if you don't write everything down?

You may think adding up sat-fat calories will take all the spontaneity out of eating. However, you probably eat a limited number of foods and a limited number of dishes (whether you cook them or eat them out). Sooner than you think, you will know their sat-fat values as well as you know the telephone numbers of your friends. Within a short time, you will learn which combinations and amounts of your favorite foods will fit into your sat-fat budget. For example, you will learn that if you want to have cheese on a bagel for breakfast, you might choose a turkey sandwich for lunch. If you want ice cream for dessert, you might choose scallops for dinner.

To help you keep track of your sat-fat intake, you may want to use the order form at the end of the book to send away for a handy, pocket-sized Sat-fat Estimator and/or a Passbook.

Another approach to determining the sat-fat content of the foods you eat is to use a computer nutrient-analysis program. Many such programs are available. The DINE System is a nutritionally comprehensive system with a database of 5500 food items. This user-friendly program will analyze the saturated fat content in the foods you eat and in recipes. It will also provide the amounts of fourteen other nutrients: monounsaturated and polyunsaturated fats, protein, complex carbohydrates, sugar, cholesterol, and key vitamins and minerals, including sodium, potassium, and calcium. The analysis compares your diet with current dietary guidelines. The DINE System is available for Apple and IBM computers. You can get more information by writing to: DINE Systems, Inc., 5 Bluebird Lane, West Amherst, New York 14228.

Monitor Your Sat-Fat Intake Every Six Months. Just as you should have your blood cholesterol level measured periodically to make sure you are maintaining a level below 200 mg/dL, you should monitor your sat-fat calories for one or two days every six months. This will help you know you are still eating within your sat-fat budget.

FOOD TABLES

The food tables at the end of the book can help you see how much saturated fat lurks in the foods you eat. This information gives you the power to take control and make your own food choices — choices that allow you to lower your blood cholesterol and enjoy eating at the same time.

The food tables are arranged in the following groups: beverages; dairy products and eggs; fast foods; fats and oils; fish and shellfish; frozen and microwave foods; fruits and fruit juices; grain products; meats; nuts and seeds; poultry; restaurant food; sauces and gravies;

sausages and luncheon meats; snack foods; soups; sugars and sweets; vegetables and legumes; miscellaneous items. Within each group, items are arranged in alphabetical order.

FOOD TABLES INDEX

To help you locate specific foods in the Food Tables, use the Food Tables Index on page 517.

Data for meats, fish, and poultry are usually given in 1-ounce amounts, to help you compare the fat contents of foods, and sometimes also in a measure commonly used for cooking or eating. For instance, if you eat 7 ounces of chicken, you would multiply the sat-fat content by 7 to determine the amount of saturated fat you actually ate.

Be careful. These food tables make meats look like low-fat foods because the fat values are given for 1-ounce amounts. Rarely does anyone eat only 1 ounce of meat.

Measuring

In order to use the food tables, you will need to measure the actual amounts of the foods you eat. In addition to measuring spoons and measuring cups, you might find an inexpensive kitchen scale useful.

Use these measuring tools to determine the size of the serving you actually eat and see how many times larger or smaller it is than the listed amount. Then calculate the actual numbers of calories you are consuming. For example, if 1 ounce of cheddar cheese contains 54 calories of saturated fat and you eat ½ ounce, then you are consuming 54 × ½ calories or 27 calories of saturated fat.

How the Food Tables Help You

By focusing on saturated fat rather than foods, the food tables allow you to choose, based on your own preferences, combinations of foods that can fit into your daily sat-fat budget.

You may be able to eat less of a certain food rather than eliminate it entirely. Since the cup of ice cream you long for contains 80 sat-fat calories, then ½ cup has only 40 sat-fat calories. Maybe your sat-fat budget can accommodate the smaller helping.

Using the food tables, you may be able to find a low sat-fat substitute for a food you normally eat. For example, during the course of a day, you may eat a total of six pats of butter — on toast, sandwiches, and a baked potato. Since each pat of butter contains 23 calories of sat-fat, butter is contributing 23 × 6 or 138 calories of sat-fat to your daily sat-fat budget. In place of butter, substitute margarine at 6 calories of sat-fat per teaspoon (equivalent to a pat). The margarine will contribute only 6 × 6 or 36 calories of sat-fat to your daily sat-fat budget at a savings of 102 sat-fat calories.

Here are some other benefits of using the food tables:

1. Hidden sources of saturated fat will jump out at you. "Wow! My nondairy, cholesterol-free coffee whitener has 26 calories of sat-fat per ounce. My daily 3 cups of coffee with 3 ounces of whitener equals 78 calories of sat-fat — that's a third of my sat-fat budget for the whole day, and I haven't even eaten anything!" You can determine if it is really worth eating those fatty foods once you know their sat-fat content.

2. You can check to see if foods that you always considered low-fat are truly low in fat. Take veal, for one: a fiction has developed that veal is less fatty than other beef. Check out the food tables and see how false this assumption is.

3. You can use the food tables to check and modify recipes. For example, a pie recipe uses 1 cup of sour cream, or 270 calories of saturated fat. Replace the sour cream with an equivalent amount of low-fat yogurt, and you only add 3 calories of saturated fat to the pie.

KEEPING A FOOD RECORD

Read pages 523–531 and get the inside scoop on keeping a food record — the KEY to lowering your blood cholesterol.

And Coming in the Next Chapter . . .

Hold on to your seats: the next chapter will tell you all the juicy gossip about the fats in the foods you eat.

Remember:

1. Budget saturated fat into your daily food intake by keeping a running total for each day or planning ahead for the week.
2. The food tables list saturated fat contents of common foods. They help you:
   a. keep track of your saturated fat intake;
   b. choose a variety of foods you like with different sat-fat values to fit into your sat-fat budget;
   c. check and modify recipes.

WHERE'S THE FAT? 7

THE FOCUS of *Eater's Choice* is on limiting saturated fat in your diet while still allowing you to make food choices that reflect your food preferences. There is no large source of saturated fat concentrated in just one food. Nearly every food contains some fat, and most of the fat is hidden. Fats added at the table, such as spreads and salad dressings, account for only about one-fourth of the fat intake, while three-quarters of the fat is invisible or hidden in foods such as red meat, dairy products, baked goods, frozen dinners, and fat used in food preparation.

To help you analyze and change your daily meal plan, the list below will focus your attention on the high sat-fat foods you may have been eating — often without realizing they are high sat-fat foods. For example, do you think of beef as full of fat, or do you think of beef as protein? Is milk on your list of high-fat foods? Do you know how much fat is in a glass of whole milk?

The Top 50 Percent. The following food items contributed about 50 percent of the total saturated fat consumed by Americans during the time period 1976–1980. In descending order of importance, they were: hamburgers, cheeseburgers, meat loaf; whole milk and whole-milk beverages; cheeses, excluding cottage cheese; beef steaks and roasts; hot dogs, ham, and luncheon meats; doughnuts, cookies, and cake; eggs.*

The Next 28 Percent. Another 28 percent (for a cumulative total of 78 percent) of the saturated fat intake was contributed by, in descending order: pork, including chops and roasts; butter; white bread,* rolls,* and crackers; ice cream and frozen desserts; marga-

---

*These foods are relatively low in saturated fat, but the large amounts consumed contribute substantial saturated fat calories to the American diet.

rine; 2% milk; mayonnaise and salad dressings; French fries and fried potatoes; salty snacks; bacon; nondairy coffee creamers; sausage.

Do these foods sound familiar? Do they contribute heavily to your saturated fat intake? Check the food tables to see how much saturated fat these and other foods actually contain. You might be surprised — even shocked. Your immediate reaction might be that you must eliminate these foods, *now*, if not sooner.

Not a Bare-Bones Eating Plan. Relax. Any food can be fitted into *Eater's Choice*. No food need be completely eliminated. The food tables will help you determine *how much* and *how often* you can eat certain foods. Of course, the higher the saturated fat content of a food, the less often or the smaller the amount you will be able to fit into your personalized daily saturated fat budget.

Use Food Tables as You Read This Chapter. As we discuss the fat contents of common foods in this chapter, check back to the food tables to compare foods. Soon, you will have learned the sat-fat contents of the foods you commonly eat and will find you no longer need to look up every food in the tables.

MEATS

Since ground beef is number one on the saturated fat hit parade, let us look at the meat category. All the meat, poultry, and fish entries in the food tables are given in 1-ounce portions to help you compare the different meats. You can easily calculate the sat-fat content by multiplying the number of ounces of meat you eat times the saturated fat contained in 1 ounce. For instance, 1 ounce of braised lean flank steak has 16 calories of saturated fat per ounce. If you eat 6 ounces of flank steak, you are consuming 6 × 16 or 96 calories of saturated fat.

Hamburger — Three Times Fattier. You're thinking about dinner. The refrigerator is bare. Should you buy round steak or ground beef? You look at the beef section of the food tables. Trimmed, lean, round steak happens to be the leanest cut of red meat. It contains 7 calories of saturated fat per ounce. Check out the broiled lean ground beef: 25 calories of saturated fat for the same portion size. If you eat 6 ounces of either meat, the round steak will contribute 7 × 6 or 42 sat-fat calories, while the ground beef will contribute

25 × 6 or 150 sat-fat calories. The round steak has less than one-third the calories of saturated fat found in the broiled lean ground beef. Would this comparison help you decide?

Admittedly, hamburger is a convenience food. It's fast and tasty. However, it is so chock full of saturated fat your arteries shudder when a mere whiff of hamburger floats under your nose. If you need to prepare a delicious meal in a hurry, sauté scallops with garlic and ginger (5 minutes), cover a white fish with lemon yogurt and bake for 5–10 minutes, or cut round steak thin and sauté with onions and green peppers (15 minutes). Or try Vegeburgers (page 347), a healthy substitute for hamburgers.

For those of you who would rather give up your right arm than give up hamburgers, here are several hints to make your hamburger healthier. Broil rather than pan-fry hamburgers so some of the fat drips away. Immediately after cooking, place hamburgers between paper towels to absorb excess fat. Mix ground beef with bread crumbs or soybean protein (GranBurger, available from Worthington Foods) to make your hamburger half as fatty.

The Veal Story. According to the newly published U.S. Department of Agriculture Food Tables, many cuts of lean veal are relatively low in saturated fat. When trimmed of fat, braised veal leg has 5 sat-fat calories per ounce. Roasted veal shoulder blade, trimmed of fat, has 7 sat-fat calories per ounce. However, you must still be cautious when choosing veal cuts that have not been trimmed. For example, braised veal breast, untrimmed of fat, contains 156 calories of saturated fat per 6 ounces — that's a pretty big chunk out of a daily sat-fat budget of 200.

RED MEATS — BIG SATURATED FAT DONORS

In general, the higher the grade of meat, the more fat and saturated fat it contains. Take note: regardless of the grade or cut, the fat of all red meats is predominantly saturated (about 50 percent of the fat) and very little polyunsaturated fat (2 percent of the fat). Although some fat is lost through broiling and some fat can be trimmed, much of the fat is marbled throughout the meat and remains in it even after cooking.

Under the Wool, a Lot of Fat. The saturated fat content of lamb is comparable to all but the fattiest cuts of beef. Even the leanest cuts of lamb — lamb leg and lamb loin — are moderately high in saturated fat, containing about 60 calories of saturated fat per 6 ounces. Lamb shoulder and rib chops contain about 84 calories per 6 ounces.

Pork, Both High and Low. Pork has a reputation as a high-fat food. But the amount of fat (sat-fat) in pork dishes depends on the cut and the way you prepare it. For example, some pork dishes are relatively low in saturated fat, such as roasted lean tenderloin (24 sat-fat calories per 6 ounces) or broiled lean center loin (54 sat-fat calories per 6 ounces), while other dishes are high in sat-fat, such as roasted center rib loin with fat (132 sat-fat calories per 6 ounces) and pan-fried loin blade with fat (204 sat-fat calories per 6 ounces).

TAKE NOTE: Trim the fat from pork before cooking and you remove half the sat-fat calories. Save another 3 to 5 calories of sat-fat per ounce of meat by braising, broiling, or roasting instead of pan-frying.

By far the worst pork product in terms of saturated fat content is bacon. Three medium slices of cooked bacon contain 30 calories of saturated fat. A healthier alternative to bacon is Canadian bacon, which has about one-sixth as much saturated fat. Thus, an amount of Canadian bacon equivalent to 3 slices of regular bacon contributes only 5 calories of saturated fat.

What If You Still Want Red Meat?

You can see that all red meat contains too much saturated fat to be healthy for your coronary arteries. But can red meats fit into your *Eater's Choice* budget? The answer is yes — a yes that depends on the cut of meat, the amount, and how it is prepared. And because red meats are so high in saturated fat, you may have to adjust your saturated fat intake from other sources.

For example, if you consume 2000 calories per day, the *Eater's Choice* 10 Percent Plan allows 200 calories of saturated fat, and the *Eater's Choice* 6 Percent Plan allows 120 calories of saturated fat. One 4-ounce lean hamburger provides 100 sat-fat calories, 50 percent of the daily saturated fat allotment on the *Eater's Choice* 10 Percent Plan and 83 percent on the *Eater's Choice* 6 Percent Plan. That leaves 100 (10 Percent Plan) or 20 (6 Percent Plan) sat-fat calories for the rest of the day. Maybe every once in a while you have to have red meat or you will bite a passing stranger. Fine, have the red meat. On the other hand, you have other choices.

Meat Leaves Center Stage

If red meats are to be eaten on the *Eater's Choice* plan, you have two choices: either you limit the rest of your saturated fat intake for that day, or you use meat as a condiment. Eventually you will stop thinking of meat as the centerpiece of the meal — a 12-ounce steak with a vegetable on the side. Instead, you will use a meat such as thinly sliced flank steak to provide taste and texture to, say, a rice-based or a vegetable-based dish or a pasta.

Good Meat: Chicken

Chicken is very low in sat-fat compared to other meats. Six ounces of roasted chicken breast without skin contain 18 calories of saturated fat, versus 42 for round steak and 150 for ground beef.

Chicken breast is the part of the bird lowest in fat and thus your best choice.

CHICKEN PART (WITHOUT SKIN)	SAT-FAT CALORIES PER 6 OZ
breast	6
drumstick	12
wing	12
leg	18
thigh	18
back	24

In addition, chicken breast is one of the most versatile of meats and can be substituted for beef or pork in many recipes. Lemon Chicken (page 213), Phyllo-Wrapped Chicken with Rice, Artichokes, and Cream Sauce (page 226), and Sesame Chicken Brochettes (page 223) are but a few of the millions of interesting, delicious, and often quick and easy recipes using chicken breasts without skin.

Skin the Beast. Chicken breast scores high as a heart-healthy food as long as it is prepared properly. Bake half a breast without skin for 4 calories of sat-fat. Bake it with the skin on, and your sat-fat calories climb to 19. Batter-dip and fry it with the skin on, and your sat-fat calories soar to 44. TAKE NOTE: skin must be removed *before* cooking or the fat from the skin will be absorbed by the meat.

Better Meat: Turkey

The leanest poultry meat is roasted turkey breast without skin (see box below) which contains only 3 calories of saturated fat per 6 ounces. Dark meat turkey, such as the leg, contains six times as much saturated fat (18 calories), but compared to even the leanest red meats, it is low in saturated fat.

Turkey breast or cutlets ground in a food processor or meat grinder make an excellent low sat-fat ground beef substitute for making burgers, adding to spaghetti sauces and chilis, etc. However, be aware that ground turkey purchased at the grocery store may be loaded with large amounts of turkey fat and skin, and thus may not be a low-fat choice. For example, one commercially ground turkey product contains 36 calories of fat per ounce. Considering that plain white turkey meat contains less than 2½ calories of fat per ounce, the food manufacturer must be adding 33½ calories of fat and skin per ounce to the ground turkey. That's a lot of fat. At about 11 calories of sat-fat per ounce (44 sat-fat calories per 4 ounces), this brand of ground turkey is a better choice than lean ground beef at 25 sat-fat calories per ounce (100 sat-fat calories per 4 ounces). However, it is a choice that should not be eaten with abandon. To make matters worse, the fat content of commercially ground turkey is often not given. To ensure that your ground turkey is low in fat, grind it yourself.

WARNING: Pay attention to turkey labels. Do not buy Butterball turkeys or turkeys that have been shot up with coconut or other hydrogenated oils. Buy plain ol' natural unadulterated turkeys. Cook them breast down and they will still be juicy.

Best Meat: Fish

All animals that live in the water — shellfish, fish, and even marine mammals — contain a special kind of fat called omega-3 polyunsaturated fat. Omega-3 polyunsaturated fats are especially potent in lowering blood triglyceride levels. So, if high blood triglycerides are your problem, eating plenty of fish may be your salvation. Omega-3 polyunsaturated fats also reduce blood clotting. It is the small clots floating through the blood stream that often get caught in clogged arteries, causing heart attacks. The fewer clots that are formed the better.

Not only do fish contain the risk-reducing omega-3 polyunsaturated fats; they also are low in saturated fat. Lean fish such as flounder and sole contain only about 1 calorie of saturated fat per ounce. Even fatty fish such as red salmon have only about 5 calories of saturated fat per ounce — and the fattier the fish the more omega-3 polyunsaturated fat they contain. However, be advised — deep-frying fish or cooking them in cream or butter sauces turns a heart-healthy food into a heart-risky one.

Eat the Fish, Not the Capsule. The best way to get omega-3 polyunsaturated fats is by eating fish. Fish oil capsules are not the answer.

- Fish oil capsules are not regulated by the Food and Drug Administration, and thus may contain either very little or a lot of omega-3 polyunsaturated fat. You have no way of judging the potency of different brands.
- All the fat-soluble contaminants found in fish are concentrated in the fish oil in the capsules.
- Fish oil capsules add unnecessary fat and calories to your diet.
- Fish oil capsules are expensive.

A TIP: tuna packed in water tastes delicious and has 12 fewer calories of saturated fat per 3½-ounce can than tuna packed in oil. The oil used is soybean oil and not fish oil. If you are only able to purchase tuna packed in oil, wash the tuna with water to remove excess oil before eating. This will remove unwanted fat and calories.

Ruining Chicken, Turkey, and Fish

We often hear protests: "I eat only chicken, fish, and turkey, and yet my cholesterol is pushing 280 mg/dL. Am I one of those people whose cholesterol isn't affected by diet?" No! Even heart-healthy foods can be made heart-risky by the way they are prepared.

Nutritious and low in fat, chicken, turkey, and fish are often transformed into cholesterol-raising high-fat foods when they are processed into frozen dinners. This is how it works: pollock is a fish with trace saturated fat — that means a tiny bit more than 0 calories of saturated fat. A food processing company takes the pollock, cuts it into fish sticks, breads it, fries it in partially hydrogenated palm oil, and packages it. Now, according to the label the serving size of 4 pollock fish sticks contains 10 grams or 90 calories of fat and 45 calories of saturated fat (calculated by the Sat-fat Estimator,* which helps you estimate the sat-fat calories from the grams of fat on a label). The food processing company took an almost totally fat-free, heart-healthy food and increased its fat content by more than 9000 percent.

Fast-food restaurants commit similar crimes when preparing chicken and fish. Foods with negligible saturated fat become sat-fat gold mines when breaded and deep-fried in saturated oils. Remember — just because it's chicken, turkey, or fish does not mean it's heart-healthy.

Low in Fat but Not Much to Eat

Supermarket freezer cases are bulging with new, healthier frozen dinners that are truly low in saturated fat. But like all frozen dinners, they are no substitutes for freshly prepared food. In addition, the factor that makes them so low in saturated fat also creates another problem. Many of these dinners contain only about 1 to 2 ounces of meat. This is not much meat and not much food. People tend either to eat several of these dinners (which doubles or triples the sat-fat calories). Or, to diminish their hunger, they fill up later on other foods that are often high in saturated fat. Low-sat-fat frozen dinners are only a solution to your cholesterol problem if you eat one dinner and enhance it with plenty of vegetables and whole grains.

Cholesterol in Meats

All the meats — fish, poultry, and red meats — contain approximately equal amounts of cholesterol, about 25 mg per ounce or about 150 mg per 6 ounces. But take a look at the differences in calories of saturated fat. (Remember, these amounts are for only 1 ounce of meat.) Thus, decisions about choosing meats are best made on the basis of saturated fat content and not cholesterol content.

Fish and white meat turkey or chicken without skin are so low in saturated fat that large quantities could be fitted into any heart-

---

*See order form on the last page of the book.

CHOLESTEROL AND SATURATED FAT VALUES OF MEAT, POULTRY, FISH, AND SHELLFISH

	CHOLESTEROL MG/OZ	SATURATED FAT CALORIES/OZ
Veal breast	36	26
Lamb loin chop, broiled	26	23
Pork chop, broiled	28	21
Sirloin steak, broiled	26	19
Chicken breast, no skin	24	1
Turkey breast, no skin	20	½
Flounder, baked	20	1
Shrimp	43*	1

*Shrimp has slightly more cholesterol than other meats, but is extremely low in saturated fat (1 calorie per ounce) and contains risk-reducing omega-3 polyunsaturated fats. How much shrimp can you eat? As much as you can afford — unless you are a shrimp fisherman or very wealthy.

healthy eating plan if it were not for their cholesterol contents. However, if you are going to stay within the American Heart Association guideline of 200–300 mg of cholesterol per day (see Chapter 5), you should not exceed 10–12 ounces per day of even the leanest fish or poultry. If your physician or dietitian has recommended a limit of 100 mg of cholesterol per day, then you should not eat more than about 4 ounces of even the leanest fish or poultry. Don't worry — you won't starve eating even this amount.

Sausages and Luncheon Meats

Sausages and luncheon meats are extremely high in saturated fat as well as extremely high in sodium. They are poor choices to fit into your eating budget.

Consider the sausage. One Polish sausage contributes over 200 calories of saturated fat to your sat-fat budget, more than is allowed for the whole day on the *Eater's Choice* 10 Percent Plan for a 2000 calorie per day intake level.

Smoked link sausages are also very high in saturated fat. Although they are small, each 2.4-ounce sausage link contains about 70 calories of saturated fat, which represents approximately 35 percent of the 200 sat-fat calories allowed on the *Eater's Choice* 10 Percent Plan and 58 percent of the 120 sat-fat calories allowed on the *Eater's Choice* 6 Percent Plan. Thus, eating only one sausage link may mean making severe restrictions in your saturated fat intake for the rest of the day. Two links would completely use up your saturated fat allowance on the *Eater's Choice* 6 Percent Plan.

What's a baseball game or cookout without a hot dog nestled in a warm bun and covered with ketchup or mustard and pickle relish? What about two or three? Beware! A two-ounce all-beef frankfurter contains 61 calories of sat-fat. If that hot dog is in addition to your regular meals, you may be in great danger of having overspent your sat-fat budget — unless you planned ahead.

MILK AND MILK PRODUCTS

Milk — A High-Fat Food

Milk is characterized by its fat content. Thus, whole milk is generally about 3.3 percent fat. This means that 3.3 percent of the total weight is contributed by fat. (This system of rating milk was established many years ago to insure a minimum fat content as a way of protecting consumers from watered-down milk.)

The amount of fat in whole milk — 3.3 percent — seems so trivial, hardly worth counting. False — do not be fooled. Most of the weight of milk is accounted for by water. In terms of calories, fat accounts for 72 of the total 150 calories in a cup of whole milk, or 48 percent of the total calories. A cup of whole milk contains 45 calories of saturated fat.

Thus, whole milk is a high-fat food. On a 2000 calorie per day eating pattern, 4.4 cups of whole milk would provide 200 calories of saturated fat and would thus account for the entire saturated fat

---

Most (about 64 percent) of the fat in milk products is saturated fat regardless of whether it is whole, 2%, or 1% milk. This is true of all milk products, including yogurt, cream, ice cream, and cheese. **Think before you eat.**

allotment on the *Eater's Choice* 10 Percent Plan. A mere 2.7 cups of whole milk would provide 120 calories of saturated fat, accounting for the entire saturated fat allotment on the *Eater's Choice* 6 Percent Plan.

Move Toward Skim Milk

Low-fat milk (2%) tastes pretty similar to whole milk. If you are a whole milk drinker, start by changing to 2% milk. Although 2% milk contains less fat than whole milk, it still contains 27 calories of saturated fat per cup. After a few weeks, try 1% milk. It contains only 14 calories of saturated fat per cup.

However, the best favor you can do your heart is to drink skim milk. "Yuk," you say, "it looks like blue water." We say, "If you don't love it now, you will. It just takes getting used to. Our kids are revolted by whole milk."

And what great benefits. Skim milk is essentially fat-free, containing at most 3 calories of saturated fat per cup. Look at these statistics:

	WHOLE MILK PER CUP	SKIM MILK PER CUP
Total calories	150	86
Sat-fat calories	45	3
Cholesterol, mg	33	4
Calcium, mg	291	302

It may take time, but it is worth working your way toward skim milk.

More Calcium in Skim Milk Than Whole Milk. Milk is an important source of calcium. Calcium is vital for developing and maintaining strong bones and preventing osteoporosis in later life. Skim milk contains more calcium than whole milk: 302 mg of calcium per cup of skim milk versus 291 mg per cup of whole milk. Most skim milk available today has been fortified with vitamins and thus contains just as many vitamins as whole milk. Skim milk is just as nutritious as whole milk *and* is heart-healthy.

Butter

The creamy sweet taste of butter is irreplaceable, but its saturated fat content is so high you must either use it sparingly or find a suitable substitute. The food industry has invested heavily in producing such substitutes. They range from whipped butter, which has about 25 percent less saturated fat than regular butter, to butter-margarine blends, with about 50 percent less saturated fat, margarines, with about 70 percent less saturated fat, and diet margarines, with about 86 percent less saturated fat.

Cream

Coffee drinkers, did you realize that adding 1 tablespoon of light cream to a cup of coffee uses 18 calories of saturated fat of your sat-fat budget? Three cups of coffee with cream provide 54 calories of saturated fat, about one-quarter of the daily allotment of saturated fat under the *Eater's Choice* 10 Percent Plan for 2000 total calories and almost half of the daily allotment under the *Eater's Choice* 6 Percent Plan. And all that for three dinky little tablespoons of cream. Mind-boggling.

Half-and-half contains half as much saturated fat as light cream while 2% milk provides about a tenth the amount of saturated fat as light cream. How about using 1% or skim milk, or drinking your coffee black?

You must be careful when using nondairy coffee whiteners. Most of the dry creamers still contain tropical oils. The serving size is a mere teaspoon and contains less than 9 sat-fat calories. (Do you use 1 teaspoon?) Even most of the "lite" powdered creamers contain coconut oil, palm kernel oil, or palm oil. One lite creamer that contains hydrogenated vegetable oil instead lists no polyunsaturated fat and no saturated fat, only monounsaturated fat. The hydrogenation process has obviously generated a lot of monounsaturated fat in the trans form (see discussion of trans fats on page 80). The frozen creamers generally contain hydrogenated vegetable oils (trans fats) and contain less than 9 sat-fat calories per tablespoon.

Cheese, Wonderful Cheese, Why Are You Almost All Fat?

The sad story about cheese is that whole milk cheeses derive 80 to 90 percent of their calories from fat. Thus, 1 ounce of cheddar cheese provides 114 calories, of which 81 are from fat. One ounce of cream cheese contains 90 calories of fat and a total of 99 calories. Over half of the fat calories are contributed by saturated fat.

You can include cheese in your *Eater's Choice* eating plan, but you will have to sacrifice other sources of sat-fat in your diet. Just plan ahead. Keep your daily sat-fat budget low and you will be able to sneak in a piece of cheese without sinking your heart-healthy diet boat. However, before you devote your entire sat-fat budget to cheese, be aware that most cheeses are extremely high in sodium.

HINT: Satisfy your cheese hunger with minimal sat-fat calories by using a cheese slicer to shave yourself a thin piece of cheese. Remember: many thin slices make one big fat slice.

Lower-Fat Cheeses. A truly low-fat cheese is 1% cottage cheese. One percent cottage cheese contains one-quarter the saturated fat calories of creamed cottage cheese and tastes just as good. Mix cottage cheese with cut-up fruit for a refreshing low-fat lunch. Cover Honey Whole-Wheat Bread (page 360) with sliced bananas and 1% cottage cheese for a filling, scrumptious breakfast. One percent cottage cheese can be used in cooking as a creamy substitute for higher-fat cheeses, as in Creamy Chicken Pie (page 231), Spinach Quiche (page 316), and Calzone (page 311).

The dairy cases in grocery stores now offer a multitude of lower-fat cheeses ranging from 9 to 45 sat-fat calories per ounce. Be careful to read the label. Just because the cheese is advertised as "low-fat," "lower in fat," or "lite" does not mean that it is actually low in saturated fat. For example, part skim milk ricotta and mozzarella are lower in saturated fat than their whole milk counterparts. One-half cup of part skim milk ricotta contains about half the saturated fat calories of whole milk ricotta: 55 versus 93. One ounce of part skim milk mozzarella contains 28 sat-fat calories versus 40 sat-fat calories for whole milk mozzarella. These cheeses may be lower in saturated fat, but they are still high enough so that you need to monitor them carefully.

And don't forget that although one piece of Kraft Reduced-Fat Swiss Cheese may contain only 27 sat-fat calories, two pieces contain 54 sat-fat calories, and three pieces contain 81. If you want to eat a limited amount of low-fat cheeses, fine. We recommend eating real (high-fat) cheeses, but rarely and in very small quantities. We guarantee you'll really taste them.

Yogurt

Several different varieties of yogurt, with vastly different saturated fat contents, are available. They include nonfat, low-fat, and regular high-fat yogurt. Some yogurts are loaded with eggs and cream. Read the label of the yogurt you choose to make certain it has a low saturated fat content.

Nonfat or low-fat yogurt makes a good substitute for sour cream in many recipes (even in a sweet dessert such as Deep-Dish Pear Pie, page 402). Whole milk plain yogurt contains about a sixth as much saturated fat as sour cream, while skim milk plain yogurt contains almost 1/100.

Do Not Skimp on Low-Fat Dairy Foods

Let us say it again: to stay healthy and to keep your bones and teeth strong, you need the calcium that dairy foods provide. Women especially need calcium to prevent osteoporosis. Children need calcium for strong bones and teeth and for growth. Eat dairy products, but eat low-fat dairy products, such as skim milk, 1% cottage cheese (creamy and good), and low-fat or nonfat yogurt.

Fit cheeses, cream, sour cream, whole milk, and whole milk yogurt into your sat-fat budget as a splurge. Cook with low-fat products. Substitute low-fat yogurt or buttermilk for cream or sour cream. We even substitute skim milk for cream (see Potato Soup with Leeks and Broccoli, page 182, or Mushroom Sauce, page 274) with excellent gustatory results.

FATS AND OILS

Two of the most important and widespread changes made by the American public to lower blood cholesterol levels are the substitution of margarine for butter and the substitution of unsaturated vegetable oils for saturated animal fats such as lard or beef tallow.

Margarine

For years, margarine has been accepted as a good substitute for butter. Whereas butter contains 65 calories of saturated fat per tablespoon, margarine contains only 18.

Enter the Villain *trans.* We still endorse margarine as a substitute for butter, but the less you use margarine and the more you use olive oil, the better. Here is the scientific explanation. Polyunsaturated fats and oils are hydrogenated (a chemical process that adds hydrogen and results in a more saturated fat) to make them more solid at room temperature and to increase their shelf life — the time they can sit on a shelf without becoming rancid. Food manufacturers use hydrogenated and partially hydrogenated vegetable oils in margarines and many other processed foods exactly because of these properties. Just read food labels to see how pervasive hydrogenated soybean, cottonseed, and corn oil are in commercial foods.

During the process of hydrogenation, a new class of chemical is produced called *trans* fats. (Fats that occur in nature are almost completely of the *cis* form. *Cis* and *trans* refer to the three-dimensional arrangement of the fat.)

Trans fats have several properties that please food manufacturers and several that won't please you. Food manufacturers like trans fats because they are even harder at room temperature than their cis counterparts. Also, because trans fats are monounsaturated, they do not contribute to the saturated fat content of the food. The food appears to be heart-healthy because the food label doesn't show a high-saturated-fat content. In fact, the manufacturer can emphasize the amount of monounsaturated fat on the label.

But the down side of trans fats is that even though hydrogenation has made them into monounsaturated fats, they affect your blood cholesterol more like saturated fats. Studies show that trans fats raise LDL ("bad cholesterol") and lower HDL ("good cholesterol").

So, while foods containing trans fats are probably less heart-risky than those containing saturated fats, it is better to limit your intake of foods containing trans fats. Better still, use more natural (versus man-made), monounsaturated fats such as olive oil. (We use olive oil almost exclusively in the *Eater's Choice* recipes, even in breads, cakes, and pie crusts). The best course of all is to limit the total amount of any type of fat (even heart-healthy monos) you eat to reduce your risk of obesity and colon and breast cancers.

The Vegetable Oil Contest

Olive Oil: Number-One Choice. Olive oil contains mainly monounsaturated fat and little saturated or polyunsaturated fat. It is the most heart-healthy of all the fats. Recent research indicates that olive oil lowers LDL-cholesterol without lowering HDL-cholesterol. In addition, by preventing the oxidation of LDL remnants, olive oil helps prevent the first step of the atherosclerotic process. Epidemiological studies show that populations (such as

Greeks and Italians) who use olive oil as the predominant source of fat in their diet have very low rates of heart disease. Choose olive oil even for baking. (Like olive oil, peanut oil is predominantly monounsaturated. However, scientific research has shown that peanut oil causes clogging of coronary arteries in some animals. Why take a chance?)

Canola Oil: Newcomer on the Food Scene. Second choice is canola oil, derived from the rapeseed plant. While it has the lowest amount of saturated fat of all the oils and a lot of monounsaturated fat, canola oil has not been people-tested for a long enough time to assure us that it has no long-term adverse health effects. Why take a chance when you can easily and safely use olive oil?

Polys Have Their Problems. Safflower, sunflower, corn, and soybean oils are primarily polyunsaturated, with small amounts of saturated fat. Safflower contains about 10 percent saturated fat; sunflower, 11 percent; corn, 13 percent; and soybean, about 15 percent. However, as we have mentioned, high intakes of polyunsaturated oils lower HDL levels and may raise the risk of cancer. So don't overdose on polyunsaturated fats.

Cottonseed oil is highly saturated for a polyunsaturated fat. It contains 27 percent of its calories as saturated fat. This is only 1 percent less than vegetable shortening (such as Crisco). Cottonseed is a favorite with food producers. Watch out for it when you buy commercial foods.

Hydrogenated vegetable oils have the problem of containing trans fats (see page 80). The fats that don't become monounsaturated (and trans) during hydrogenation become saturated. Even safflower oil, one of the least saturated fats, loses much of its heart-healthy properties when it is hydrogenated.

Coconut Oil: The Pits. Coconut oil is given to lab rats and other animals normally resistant to developing elevated blood cholesterol levels to produce atherosclerotic plaques and heart disease. With 106 sat-fat calories per tablespoon, it is the most heart-risky fat known. If you are smarter than a rat, you will avoid coconut oil at all costs. Following close is palm kernel oil (100 sat-fat calories/tablespoon) and palm oil (60 sat-fat calories/tablespoon). You should avoid all of these tropical oils. We happily report that tropical oils have almost been entirely eliminated from commercial food products. But, just to be safe, *read the list of ingredients on food labels.*

All Oils Have Equal Calories

You will note that all the oils are really mixtures of polyunsaturated, monounsaturated, and saturated fats. (See Figure 11, page 40.) None contains only one type of fat. We refer to an oil as polyunsaturated or monounsaturated or saturated because it contains predominantly that type of fat. Regardless of the type of oil, they all contain the same number of calories because they are 100 percent fat, and all fats contain 9 calories per gram. All are high in calories and should be avoided as much as possible, especially by people trying to maintain their desirable weight.

Lard, Chicken Fat, and Other Animal Fats

All animal fats contain large amounts of monounsaturated fat, relatively small amounts of polyunsaturated fat, moderate to large amounts of saturated fat, and moderate amounts of cholesterol. Of the animal fats, chicken fat is the least heart-risky and beef tallow is the most heart-risky. *But no animal fats can be recommended for persons trying to lower their blood cholesterol levels.* The heart-healthy alternative is olive oil.

Keep Short on Shortening

Your mom may have used shortening to bake the flakiest pie crust imaginable, but in this case, don't follow in her culinary footsteps. One tablespoon of shortening has from 30 to 47 calories of saturated fat. For the sake of your heart-health, don't use shortening at home or buy it baked into commercial goods.

Mayonnaise

You will be happy to find something you know and love but do not have to avoid completely: mayonnaise. If you budget carefully, you can fit real mayonnaise into your diet at 11 to 14 sat-fat calories per tablespoon. A better choice is reduced-calorie mayonnaise at 9 sat-fat calories per tablespoon.

Before you feel too happy, take heed. All mayonnaises are almost pure fat and so are high in fat calories. Even reduced-calorie mayonnaises with half the total fat calories contain 45 fat calories per tablespoon, which is still a lot of fat. Use mayonnaise in moderation.

Salad Dressings

Many salad dressings are high in saturated fats as well as total and polyunsaturated fats. A tablespoon of blue cheese dressing or French dressing has 14 calories of saturated fat. Russian has 10, followed closely by Italian with 9, and Thousand Island with 8. One problem with using salad dressing is that one never delicately sprinkles only a tablespoon of salad dressing on one's salad. Another problem is that salad dressings are often high in sodium. Do not ruin the health value of your salad by drowning it in highly fattening and fatty salad dressing.

THE FORK METHOD

Use the fork method to retain the taste of salad dressing without consuming all the fat calories. Have your salad dressing served on the side or pour a small amount into a bowl. Dip your fork into the dressing, then spear your salad greens or vegetables. Voilà! — a tasty low-sat-fat forkful.

A more heart-healthy alternative is to use commercial low-fat dressings. Or make your own: in a jar, combine olive oil, vinegar, minced garlic, some herbs (oregano, thyme, or basil, for example), a little Dijon mustard, salt, and pepper — and shake.

DESSERTS

Many Americans enjoy having a sweet, rich dessert to top off their dinner and often their lunch, too. Unfortunately, many of our favorite desserts are rich in saturated fat. A cup of ordinary vanilla ice cream contains 80 calories of saturated fat. Compare this with a cup of vanilla ice milk (32 calories of saturated fat), a cup of orange sherbet (21 sat-fat calories), and a cup of low-fat frozen yogurt (12 sat-fat calories). The low-fat frozen yogurt has less than one-sixth as much saturated fat as the ice cream. Even better are the new nonfat frozen yogurts (such as Colombo Lite) that eliminate all sat-fat calories while retaining the creamy texture and delicious taste.

Fortunately frozen yogurt is becoming increasingly more available in ice cream parlors, restaurants, and grocery stores. But be advised.

Yogurt is not a synonym for *low-fat*. Ask about the fat content and the ingredients. Many yogurt vendors can provide nutritional information. For example, one popular brand contains 2 grams of fat per 4 ounces. The primary fat is butterfat. This works out to 18 calories of total fat and about 12 sat-fat calories. Another brand contains 0.9 grams of butterfat per ounce. If you eat 4 ounces (about half a cup), you will be eating (4 × .9) 3.6 grams of total fat or about 32 fat calories and about 22 sat-fat calories.

But before you dash over to your frozen yogurt shop, keep in mind that Oreo cookie bits, Heath crunch, Reese's Pieces, chocolate chips, shredded coconut — all the toppings you love to eat — don't become less heart-risky just because they sit atop a nonfat frozen yogurt. Choose a fruit topping (or no topping) to adorn your treat.

The Fat Impact of Desserts

A single cake-type doughnut contains 25 calories of saturated fat. A piece of chocolate devil's food cake made with butter and iced with chocolate contains 56 calories of saturated fat. Coconut custard pie contributes about 51 calories of saturated fat per slice. Apple pie made with vegetable shortening, lemon meringue pie, and cherry pie each contain about 30 calories of saturated fat per slice. A piece of Boston cream pie made with butter contains 27 calories of saturated fat.

Commercial cookies are the downfall of many sat-fat counters. Like crackers and nuts, cookie consumption is a miraculous occurrence. Somehow, scores of cookies get from the plate or the box into the mouth without the cookie consumer having put them there. Cookie eaters must pay attention. Cookie packages generally list the amount of saturated fat for one cookie. The only person in the world who ate just one cookie is listed in the *Guinness Book of World Records*. Most people begin with one cookie and end with many cookies. Even at less than 1 gram of saturated fat each (which may mean 8 sat-fat calories), cookie sat-fat calories quickly add up. If you are not a cookie monster and have enough self-control, give yourself a treat and fit just one or two cookies into your sat-fat budget. Otherwise, leave the cookie box in the grocery store.

Being on a low sat-fat diet does not mean you must give up delicious desserts. Why not bake your own? Try the desserts beginning on page 378. Nothing could be simpler or more delicious than Cinnamon Sweet Cakes (page 403) at 8 sat-fat calories per square. What about Deep-Dish Pear Pie (page 402) at 11 sat-fat calories per slice, or Tante Nancy's Apple Crumb Cake (page 396) at 15 sat-fat calories for a trip to the sublime?

Just a note of caution: even desserts that are low in saturated fat are generally more caloric and fat-filled than other parts of your meal. You are not going to stay thin by eating baked or frozen desserts at every meal. How about fruit?

Read labels for hidden coconut, palm kernel, palm, or hydrogenated vegetable oil in commercial desserts.

The Good Guys

Many Europeans finish their large meal of the day with a piece of fruit. How about a delicious (and heart-healthy) dessert of sliced fruit mixed with low-fat yogurt? You will see the advantages fruits offer when you consider the saturated fat content of most fruits. An apple contains less than 1 calorie of saturated fat, 3 apricots less than 0.2, a banana about 2, 1 cup of cherries about 0.7, an orange about 0.4, a peach less than 0.1, a pear about 0.3.

Substituting fruits for rich, sweet desserts will allow you much greater freedom in choosing meats, dairy products, and other foods that contain saturated fats. The choices are yours to make . . . as long as you stay within your own saturated fat budget.

SNACKS

High-fat snacks can be the downfall of any healthy eating plan. Because they are habit-forming, you eat a lot of them. What may start out as a few sat-fat calories per bite quickly ends up bankrupting your sat-fat budget. Even if the sat-fat content is just moderately high, the fat content of most snacks is almost always sky-high. And, remember, eating a diet high in fat increases your risk for cancer, heart disease, diabetes, and obesity.

Of course, all snacks are not high-fat. Read on to find snacks you can eat with moderate abandon.

Popcorn

Potentially Ideal Snack. One of the greatest snacks known to mankind since some ancient American Indian threw dried corn kernels into a fire is popcorn. Fat-free, air-popped* popcorn is high in both insoluble fiber (important for effective bowel function and reducing risk of colon cancer) and soluble fiber (helps to lower blood cholesterol and risk of heart disease). It is filling without being fattening, and it satisfies the hand-to-mouth craving without punishing your budget. Popcorn is truly a treat.

But Easily Ruined. Drench it in butter at 65 sat-fat calories per tablespoon (would 1/4 cup, or 260 sat-fat calories, be more like it?), and popcorn becomes an ultra-high-sat-fat snack.

Go to the movies and buy a box. Movie popcorn is almost always made with coconut oil. You can eat up your sat-fat budget for a day (the small size), for two days (the medium size), or blow your budget for the week (the large, 22-cup tub).

And as for total fat, pop popcorn in your microwave and you are probably eating from about 24 to 30 fat calories per cup or, more realistically, 240 to 300 fat calories per 10 cups. (The typical serving size of microwave popcorn is 3 cups. But who stops at 3 cups?)

Buy it already popped from the grocery store, and even air-popped popcorn is filled with fat. Take Bachman air-popped popcorn at 99 fat calories per 1-ounce serving (about 5 cups). Look at the label and try to figure out how a fat-free food (air-popped popcorn) gained 99 fat calories per ounce. The answer: fat was poured on *after* the popcorn was air-popped.

For your best buy, both in terms of health and your wallet, stick with the plain air-popped popcorn you pop at home. At first it tastes a bit like cardboard, but keep eating it and soon you'll even crave it.

HINT: Store popcorn kernels in the refrigerator to keep them fresh and pop-worthy.

Chips and Other Addictive Crunchies

First, if the package has no nutrition label, you don't want it. When you read the ingredient list you will discover why. A good

---

*Air-poppers are inexpensive and easy to care for. They require no cleaning after use. Just drop about 1/2 cup of popcorn kernels into the machine, and in 2 to 3 minutes 12 cups of delicious, healthy popcorn will tumble out.

example is Fiddle Faddle. It still contains coconut oil, but you'll never know how much. Or read the ingredients contained in Durkee potato sticks: potato and partially hydrogenated vegetable oil. Is coconut the vegetable? How much oil and how much potato? Or you may ask why Utz has no listing of fat calories on its cheese-flavored curls but lists fat calories on its other products.

Even if chip-type snacks do have nutrition labeling, you must be wary. Chips are so easy to eat, you swallow one and crave another and another and another. It takes no effort to inhale an 8-ounce bag all by yourself. The sat-fat and fat calories add up. Look at General Mills Bugles. At 64 calories of saturated fat for 1 ounce, Bugles might help you to see the wisdom of eating a carrot. Pringle's Original chips have 27 sat-fat calories per ounce (108 total fat calories!), but who eats 1 ounce of chips? Most of the smallest deli bags contain more than one ounce of chips. Pringles Light, at about 17 sat-fat calories per 14 slender little crisps, is not much of a bargain, either, fatwise. If you have enough self-control to eat just a few chips, fit them in. But don't even open the bag if you and your arteries will regret it later.

Crackers

Since the last edition of *Eater's Choice* was published, hydrogenated and partially hydrogenated vegetable oils have replaced tropical oils in most crackers. This change has lowered the saturated fat content on the food label but has raised the trans fat content of the crackers, and trans fats are no friend to your arteries. Crackers have three additional problems. First, they are usually so small, you hardly notice that you have eaten ten (or more) in one sitting. And, of course, the fats add up, as one cracker after another disappears into your mouth. Next, most crackers are high in total fat. And, finally, crackers prefer not to be eaten alone. When you add up the sat-fat calories of the Cheddar cheese or sour cream and onion dip that tops your cracker, you have a mighty high sat-fat snack.

Nuts

Nuts are a popular snack choice. The trouble with nuts is that they are very high in total fat and thus high in fat calories: about 126 to 196 calories per ounce. (Only 35 shelled peanuts, a small handful, weigh an ounce.) Nuts are also addictive. Who ever heard of eating one peanut? A couple of handfuls disappear without notice — but you and everyone else will notice soon enough if you overdose on nuts. Eat nuts sparingly.

If you must eat nuts, the ones with the least amount of saturated fat are walnuts, pecans, almonds, pistachios, and hazelnuts (about 13 to 17 sat-fat calories per ounce of dry-roasted shelled nuts).

The Bad Guys

Cashews, macadamia nuts, brazil nuts, and coconut contain, in increasing order, greater amounts of saturated fat. Coconut is almost purely saturated fat and should be avoided like the plague.

Peanut Butter

Pure, unadulterated peanut butter is a high-protein food, composed mainly of monounsaturated fats and a relatively small amount of saturated fat (12 sat-fat calories per tablespoon). All-natural peanut butters made from peanuts only, no salt added, are often ground and packaged in your local grocery stores. That is the good news. The bad news is that peanut butter is a high-fat food. It derives 72 of its 95 total calories (per tablespoon) from fat. And, in addition, experiments implicate peanut oil in clogging the arteries of some animals. Beware of familiar brands of processed peanut butters, which are filled with added salt, sugar, and partially hydrogenated vegetable fats. Eat peanut butter in moderation.

Seeds

Sunflower seeds are often considered healthy. Any food that contains 36 sat-fat calories (and 135 fat calories) per ounce should not be mistaken for health food. Seeds naturally contain a lot of fat, but when stuck into a little bag with added salt and fat, seeds are a particularly poor choice.

Veggies

Tasty, healthy, and filling, but often overlooked as snacks, are cut-up vegetables. Carrots, cauliflower, broccoli, celery, and cucumbers may be eaten raw or with a low-fat yogurt dip.

Yogurt

A carton of yogurt is a refreshing snack. (See page 79.) Choose nonfat, flavored yogurts. They give you gustatory pleasure without adding a single sat-fat calorie to your sat-fat budget. (Ron says eating Colombo Lite Vanilla is like eating ice cream.)

Pretzels

A real treat is a large twisted pretzel with 0 fat and 0 sat-fat calories. (Pretzels vary in fat content, so be sure to check the nutrition label.) You might want to scrape off some of the salt before you begin to munch. Do be careful. A few pretzels are a great snack, but stop at a few. Better to fill up on fruit, vegetables, or whole grains, which provide vitamins, minerals, and fiber.

Muffins, Bagels, Etc.

An Eater's Choice Oat Bran Muffin (pages 370–372) with coffee, a slice of Honey Whole-Wheat Bread (page 360) with a glass of skim or low-fat milk, or half a bagel with margarine make excellent snacks. Of course, you know any snack should be eaten in moderation — even healthy ones.

FAST FOODS

You lead a busy life. Fast-food restaurants offer the chance to pop in and get a filling and tasty meal at a moderate price. But is it healthy for your heart?

The road to heart-health does not run through a fast-food restaurant. The bulk of fast-food offerings are high-sat-fat and high-fat. For example, a Burger King Double Whopper with Cheese has a whopping 216 sat-fat calories (and 549 total fat calories!), Jumbo French Fries at Jack in the Box contain 142 sat-fat calories, and a KFC (Kentucky Fried Chicken) Chocolate Creme Parfait has 97 sat-fat calories. Even though some new offerings can easily fit into your sat-fat budget, it is difficult to resist all the other high-sat-fat and high-fat goodies available.

In addition, what happens to family togetherness when dinner time consists of grabbing a bite to eat at a fast-food restaurant? What are you teaching your children?

- It doesn't matter what you eat as long as it's quick.
- High-fat food tastes great and is good for you.

And what aren't your children learning?

• Vegetables, fruits, and whole grains taste great and are essential for a balanced and healthy diet.

Fast-food restaurants must be approached carefully and rarely. But, if you happen to find yourself in a city that has nothing but fast-food restaurants and you haven't eaten in a week, here are some low-fat choices to consider.

The New Fast-Food Rage — Chicken

Responding to the fat-conscious market, fast-food moguls have introduced a food that people associate with low-fat — chicken. McDonald's says its Grilled Chicken Breast Sandwich has only 9 sat-fat calories; and Carl's Jr. claims its Charbroiler BBQ Chicken Sandwich has 18 sat-fat calories. Jack in the Box lists its Chicken Fajita Pita as containing 26 sat-fat calories. Other chicken offerings (such as Burger King's Broiler Chicken Sandwich at 27 sat-fat calories or Arby's Chicken Breast Sandwich at 35 sat-fat calories), while not extremely high in saturated fat, are very high in total fat and thus not a buy, healthwise. Arby's Chicken Breast Sandwich contains 232 total fat calories. That's 75 percent of a 130-pound woman's total daily fat budget. Be careful. Check the *Eater's Choice* Food Tables before you go to a fast-food restaurant and order. Just because the dish is chicken does not mean it is low in sat-fat and/or low in total fat.

Low-Fat Fish + Fat = High-Fat Fish

Likewise, f-i-s-h does not always spell low-fat. The Long John Silver catfish fillet* at 23 sat-fat calories is a choice that can easily fit into your sat-fat budget, but the Dairy Queen fish fillet sandwich, with no cheese (27 sat-fat calories) has too many total fat calories (144) to make it a wise choice. Except for Dairy Queen's fish fillet, fish fillet sandwiches range from a low (which is really quite high) of 216 fat calories at Hardee's to a high of 288 total fat calories at Jack in the Box. Consider other options before you order a fish fillet sandwich.

Salad Bars

Many fast-food restaurants offer salad bars. All the dangers of any salad bar exist (see discussion, page 101), but if you stick to fresh

---

*The catfish fillet weighs about 1 ounce, which is not much to eat.

fruit and vegetables and a minimal amount of dressing (note: the small ladle in a fast-food restaurant holds 2 tablespoons of dressing, the large one holds 4 tablespoons), you will not break your sat-fat bank. However, you won't be getting much to eat and may be tempted to supplement your salad with high-fat snacks later.

Overdose on Sodium

In addition to containing large amounts of saturated fat, fast foods contain very large amounts of sodium: a Big Mac contains 1010 mg of sodium, a Dairy Queen Super Brazier hot dog with cheese contains 1986 mg of sodium, Arby's club sandwich contains 1610 mg. Your intake of sodium should be between 1100 and 3300 mg for the whole day. (See Chapter 9.) Each of these items contains more than enough sodium to catapult you over the daily minimum without any additional sources of sodium for the day. With sodium from other foods eaten that day, you are likely to exceed even the maximum allotment of sodium. This is especially a problem if you have high blood pressure.

Underdose on Health

Be sure to check the Food Tables at the back of the book before going to a fast-food restaurant. Do not stray from your original choice when temptation rears its ugly head. And remember, although fast-food restaurants are using fewer saturated fats, the total fat and sodium poured into their offerings are enough to add pounds to your body and subtract years from your life.

FROZEN DINNERS

Take a look at the frozen foods section of your grocery store to get a picture of our changing lifestyle. The freezer cases are jam-packed with microwave dinners for people who don't want to take time to cook. Frozen dinners may be quick, but what are you saving time for? You pay for convenience both in money and health. When you buy a beef sirloin tips dinner (Healthy Choices) you are paying about $28 a pound for the beef and about four times more for the dinner than if you made it yourself. To save a few minutes in the kitchen costs you about 85 sat-fat calories when you stick Le Menu's Chicken Parmigiana in your microwave. If you bread a boneless chicken breast without skin and bake it in your oven, it will cost you 19 sat-fat calories and perhaps 10 minutes of preparation time. Steam some broccoli or carrots, bake *Eater's Choice* Potato Skins or a sweet potato, and you have a real feast at a cost of $1.50 (if the chicken is not on sale). For very little expenditure of time and money you will have created a dinner you and your arteries can truly enjoy.

THE JOYS OF REAL FOOD

Perhaps you have to go to a fast-food restaurant or grab a frozen dinner every once in a blue moon. But, on the whole, why not eat real food? Every recipe need not be time-consuming. Try the starred recipes in this book, for starters. They are quick and easy. Sitting down with your family in relaxed surroundings is more heart-healthy than spending ten seconds at a fast-food joint, stuffing your mouth with a highly saturated piece of rubbery, salty meat surrounded by airy white bread. Your dinner will also be much more delicious and filling than the contents of a little box heated up in your microwave.

This sentiment needs repeating: take time to make real food. One hour a day to prepare dinner is a small amount of time to devote to an activity that will lengthen and improve the quality of your life.

Remember:

1. Red meats such as beef, veal, lamb, and some pork products are extremely high in saturated fat. The higher the grade of meat, the more saturated fat it contains.
2. Turkey and chicken with the skin removed and fish are all low in saturated fat. (Always remove the skin *before* you cook poultry.) Beware of sat-fat added in preparation.
3. Dairy products are excellent sources of calcium but many are high in fat and saturated fat. Whole milk derives almost half its calories from fat. Most cheeses derive about 80 percent of their calories from fat. Choose low-fat dairy products, such as low-fat yogurt, low-fat cottage cheese, and skim milk.
4. Recent evidence indicates that olive oil, rich in monounsaturated fatty acids, may be the most heart-healthy oil. But before you chug-a-lug a glass of olive oil each morning for breakfast,

remember that all fats and oils are fattening and increase your risk for certain cancers, diabetes, and obesity. For long-term good health, reduce all the fats in your diet.

5. Coconut oil, which is found in many commercial foods, is one of the most heart-risky foods you can eat. *Avoid it diligently.*

6. Most fast foods are loaded with sat-fat and sodium. Do your coronary arteries a lifelong favor by staying clear of fast-food restaurants.

7. The cost of frozen dinners can be high in terms of dollars, health, and real enjoyment of food. Cooking from scratch can be quick, easy, healthy, and truly delicious and satisfying.

FROM THEORY TO PRACTICE 8

YOU ARE NOW ready to act. You have already figured out your ideal caloric intake and your daily sat-fat budget. Now you must look at your own eating pattern to see how much saturated fat you actually eat and how to reduce it.

Keep a Record. The best way to find out what you actually eat is to write down everything you consume for two or three days. Include a typical week day and a weekend day. *Write down everything.* Be sure to include that glass of orange juice you drank in the afternoon and that handful of peanuts you grabbed before dinner. Measure everything. (See "The Nitty-Gritty of Keeping a Food Record," page 523.)

Next, use the food tables to find the total calories and sat-fat calories for the foods you ate and add them up.

This very important exercise may surprise you. You may discover that the Danish pastry you usually eat for breakfast squanders 47 sat-fat calories, without giving you any nutritional value. You may find that most of the saturated fat you eat is concentrated in a few foods, which you can easily change. Analyzing your eating pattern will allow you to make the most effective and enduring changes in the way you eat.

Slow, but Enduring. Having discovered the sat-fat pitfalls in your daily food record, you may be eager to take immediate action and completely revamp your eating pattern. However, slow down! If you make too many changes too fast, you are not likely to stick with them. The changes in your eating pattern will do you and your heart good only if they are permanent.

Remember, it takes years to develop the atherosclerotic plaque that blocks the coronary arteries. Taking a few months to modify your lifelong eating patterns should not cause any harm and will result in more lasting changes.

APPROACH I

One approach to making gradual changes is to focus your attention on the worst culprits. Can you eat these less often, in smaller amounts, or even not at all? Go for the worst first. Change one or a few things at a time.

First, write down your menu for yesterday. Say it looks like this:

FOOD ITEM	CALORIES	
	TOTAL	SAT-FAT
Breakfast		
Soft-boiled egg	79	15
3 slices bacon	109	30
1 slice whole-wheat toast	60	1
1 pat butter	36	23
Coffee + 1 tbsp half-and-half	20	10
Lunch		
Burger King Whopper with cheese	706	144
_____		
_____		
_____		
10 French fries	220	33
Pepsi Lite	1	0
Dinner		
6 oz sirloin steak	372	72
1 small baked potato	105	0
1 pat butter	36	23
_____		
_____		
_____		
1 cup ice cream	270	80
Coffee + 1 tbsp half-and-half	20	10
Snack		
_____		
1 cup whole milk	150	45
Total	2184	486

Interesting. If your total calorie intake for the day was supposed to be 2000, 486 is way over your sat-fat allotment of 200 calories allowed on the *Eater's Choice* 10 Percent Plan. You need to eliminate 286 calories of saturated fat to get down to your 200 calorie sat-fat budget.

REPLACEMENT FOOD ITEMS	CALORIES		SAVINGS IN SAT-FAT CALORIES
	TOTAL	SAT-FAT	
Breakfast			
1 waffle	86	6	9
2 slices Canadian bacon	86	12	18
2 slices whole-wheat toast	120	2	(1)
2 tsp margarine	60	10	13
Coffee + 1 tbsp 2% milk	8	2	8
Lunch			
Turkey sandwich			
3 oz turkey breast	114	3 ⎫	
2 slices whole-wheat bread	120	2 ⎬	145
1 tsp mayonnaise	33	5 ⎭	
10 French fries	220	33	0
Orange juice	110	0	0
Dinner			
6 oz sirloin steak	372	72	0
1 medium baked potato	146	0	0
1 tsp margarine	30	5	18
Steamed broccoli w/lemon	53	1	(1)
Mixed salad	8	0	
1 tbsp Italian dressing	69	9	(9)
1 slice whole-wheat bread	60	1	(1)
1 tsp margarine	30	5	(5)
1 cup ice milk	184	32	48
Coffee + 1 tbsp 2% milk	8	2	8
Snack			
1 oz Cheerios	110	3	(3)
1 cup 2% milk	121	27	18
Total	2148	232	265

What contributes the most saturated fat for the day? The Burger King Whopper with cheese at 144. How about having a ham and cheese sandwich at 81, or better yet tuna or turkey breast (3 ounces of either, with 1 teaspoon of mayonnaise) at 10 sat-fat calories each? Even with the ham and cheese, your total sat-fat for the day is reduced to 423. With the tuna or turkey breast, the total becomes 352. That's beginning to look a lot better.

Can you do without those fatty strips of bacon? Replace the bacon with Canadian bacon and reduce your sat-fat calories from 30 to 12. Why not eat that egg on a day when your cholesterol intake is not so high? How about eating ice milk (32 sat-fat calories) instead of ice cream (80 sat-fat calories)? And margarine instead of butter (20 sat-fat calories for the day instead of 46)? And 1 cup of 2% milk instead of whole milk, for 27 instead of 45 sat-fat calories? All these changes together bring your daily total sat-fat intake to 232 calories (see meal plans). Great! You are almost there. And there is always tomorrow to make more changes.

Great news for all you food lovers. You can see in the meal plans that by reducing your sat-fat calorie intake, you are actually eating *more* — more foods, more variety, more bulk, a more balanced and healthier menu. Reducing your sat-fat intake will not make you hungry; just the opposite — the fruits, vegetables, and grains you substitute will make you feel blissfully full.

A Few "Sacrifices" for the Old Bod'

By evaluating your eating habits and figuring out what foods you can do without or replace with less fatty substitutes, you can bring your saturated fat total down with little pain. The next stage is to make a few sacrifices. (You will find that these so-called sacrifices are not sacrifices at all. You are substituting foods that are just as satisfying or *more* satisfying than those you ate before.)

Try drinking 1% milk instead of 2%. That's a reduction of 13 calories of saturated fat per cup. How about skipping fatty desserts every day but Sunday? Wow. Watch that sat-fat total drop.

Use small amounts of beef as a condiment with rice or pasta. Choose leaner cuts of beef, such as trimmed round. Instead of having beef four times a week, eat it only twice a week. Perhaps not at all.

Replace some or all of your red meat meals with chicken, turkey, or fish. (This book is filled with scrumptious recipes for chicken, turkey, and fish. Try them.) Notice how much impact the substitution of fish or poultry for beef has on your daily saturated fat intake. Also notice how eliminating sat-fat calories from meat frees up calories that you can spend on a wide variety of foods — foods that are tasty, nutritious, and low or moderate in fat content.

REMEMBER: as you reduce your fat intake, increase your complex carbohydrate intake. Eat more whole-grain cereals and breads, rice, and pasta. Eat more fruits and vegetables. You will feel less lethargic after meals, you will be more regular, you will undoubtedly lose weight, and, who knows, you might have a better sex life.

APPROACH 2

An alternative approach to changing your eating habits is to focus on changing one meal at a time. For example, for the first few weeks only make changes in your breakfast menu. Get rid of that bacon and sausage. Eliminate those doughnuts at 24 calories of saturated fat each, not to mention all that sugar. Avoid granola: it is billed as healthy but look how saturated it is. Notice the coconut they add. It is not worth clogging your arteries for a little crunch.

New Breakfast

How about toast and margarine or jelly? Try low-fat Cinnamon French Toast (page 377) or Buttermilk Pancakes (page 375), 1% cottage cheese in half a cantaloupe, strawberries and nonfat yogurt, oatmeal or oat bran with raisins and cinnamon, or a carton of flavored nonfat yogurt.

Oat bran, which became a national fad several years ago and then faded, is a rich source of soluble fiber. All foods that are high in soluble fiber, such as dried beans and peas, have a modest effect on lowering cholesterol.

If you enjoy hot oat bran cereal or oat bran muffins you bake at home (see Chapter 23 for a variety of tasty muffin recipes), eat away. (Warning: some commercial oat bran muffins contain so much saturated or total fat, they make doughnuts look like health food.) However, before you sprinkle oat bran in your orange juice and eat nine oat bran muffins a day, fill up on oat bran pretzels and oat bran beer, be forewarned that eating oat bran will not save you from the cholesterol-raising effects of a diet high in saturated fat. **A low sat-fat diet is the most effective way to maximize your cholesterol-lowering.**

WHERE TO FIND SOLUBLE FIBER*

FOOD	SERVING SIZE	SOLUBLE FIBER (G)
Grains		
Oat bran	⅓ cup dry	2.0
All-Bran	⅓ cup	1.7
Oat bran muffin	1	1.6
Oatmeal	¾ cup, cooked	1.4
Rye bread	2 slices	0.6
Whole-wheat bread	2 slices	0.5
Dried Beans and Peas		
Black-eyed peas	½ cup, cooked	3.7
Kidney beans	½ cup, cooked	2.5
Pinto beans	½ cup, cooked	2.3
Navy beans	½ cup, cooked	2.3
Lentils	½ cup, cooked	1.7
Split peas	½ cup, cooked	1.7
Vegetables		
Peas	½ cup, cooked	2.7
Corn	½ cup, cooked	1.7
Sweet potato	1 baked	1.3
Zucchini	½ cup, cooked	1.3
Cauliflower	½ cup, cooked	1.3
Broccoli	½ cup, cooked	0.9
Fruit		
Prunes	4	1.9
Pears	1	1.1
Apples	1	0.9
Bananas	1	0.8
Oranges	1	0.7

*From: Nutrition Action Healthletter, Center for Science in the Public Interest, December 1985.

NOW FOR LUNCH

After you have established new and lasting changes in your breakfast, you will be ready to make changes in lunch. If you often eat this meal out, you have an additional challenge. You will have less control over the foods available than if you bring your lunch from home. (See Chapter 10 for tips on how to eat out.)

You might want to consider these options: eating out less often and bringing lunch from home more often; choosing low-fat, low saturated fat items from the menu and passing up the high-fat, heart-risky items; choosing restaurants that offer more low-fat, low saturated fat menu choices. The last option may be especially necessary if you are used to eating lunch in a fast-food restaurant.

If you have to eat at a fast-food restaurant, check the Food Tables first for the choices with the lowest amount of saturated fat. If that is impossible, stick to the salad bar, but be wary.

The Salad Bar: Lettuce, Tomatoes, and Fat

Don't assume that just because salads are composed of vegetables, fruits, and sometimes pastas, they are always healthy choices. The amount of saturated fat and total fat in many salad bar offerings — red potatoes in sour cream dressing, mayonnaise salad with a bit of macaroni, cold cuts swimming in oil — overrides their nutritious

---

YOUR MOTHER WAS RIGHT

Many adults have established the pattern of eating no breakfast and no lunch or a very light lunch. For some, the mistaken notion is that this is a good way to lose weight. For others, breakfast and lunch may be the casualties of life in the fast lane. In any case, it is much healthier to eat three well-balanced meals than to starve yourself all day. Stuffing into one meal all the calories and nutrients needed for functioning at peak efficiency makes for very low efficiency peaks.

The chances are that if you eat only one or two meals a day, you will get hungry and eat snacks. Most snacks are notoriously high in fat, saturated fat, sodium, and/or sugar and appallingly low in vitamins, minerals, and fiber.

The best policy is to make your three meals low-fat (see the meal plans in Chapter 13 for a variety of low-fat meal suggestions) and see if you don't feel better and function at an optimum.

benefits. Even plain salad greens and vegetables become high-fat fare when sprinkled with bacon bits, shredded cheese, and sesame seeds, and covered with a ladle or two or three or four (2 to 16 tablespoons) of high-fat and high-sat-fat dressing. Choose fruits and plain vegetables. Choose low-calorie dressings or make your own dressing with oil and vinegar. If you must use regular salad dressings, use the fork method (see page 84).

But consider a salad — even a low-fat salad — a side dish. A truly low-fat salad for lunch is not enough to eat. It may make you feel virtuous, but it can also leave you very hungry. Better to eat a satisfying, low-sat-fat lunch than to starve yourself on a bowl of rabbit food and fill up on high-fat snacks later.

Lunch Options

How about a turkey breast sandwich for lunch (not on a croissant, which is loaded with butter)? Most delis and sandwich shops carry white meat turkey sandwiches. Even with mayonnaise, a turkey sandwich contains a mere 10 calories of saturated fat. How about a bowl of chili *non* carne (peas and beans are rich in protein and fiber and low in fat)? How about a big bowl of sliced fresh fruit mixed with low-fat yogurt or low-fat cottage cheese? How about a chef's salad (hold the cheese) with turkey and ham (optional) and low-fat dressing? Your coronary arteries are looking better and better.

How about filling a pita with last night's dinner and eating it for lunch? How about a pita sandwich of Chili Non Carne (page 320) topped with chopped green pepper, onion, tomato, and lettuce? What about a Bar-B-Que Chicken sandwich? Place Bar-B-Que Chicken (page 242) on a slice of bread, heat the sauce and spoon it over the chicken, cover with tomato and onion slices, and top with a second slice of bread. And, would you believe cheeseless pizza? You can order a vegetarian pizza without cheese at almost any pizza parlor for a real taste treat that is low in sat-fat.

One of the advantages of changing from a high-fat to a low-fat lunch will become evident immediately. You will not feel tired and sluggish after a low-fat meal, so you will be at your peak during the afternoon. You may be so energetic your boss will give you a raise. If you are the boss, you might give yourself a raise.

THE DINNER TACKLE

Finally, after you have both breakfast and lunch under control, you are ready to tackle dinner. Try beginning your meal with a low-fat soup, such as Cucumber Soup (page 190) at 2 sat-fat calories per bowl. Not only is it low in saturated fat, it is cooling, delicious, and one of the easiest-to-make soups known to modern man. Soups help fill you up so you are less tempted to gorge on the higher-fat foods in the main course and in dessert. If you make your own soups, you can control the amount of salt and fat you use. Make a large pot of soup and freeze part for future meals.

Why not eat a low-fat chicken or fish dish? Try Apricot Chicken Divine (page 221) or Shanghai Fish (page 276). Try Turkey Scaloppine Limone (page 256) or Kung Pao Chicken with Broccoli (page 232). There are so many delicious recipes for chicken, turkey, and fish it will take you years to try them all. Vegetable dishes should be explored. As an important part of the meal or as the main dish, vegetables offer interesting flavors and textures as well as vitamins, minerals, and fiber. When not drowned in fat, vegetables fill you up without filling you out. Pastas or rice mixed with a small amount of meat or poultry can make a tasty main dish low in sat-fat calories.

"But I must have beef, too," you cry. *Eater's Choice* allows you to fit beef into your sat-fat budget — perhaps not as often as before, perhaps in smaller portions. Perhaps rather than eating a big fat steak four nights a week, you might eat steak one night, rice mixed with small pieces of beef another, vegetarian chili yet another, and fish, chicken, and turkey the rest of the week.

If you eat dinner in restaurants, many of the same considerations that applied to lunch are relevant.

Togetherness in Health

Since dinner is often the one meal that the whole family eats together, the question arises whether the whole family should eat low-fat, low–saturated fat meals. The simple answer is a loud YES. The American Heart Association recommends that all Americans over the age of two years adopt this new low-fat eating pattern. Both the American Heart Association and the National Cancer Institute recommend it to help prevent heart disease and certain cancers. (For more information about children and diet, read Chapter 12.)

Establish Good Eating Habits Early. If you or your spouse have high blood cholesterol levels, there is a good chance that your children will also have high blood cholesterol levels. Heart-healthy meals will benefit *everyone* in the family. The eating habits that will help you control your blood cholesterol will help your children avoid developing atherosclerosis in the first place. As you have probably already realized, it is hard to change long-established, deep-rooted eating habits. It will be much easier for your children to establish healthful eating habits when they are young than to change them halfway through life.

If everybody in the family eats the same way, you are more likely to stick to the new eating pattern. Of course, this means everyone must learn to eat new foods and recipes and gradually modify their eating pattern. It will be worth it. You will be doing your children and spouse a lifelong favor.

A BALANCED DIET; OR, MAN DOTH NOT LIVE ON LESS SATURATED FAT ALONE

Although *Eater's Choice* focuses on saturated fat, you must take care to eat foods from all major food groups: whole grains and cereals; vegetables; fruits; dairy; meats, fish, and poultry. It cannot be overemphasized that good long-term health depends on eating a variety of foods. You need about 40 different nutrients to stay healthy. These nutrients are in the foods you normally eat — as long as you eat many different types of foods.

See Chapter 11 for examples of foods in each food group and what nutrients they contain.

Tips to Keep Your Eating in Balance

Here are some important tips you should keep in mind as you change your eating habits:

1. Replace fats with filling, fiber-rich nutritious foods, such as whole grains, fruits, and vegetables (not sugars, which have no nutritional value beyond calories).
2. Under normal eating conditions, all the carbohydrates you eat are burned. None is stored as fat. It is not the carbohydrates

(such as potatoes or bread) but the fats (such as butter) added to them that cause weight gain.

3. Peas and beans (complex carbohydrates) are rich in protein and fiber and low in fat.

4. Choose whole-grain (such as whole-wheat bread) rather than refined-grain products (such as white bread); refining removes vitamins and fiber from the food.

5. Dried peas and beans and whole-oat products, such as oat bran, are high in soluble fiber and have been shown to lower blood cholesterol levels.

6. Be sure to include adequate amounts of calcium in your diet. Choose low-fat milk products, such as skim milk, low-fat yogurt, and low-fat cottage cheese. They are rich in calcium and low in saturated fat.

7. Certain polyunsaturated fats are required for good health and must be obtained from the diet (just like vitamins); you should not eliminate all sources of fat from your diet.

8. Choose cooking methods that do not add fat to otherwise low-fat, low saturated fat foods. Baking, roasting, grilling, broiling, poaching, and steaming are preferred to frying (especially deep-frying). Try sautéeing in a wok to reduce fat absorption.

9. Avoid fad or crash diets. Even though you are concentrating on removing saturated fat from your diet, you must consume an adequate supply of calories to maintain your desirable weight. It is important to realize that if you consume too few calories (fewer than 1000), your basal metabolic rate will slow down to prevent starvation (your body doesn't know you are starving on purpose) and frustrate your weight loss attempts. Also, if you eat fewer than 1000 calories a day you may not get an adequate supply of vitamins, minerals, and fiber. If you have any doubts about the adequacy of your daily dietary intake, consult a physician or registered dietitian.

Plan Ahead

As we mentioned above, you may find it helpful to develop meal plans for a whole week at a time. It will make shopping easier. But in any case, bring home a variety of foods that provide adequate amounts of vitamins, minerals, and fiber and are not overloaded with calories, refined sugars, sodium, and fats.

Heart-Healthy Storage. Today your cupboard is probably filled with all sorts of horrible, high sat-fat foods that make the new you shudder in disgust. Eventually, you will stock your larder (terrible term) with low-fat foods, herbs, spices, whole grains, and your refrigerator with fresh fruits and vegetables. (See Stocking Up, page 176, for suggestions of foods to keep on hand.)

In fact, the contents of your cupboard and refrigerator are good indicators of how seriously you are taking your cholesterol-lowering. When you are able to throw away that box of cheese crackers that you have been hoarding or that small carton of whipping cream that you just might need for a special occasion, you will know that you have really changed your lifestyle and are waltzing down the path of good living and heart-health — the ultimate goal of *Eater's Choice.*

Honesty Is the Best Heart-Healthy Policy

Eater's Choice only works if you follow it faithfully. Do not fool yourself. "Only one little bite . . . just this time" is the theme song for those who have elevated cholesterol levels. You may fool yourself, but you will not fool your blood cholesterol or your arteries.

Check and Recheck Blood Cholesterol Level

You should have your blood cholesterol level checked at frequent intervals to monitor the effectiveness of the changes you have made in your eating habits, especially at the beginning.

To help you and your physician interpret your numbers, you should also keep a three-day food record some time in the two-week period before your cholesterol test. (Read "The Nitty-Gritty of Keeping a Food Record," page 523.)

By analyzing these records you will see how your sat-fat intake has affected your blood cholesterol level. You might find that your cholesterol dropped to 188 mg/dL because you eliminated fast-food restaurant-hopping. Or that your cholesterol rose by 50 points because you spent the last two weeks splurging and making exceptions. Or that a 10 percent sat-fat budget is too high to bring your cholesterol number below 200 mg/dL, so you lower your sat-fat budget to 6 or 7 percent. Or that you lowered your cholesterol by 30 points and are now ready to make more changes that will ensure another 30-point drop.

Each blood cholesterol check and food record review will give you insight. You might pat yourself on the back and continue to eat within your sat-fat budget. Or you might shake your head in disgust or disappointment and rethink your diet.

The frequency of blood checks will be determined by your physician. After your blood cholesterol has been stabilized below 200 mg/dL, you probably will not need to have your level checked more than once a year.

Remember:

1. Easy does it. Make changes in your eating pattern *slowly* so that they will be *permanent* changes.
2. To make gradual changes:

   Approach 1: Reduce or change the foods in your daily menu that contribute the most saturated fat. If this does not lower your blood cholesterol level to below 200 mg/dL, make more changes.

   Approach 2: Focus on one meal at a time. First eliminate those highly saturated breakfast foods you can do without and replace them with foods low in saturated fat. After you have established new and lasting changes in breakfast, make changes in lunch and then dinner.

3. Be sure to choose foods from all major food groups: whole grains and cereals; vegetables; fruits; dairy; meats (meat, poultry, fish, dried peas and beans, eggs, and nuts). Only a well-balanced diet will provide all the essential minerals, vitamins, fiber, and calories.
4. Dried peas and beans and oat bran have been shown to have a modest effect on lowering blood cholesterol levels.
5. Have your blood cholesterol measured periodically to learn how much your new eating habits have lowered your blood cholesterol level.

9 OTHER RISK FACTORS FOR CORONARY HEART DISEASE

WE HAVE WRITTEN this book out of our zeal to see coronary heart disease go the way of diphtheria and polio, to see it become a medical curiosity of the past. Our emphasis is on one of the most important risk factors for heart disease: blood cholesterol. Of course, there are other risk factors for coronary heart disease.

Heart disease is the leading cause of death in the United States. It kills three times as many people as all forms of cancer combined. Think of the people you know. According to national statistics, on average, half of the people you know will die of coronary heart disease.

Scientists have identified the major factors that increase risk of heart attacks. You have no control over some of these risks. However, you can affect their influence by modifying those risk factors over which you do have control.

RISKS YOU CANNOT CONTROL

Family History

Heart disease tends to run in families and thus has a genetic or inherited component. If one or both of your parents had a heart attack before the age of sixty, your chances of having one are increased by twofold.

Sex

Men have a greater chance of having a heart attack than women. Fifty-year-old men have a fivefold greater risk of having a heart attack by the age of sixty than do fifty-year-old women. Women seem to be protected from heart disease before menopause by their sex hormones. At the onset of menopause, a woman's risk of heart disease begins to rise. Whereas the rate of heart attacks in men begins to rise at about age forty-five, in women comparable rates are not seen until about age sixty. Lest women feel too complacent about their low rates of heart disease in middle age, they should know that heart disease is the leading cause of death for older women.

Age

In America, risk of heart disease increases with age for both men and women. For men thirty-five to sixty-five years old, risk of heart attack increases twofold for each decade of life. For women forty-five to sixty-five years old, risk increases threefold for each decade of life. In both cases, this increase is *not* a natural result of aging. It is a result of lifestyle. In cultures where a low-sat-fat diet is the norm, both men and women live to ripe old ages unaffected by heart disease.

While heart disease strikes beginning in middle age, it is never too early to change your lifestyle to lower your risk. Remember: the underlying disease process (clogging of the coronary arteries) begins in childhood. Don't let the lack of symptoms fool you into complacency. On the other hand, if you are already middle-aged or older, do not lose hope. It is never too late to lower your blood cholesterol and slow down, stop, or even reverse the blockage of your coronary arteries.

DON'T JOIN THE ODDS, BEAT THEM!

Do not use the fact that you have a bad family history, that you are old, or that you are a male as an excuse to die of a heart attack. Bringing down your blood cholesterol level to below 200 mg/dL by eating a diet low in saturated fat gives you the same odds as people without those risks.

RISKS YOU CAN CONTROL

The fact that you cannot change your age, sex, or parents should not discourage you. The uncontrollable risk factors account for only a part of the total risk. The rest is accounted for by three powerful risk factors over which you do have control: cigarette smoking, high blood pressure, and high blood cholesterol.

Smoking

Most people associate cigarette smoking with lung cancer. While it is true that most lung cancer is caused by smoking, cigarettes cause more coronary heart disease than lung cancer. Smoking one pack a day doubles the risk of a heart attack, while smoking more than one pack a day triples the risk. In addition to heart disease, smoking causes serious diseases of the lungs, such as emphysema and chronic obstructive lung disease, resulting in an estimated 50,000 preventable deaths each year.

If you smoke, you should realize that it is never too late to benefit from quitting. Your risk of coronary heart disease begins to decrease immediately upon stopping. If you smoke one pack a day, your risk of heart disease one to five years after stopping is only 20 percent higher than that of a person who never smoked. Ten years after stopping, you are at no higher risk for heart disease than if you had never smoked. If you smoke more than one pack a day, your risk of heart disease is three times higher than that of a person who never smoked. One year after stopping, your risk drops to one and one-half times higher than that of a person who never smoked. By twenty years after quitting, you are at no higher risk for heart disease than if you had never smoked. So take control of your life and give up the weed. Reduce your risk of heart disease, lung disease, and cancer all in one fell swoop by quitting smoking once and for all.

High Blood Pressure

Both high blood pressure (often called hypertension) and high blood cholesterol are silent killers. They are called silent because there are usually no symptoms or telltale signs. You will not know if you have these risk factors unless you have them measured. Yet they are both deadly. High blood pressure can cause strokes, aneurysms (the weakening and bursting of an artery wall, which causes massive internal bleeding and often sudden death), and coronary heart disease.

About 60 million Americans, or 1 out of every 4 adults, have high blood pressure. High blood pressure is a leading cause of the 500,000 strokes, 175,000 stroke deaths, and 550,000 heart attack deaths each year. High blood pressure is most common in blacks, the obese, diabetics, the elderly, and women taking oral contraceptives. The presence of high blood pressure doubles the risk of coronary heart disease and raises the risk of stroke by sevenfold.

The Joint National Committee of the High Blood Pressure Education Program recommends that blood pressures should be lower than 140/90 mm Hg. The lower the blood pressure, the lower are the risks of strokes, aneurysms, and heart disease.

Like high cholesterol, high blood pressure is under *your* control. Regular aerobic exercise and, when necessary, weight reduction* are potent medicine against hypertension. In addition, people whose blood pressure is sodium-sensitive should reduce their intake of sodium to about 1100 mg per day (see your doctor for a recommendation). Everyone else should reduce intake to between 1100 and 3300 mg per day. (For reference, 1 teaspoon of table salt contains 2132 mg of sodium.) In general, Americans consume far too much sodium. Currently, the average American consumes 4000 to 5000 mg of sodium each day. *The Sodium Content of Your Food* (*Home and Garden Bulletin* Number 233, U.S. Department of Agriculture) is a useful publication to help you keep track of your sodium intake. It is available from the Government Printing Office, Washington, D.C. 20402.

Risks Are Additive

The presence of any one of the three controllable risk factors (high blood cholesterol, high blood pressure, smoking) doubles your risk of heart disease (see Figure 1, Chapter 1). The simultaneous presence of two of these risk factors quadruples your risk. The addition of the third risk factor increases the risk yet another twofold, resulting in an eightfold higher risk of heart disease. The elimination of a risk factor has an equal but opposite effect on risk as does its addition. Thus, smokers with high blood pressure and high blood cholesterol who quit smoking and reduce their blood pressure and blood cholesterol to healthy levels can cut their risk of heart attack by up to eightfold!

The Choose to Lose Diet: A Food Lover's Guide to Permanent Weight Loss provides a simple, flexible, and effective plan to lose weight and thus reduce hypertension.

OTHER RISK FACTORS

Diabetes Mellitus

Diabetics have a twofold greater rate of coronary heart disease than do normal people. Moreover, diabetics who survive a heart attack have a poor long-term prognosis. Finally, heart disease is more likely to be fatal in diabetics than in people with normal glucose tolerance. The increased risk of coronary heart disease due to diabetes is independent of the other major risk factors, high blood cholesterol and high blood pressure. But diabetics can lower their risk of coronary heart disease by lowering their blood cholesterol and blood pressure. For diabetics as well as nondiabetics, diet is the first line of treatment for lowering blood cholesterol and blood pressure.

The new dietary recommendations for diabetics are similar to those recommended in this book for persons who want to lower their blood cholesterol levels. Thus, diabetics should reduce their intake of saturated fat and cholesterol and increase their intake of complex carbohydrates and fiber. They should limit their intake of simple or refined sugars.

Obesity

Obese people suffer significantly higher rates of illness and death than people of the same age who are not overweight. Obesity is associated with higher rates of angina pectoris, stroke, and sudden death. High blood pressure and diabetes, risk factors for heart disease, are three times more common in obese people. Death rates from heart disease are 50 percent higher for obese people. In general, the risk of death increases about 2 percent for every pound over "desirable" weight (National Institutes of Health Consensus Conference on Obesity).

Obesity also increases the risk of developing arthritis, respiratory disorders, cancer of the uterus, breast, and cervix in women, and cancer of the colon, rectum, and prostate in men.

An effective way to combat obesity is to follow *Eater's Choice*. Although not designed as a weight-loss diet, responses from readers have shown us that the *Eater's Choice* system often results in weight loss (15–20 pounds is typical; more than 40 pounds has been reported). This is easy to understand. Following *Eater's Choice*, the eater learns to make choices that are heart-healthy — and coincidentally low in fat. And scientific research has shown that fat makes fat. The only drawback in following *Eater's Choice* for weight loss is that it is possible to eat a diet low in saturated fat and not lose weight. This is because some foods, such as olive, safflower, sunflower, and corn oils and margarine, may be low in saturated fat and thus heart-healthy, but are extremely high in total fat, and thus fattening. *The Choose to Lose Diet* focuses on reducing total fat for weight loss. Fat has more calories (9) per gram of weight than protein (4) or carbohydrates (4). The fat you eat immediately becomes the squishy, soft pads on your body. The *Choose to Lose* method uses a fat budget similar to the *Eater's Choice* sat-fat budget. Based on a diet low in fat, daily aerobic exercise (walking), and an increased consumption of complex carbohydrates (fruits, vegetables, and whole grains), *Choose to Lose* allows you to fit in your favorite high-fat foods, eat loads of delicious low-fat foods, and feel better than ever while your body gets leaner and leaner.

Lack of Physical Exercise

Exercise is an important part of a healthy lifestyle and is essential for cardiovascular fitness. While it may not prevent you from having a heart attack, data suggest it will increase your chances of survival. Regular exercise helps control weight and lower blood pressure.

Most experts recommend moderate aerobic exercise for the maximum cardiovascular benefit. Aerobic exercise involves continuous exertion, usually in a repetitive or rhythmic motion. Examples include running or jogging, walking, rowing, swimming, bicycling, aerobic dancing, and jumping rope. When exercise is aerobic and performed with sufficient intensity and duration, it will raise HDL-cholesterol. But before you wear yourself to a frazzle running fifteen miles a day so you can eat lardburgers at every meal, be advised that exercise does not negate the ill effects of a high-fat diet. The best way to lower your LDL-cholesterol and thus your risk of a heart attack is to reduce your intake of saturated fat.

Aerobic exercise also aids in weight control by building and preserving fat-burning muscle mass. The more aerobic exercise you do, the more fat you will burn from your fat stores and the leaner you will become. Regular aerobic exercise also has many other benefits, such as an improved feeling of well-being, more energy, and reduced risks of osteoporosis and certain cancers.

A WORD OF CAUTION: Exercise may increase the risk of sudden death in people with advanced coronary atherosclerosis. If you are forty or older and have a sedentary lifestyle, it is highly advisable to have a physical examination by a physician, including an electrocardiogram (and even an exercise electrocardiogram) before starting an exercise program. It is also helpful to get professional guidance in designing your exercise program, to ensure that the exercises you choose are not harmful or dangerous, that you start off slowly and intensify your efforts at the appropriate rate, that you vary your exercise program to prevent fatigue, boredom, and drop-out, and, finally, that you get the most cardiovascular benefit from the time and effort you invest.

Like other lifestyle changes that you might be making at this time, exercise will only benefit your cardiovascular system and your overall health if you continue to do it faithfully. It cannot be a sometime thing. Excuse the pun, but it is for life.

High Blood Triglycerides

Many medical experts consider triglycerides to be normal up to 250 mg/dL. However, the combination of triglycerides of 150 or higher with a very low HDL level — below 40 mg/dL — puts you at high risk for heart disease. Generally, people with triglyceride levels above 250 mg/dL have a low HDL and are at increased risk of cardiovascular disease. Those with levels above 500 mg/dL are at additional risk of pancreatitis. For most people, lowering their triglyceride levels will raise their HDL levels and thus reduce their risk of heart disease.

Elevated triglyceride levels can be reduced by the following lifestyle changes: weight loss (if overweight), regular aerobic exercise, restriction of alcohol consumption, and reduced intakes of simple sugars (sweets) and saturated fats (as recommended by *Eater's Choice*). Some people may have to use drugs if diet does not normalize their triglyceride levels.

Stress

It is a commonly held belief that stress increases the risk of coronary heart disease. Scientists have not been able to confirm or deny this relationship. They are hampered by the difficulty in measuring and quantifying stress. What is stressful to you may not be stressful to others. Furthermore, people react to the same stress in different ways.

It is unclear whether stress increases heart disease directly. What is true is that people under stress often give up healthy lifestyle behaviors and thus increase their risk for heart disease. They abandon exercise and eat a diet high in saturated fat. An often quoted study examined accountants at tax time to determine if stress elevates cholesterol. The study was flawed. Yes, cholesterol levels did rise at tax time, but the study neglected to record food intake. Were the accountants stuffing down a Big Mac or two enhanced by french fries and nachos because they felt too stressed to take time out for a real meal?

Type A Behavior Pattern

People with Type A behavior patterns are characterized as hard-driving, impatient, and time-conscious. Type B people, on the other hand, are easygoing. Numerous studies have shown Type A behavior pattern to be a risk factor for developing coronary heart disease. But in all fairness, it must be said that other studies have not confirmed this observation, and so the jury is still out on the importance of Type A behavior in the development of heart disease.

Remember:

1. The major risk factors of heart disease you cannot control are family history of heart disease, sex, and age.
2. The major risk factors you *can* control (in addition to high blood cholesterol) are high blood pressure and cigarette smoking.
3. Other risk factors include diabetes mellitus, obesity, lack of physical activity, and high blood triglycerides.

10 THE REAL WORLD

YOUR NEW eating pattern is for life — in two ways. It will improve your chances for a long and healthy life, and you must follow it for the rest of your life. Following *Eater's Choice* is easy, and you will find that eating heart-healthy foods can be more satisfying than eating your old heart-risky ones.

HONESTY IS THE HEALTHIEST POLICY

Remember: you *must* be honest with yourself. Don't make exceptions — even for special occasions — or before you know it you will be off the eating plan. Face it: we all have an almost infinite capacity to fool ourselves about how much and how often we eat certain foods. We constantly underestimate the calories, fat, and sugar we consume. We make a small change in our diet and feel so sorry for ourselves that we reward ourselves with treats that negate our progress. We don't want to make a fuss or feel embarrassed, so we eat foods we should avoid when we dine out. We see special occasions deserving of exceptions in everyday occurrences, such as office parties, weekends, birthdays, going out to eat, even when this is a weekly or more frequent event. The favorite expressions of the cheater-eater are "Just this one time" and "This little bit couldn't possibly matter."

These problems do not have to be yours. Be strong. It's your life. Cheater-eaters only cheat themselves. *Eater's Choice* eaters don't need to cheat. They plan ahead. *Eater's Choice* is a flexible plan that allows you to eat your favorite foods as well as enjoy an occasional splurge. (See Chapter 13.)

Heart-Healthy Tips

- Avoid eating on the run, which may necessitate eating fast foods or junk food from vending machines. The time you save in the present may cost you dearly in the future.
- To save yourself from a massive pig-out attack, eat *before* you attend a party where you know high sat-fat foods will be served.
- Try to avoid grocery shopping when you are hungry. In a fit of hunger you might satisfy your craving with a tub of ice cream.
- When you feel like eating something sweet, give yourself a cool, refreshing treat. Create a Frothy Fruit Shake in your blender (see page 348).
- Instead of snacking on high-fat foods, make Bagel Chips. They taste great plain or dipped in Faux Guacamole. (See page 345 for both.)
- Make popcorn (with polyunsaturated oil or air-popped with no butter added) for a snack while watching TV or visiting friends. Popcorn is a low-fat, low-calorie, high-fiber food, and it's cheap.
- Turn off the TV or leave the room when food ads appear. (Do not go to the kitchen!) Many of the ads on TV are devoted to glorifying the fattiest, most heart-risky foods available to mankind. Watching food ads will make you hungry for these artery cloggers.

BE PROUD OF THE NEW YOU

You should not be ashamed that you are watching your fat intake. By letting your friends, colleagues, and family know that you are serious about your new eating pattern, you can solicit their support. Do not let them make you feel guilty because you are eating healthfully and they may not be.

Truly good friends *will* help, by cooking or serving foods low in saturated fat for you, encouraging you to stay on your new eating plan, suggesting restaurants that offer low-fat entrees. You should never feel pressured either by words or by the situation to stray from your eating plan. Say no politely, but firmly. You'll be respected for your self-control. And who knows, perhaps your friends and relatives will begin to see how good you look, how great you feel, and how well you are eating. You might just have a positive influence on their lifestyles.

EATING OUT

Eating out is no longer a rarity, a twice-a-year entertainment or treat. Eating at home has become the rarity. For those of you who haven't been cooking long or at all, don't give up before you try. You may even enjoy it. For those of you who are veteran cooks and want to retire, don't give up now. Your family's health and taste buds, as well as your own, are counting on you.

When you cook your own food, you control the ingredients. When you eat out, even when you think you are beating the high-fat system, fat sneaks in. Butter is stirred into the rice, chicken is baked with the skin, the yogurt dressing is high in fat. And, really, does the food taste that good? You will do yourself a gigantic favor by cooking food from scratch at home. This does not mean bringing carry-out or frozen dinners home. This means cooking all of the scrumptious *Eater's Choice* recipes and really enjoying eating while making your coronaries croon with joy.

Tips for Survival

For the few, rare times that you eat out, here are a few tips that will help you enjoy yourself and eat within your sat-fat budget.

- First, choose your restaurant wisely. Learn which restaurants serve foods low in saturated fat. Avoid restaurants where you have no choices.
- Be prepared to ask lots of questions. Most restaurants that serve chicken and fish can prepare them without butter, cream sauces, or other added fats. Do not be afraid to ask what the ingredients are and how the dish is prepared. Perhaps you can eat the cream sauce: just ask what's in it.

At the Restaurant: Plan of Action, or Taking Control

1. Ask the maître d' for the menu. Review it for low-sat-fat options before you sit down at a table. (To save yourself a trip, call the restaurant and ask questions *beforehand*.) Do you see any low-sat-fat foods you can eat? Can adaptations be made to reduce saturated fat? If you find no dish acceptable or even adaptable to your needs, leave and find another restaurant.
2. If you decide to stay, you will want to study the menu more thoroughly when you sit down.

a. Unless you have saved for a splurge, eliminate the foods that have absolutely no potential for low sat-fat adaptation, such as a New York sirloin, leg of lamb, duck à l'orange (the saturated fat in duck will demolish your sat-fat budget for a week), blanquette of veal, spare ribs, and breaded pork chops.

b. Next, find the dishes that are composed of foods naturally low in saturated fat, such as chicken, fish, or turkey, and try to determine how they are prepared. Was the dish grilled? or poached? or baked? or broiled? fried? deep-fried?

c. If you are not satisfied with the type of preparation, ask if the dish may be prepared in a different way. Can it be grilled with olive oil instead? Or baked with no fat? Can the skin be taken off the breast *before* cooking?

d. Ask about the ingredients. What's in the creamed soup? What's in the white sauce? What was the chicken marinated in?

e. See if adaptations can be made. Can the sauce be served on the side? Can the sauce be made with whole or 2% milk instead of cream? Can the French onion soup be made without cheese?

f. Ask about the vegetables, too. An overdose of butter is a natural addition to most restaurant rice and vegetables. Are the vegetables cooked with butter? Can margarine be used instead? Can they be steamed without fat? Can the rice be made without fat? The baked potato served plain? The sour cream, butter, or margarine served on the side?

g. Ask for fruit for dessert even if it's not on the menu. A bowl of fresh strawberries (without cream) or a fruit plate make a delightful dessert. To satisfy your sweet tooth, ask your dining companion for a tiny bite of his/her high-fat dessert.

3. When your order arrives, if your chicken comes with skin, your fish swimming in butter, or your potato drowning in sour cream, send it back. That's not what you ordered. Don't be shy. After all, they're your arteries, not the waiter's.

If a restaurant is unable or unwilling to satisfy your low-fat needs, you might consider taking your business elsewhere in the future — and letting them know why.

You can clearly see that the secret to eating out is to *ask*. As you and others ask for low-fat options with increasing frequency, restau-

CHINESE RESTAURANTS: THE MYTH

For years we thought Chinese restaurants were a perfect choice for healthy eating — small amounts of meat and lots of vegetables. However, our awareness of total fat and the resulting health risks have changed our opinion. Although the type of fat used is not heart-risky (Chinese restaurants normally use soy oil), the amount of fat is. Chinese chefs often blanch the meat in oil first. Then they sauté it in oil. They may add oil to the finished dish to make it shiny. That's a lot of fat. Not only does fat make you fat, it also puts you at risk for a multitude of diseases.

Look at some of these sat-fat numbers if you want to choke. These estimated* values are for the whole dish. You have to figure out what part of a dish you eat and how the sat-fat adds up.

DISH	ESTIMATED* TOTAL CALORIES	ESTIMATED* SAT-FAT CALORIES
Barbecued Pork (not fried)	1374	355
Barbecued Spareribs	1863	480
Beef with Vegetables	1572	263
Chicken with Vegetables	1224	102
Chicken with Cashews	1765	186
Egg Roll (each)	152	30
Hunan Shrimp	1068	100
Kung Pao Beef	2458	444
Kung Pao Chicken	1806	158
Kung Pao Shrimp	1068	115
Lemon Chicken	1003	103
Moo Shu Beef	1310	258
Moo Shu Pork	1383	292
Orange Beef	1710	342
Pork with Vegetables	1574	338
Sweet and Sour Pork	1845	389
Sweet and Sour Shrimp	1069	130
Szechuan Pork	1694	356

Gorging is normal behavior at a Chinese restaurant. If you can eat sparingly and carefully, you may want to make Chinese restaurants an occasional splurge.

---

*These estimates are derived from analyses of recipes in Chinese cookbooks and interviews with Chinese cooks. But, beware. Values will vary from restaurant to restaurant.

rants will begin to realize that there is a market for such foods and will respond.

Your Choice. Steering clear of high-fat choices at a restaurant is not easy, but it is not impossible — unless you want it to be. If you insist that you were forced to eat the sour cream in the potato and the chicken "came breaded and deep-fried so what could I do?" you are only fooling yourself . . . not your arteries. Don't blame the restaurant. You chose to eat there and you chose what to eat. If you have no self-control at a restaurant and you really want to lower your cholesterol, don't go out to eat. In fact, even if you have self-control, for the sake of your heart, make your restaurant visits a rarity.

Flying? Call Ahead

Frequent airline travelers know how rarely heart-healthy food graces the airline menu. High-fat meats, sauces, cheeses, butter, and desserts abound, and once up in the air, there are no choices to be had. However, a little forethought may provide you with food you can eat without qualms. At least twenty-four hours before your flight, call the airline reservations clerk and order a special meal. Be as specific as you can in making your request. We usually ask for fish or a chicken breast without skin, and fruit for dessert. You might request a fruit plate for lunch. We also explain that we are on a low-fat diet.

THE ART OF READING FOOD LABELS

"Lite!" "Lean!" "Low-fat!" "Cholesterol-free!" What do all the bright letters blazing across the packages really mean? Fortunately you can ignore the hype and focus exclusively on the nutrition label. Nutrition labels contain all the information you need to determine whether a food fits into your sat-fat budget. Understanding food labels is a survival skill you must master if you plan to eat commercial foods.

Ingredients

Here's how to become a label-reading expert. First, select a can or package from your kitchen so you can examine the label. Find the list of ingredients.

Ingredient List. Most packaged foods have nutrition information printed somewhere on the package (even if you need a magni-

---

LABELING REGULATIONS

At this writing, the FDA and USDA are in the process of changing the rules governing food labels and health claims on food packages. As the rules are instituted, we will update this section in *Eater's Choice*. But regardless of any changes that are made, you can always interpret food labels and evaluate health claims if you know your budget and the amount you eat relative to the serving size.

---

fying glass to read it). The ingredients are always listed in descending order by weight. For example, the raspberry sherbet I have before me has these ingredients listed: "Skim milk, sugar, water, corn syrup, red raspberries, cream, raspberry juice concentrate, carob bean gum, mono- and diglycerides, natural raspberry flavor, guar gum, dextrose, whey, citric acid, polysorbate 80, pectin."

This label tells you there is more skim milk than any other ingredient in the carton. Unfortunately, since the actual weights of ingredients are not provided, you have no way of knowing if the skim milk is 49 percent or 20 percent of the weight of the sherbet. You know there is less sugar than skim milk, and more cream than raspberry juice concentrate, but you don't know the actual amount of sugar or cream or any other ingredient.

Ingredient lists can be very beneficial even when they are not quantitative because they may list ingredients you want to avoid. If the first ingredient listed on your package of cereal is sugar, you might want to avoid eating that cereal. If coconut oil is listed second on the label of your bag of potato chips, you might decide to leave that package of potato chips in the store.

Nutrition Information

Soon, if not now, it will be mandatory for almost all food products to have nutrient information in addition to a list of ingredients. This information will include grams of saturated fat and grams and calories of total fat per serving.

Although the nutrition labels look complicated, deciphering them is simple. Keep your sat-fat budget in mind. The two numbers on the label that should interest you most are the grams of saturated fat per serving and the serving size. You will also need to read the list of ingredients to find the sources of saturated fat.

Let's analyze the label of a typical frozen food. First let's look at the information that is most important to you.

```
NUTRITIONAL INFORMATION PER SERVING
SERVING SIZE: 10.0 OZ.                        SERVING PER CONTAINER: 1
CALORIES ......................... 280   POLYUNSATURATED FAT ............... 2g
PROTEIN ............................ 14g  SATURATED FAT ..................... 2g
CARBOHYDRATE ..................... 47g   CHOLESTEROL ..................... 15mg
FAT ................................. 4g  SODIUM ......................... 260mg
PERCENT OF CALORIES FROM FAT .... 13%    POTASSIUM ...................... 510mg
PERCENTAGE OF U.S. RECOMMENDED DAILY ALLOWANCE
PROTEIN ........................... 20    RIBOFLAVIN ........................ 15
VITAMIN A ......................... 15    NIACIN ............................ 10
VITAMIN C ......................... 70    CALCIUM ............................ 6
THIAMINE .......................... 25    IRON .............................. 15
THIS MEAL IS NOT A CURE FOR HEART DISEASE. AND IS ONLY ONE PART OF A DAILY
REGIMEN FOR HEALTHY LIVING
```

SATURATED FAT . . . . 2 g. Saturated fat is listed in grams. There are 9 calories per gram of saturated fat, so multiply by 9 to determine the calories of saturated fat. This spaghetti with meat sauce has 2 grams, or 18 calories, of saturated fat.* (2 grams × 9 calories of fat = 18 calories of fat.) You should also check the total fat content: if it is extremely high, you may want to choose another product.

SERVING SIZE: 10.0 OZ   SERVING PER CONTAINER: 1. It is most important to check the serving size. The manufacturer's idea of a serving size and the amount you actually eat may differ. In this case, 10 ounces is the whole package and probably the amount you will eat.

These listings may also be useful.

FAT . . . . 4 g. If fat is listed in gram amounts, multiply by 9 to determine the calories of fat. This food has 36 fat calories.

CHOLESTEROL . . . . 15 mg. This number is useful, *not* because you should be concerned with cholesterol content, but because knowing the cholesterol content can help you determine the amount of meat in the package. For example, since 1 ounce of beef contains approximately 25–30 mg of cholesterol, you can see that

---

*To determine calories of saturated fat from labels that list only grams of total fat, we have developed an inexpensive "pocket companion" called a Sat-fat Estimator. See the last page of the book for ordering information.

this spaghetti dish contains about half an ounce of beef. Of course it is healthier to eat less meat, but you might be annoyed that you paid as much as you did for so little food.

CALORIES . . . . 280. Manufacturers often capitalize on the public's confusion about the impact of total calories on weight gain. They advertise a product as being low in total calories even though it is very high in fat calories. You need not be concerned about total calories because only fat calories make you fat.

Beguiled by the Health Guidelines

The food industry has gotten the message that the public wants to eat healthfully. Don't be misled by this label:

NUTRIENT	NATIONAL CHOLESTEROL EDUCATION PROGRAM RECOMMENDATIONS (DAILY AVG) FOR ADULTS WITH HIGH BLOOD CHOLESTEROL	SPAGHETTI WITH MEAT SAUCE
TOTAL FAT	LESS THAN 30% OF CALORIES	13% OF CALORIES
SATURATED FAT	**LESS THAN 10% OF CALORIES**	**7% OF CALORIES**
POLYUNSATURATED FAT	UP TO 10% OF CALORIES	7% OF CALORIES
CHOLESTEROL	LESS THAN 300 MG	15 MG

The package boasts that although the National Cholesterol Education Program recommends that saturated fat should be less than 10 percent of calories, this product derives a mere 7 percent of calories from saturated fat. This information is true but irrelevant. The NCEP has recommended that fat should be less than 10 percent of calories for the *whole day's food intake,* not for individual foods.

Here's an example that should help clarify the difference between percentage of sat-fat calories for a whole day versus percentage of sat-fat calories for an individual food. A Dairy Queen float contains 410 total calories, 41 of them, or 10 percent, from saturated fat. Dairy Queen could boast that its float meets the NCEP guidelines because only 10 percent of the float's calories come from saturated fat. However, if you drink two of these floats you are consuming 82 sat-fat calories, or 39 percent of a sat-fat budget of 210. If you drink three floats, you are consuming 123 sat-fat calories, or 58 percent of a sat-fat budget of 210. The fact that each drink is only 10 percent sat-fat is beside the point. What matters is that you are consuming 123 sat-fat calories, which amounts to a large chunk of anyone's sat-fat budget, and you haven't had much to eat. All you need to know is how many calories of saturated fat a food contains and how it fits into your sat-fat budget.

You will also find the dietary recommendations on this frozen dinner label irrelevant.

THIS ENTREE	DAILY GUIDELINES*	MEN	WOMEN	DIETERS
230	Calories	2400	1800	1400
70 (30%)	Calories from Fat (30% /DAY OR LESS)	720	540	420
8g	Fat (30% OF CALORIES PER DAY FROM FAT)	80g	60g	47g
3g	Saturated Fat (10% OF CALORIES/DAY FROM SATURATED FAT)	27g	20g	16g
50mg	Cholesterol	—Less than 300mg—		
510mg	Sodium	—Less than 2400mg—		

*INDIVIDUAL CALORIE NEEDS VARY. CHART SHOWS SEVERAL NATIONAL RESEARCH COUNCIL DIETARY RECOMMENDATIONS APPLIED TO THREE EXAMPLE CALORIE LEVELS. THE NATIONAL RESEARCH COUNCIL DOES NOT ENDORSE ANY PARTICULAR PRODUCT.

The label lists the total calories, fat calories, fat grams, saturated fat grams, and milligrams of cholesterol and salt recommended for men who eat 2400 calories per day, women who eat 1800 calories per day, and dieters who eat 1400 calories per day.

What do these numbers mean to you? First, the total calories and sat-fat calories recommended on the package for men, women, and dieters are unlikely to be the amount you determined for yourself. Using the total caloric intake numbers listed on the label for generic "women" or "dieters" or "men" is like basing your personal expenditures on an arbitrary family income rather than on your own personal income. It is as preposterous that everyone who eats this frozen dinner earns $50,000 a year as that his daily total caloric intake is 2400 or 1800 calories per day.

Second, the label assumes that the dietary guideline specifying 10 percent of calories from saturated fat is a target and not a ceiling. The health guidelines recommend "eat *no more than* 10 percent of calories from saturated fat," not "eat 10 percent of calories from saturated fat." There is a difference. The fewer calories you eat from saturated fat, the better. Some of you may need to lower your sat-fat budget to 8 percent or 6 percent to reduce your cholesterol to a desirable level. Eating 10 percent of your calories from saturated fat would make reaching this level impossible.

Thus, according to the label, assuming 10 percent of the total calories come from saturated fat, men are allowed 243 sat-fat calories, women 180, and dieters 144. A moderately active, 6 foot 2 inch man whose ideal weight is 165 has a 10 percent sat-fat budget of 243. But what if you are a 5 foot 7 inch male who weighs 150 pounds and describe yourself as very sedentary? More important, does a sat-fat budget of 243 fit you? A sedentary 5 foot 8 inch female whose ideal weight is 145 has a 10 percent sat-fat budget of 180. What if you are a superactive woman who is 5 foot 3 inches and weighs 115? Obviously the only sat-fat budget that will fit you is the one you determined, based on your height, frame, ideal weight, and activity level.

CORN CHIPS
NUTRITION INFORMATION
(Per Serving)

Serving Size 1 ounce
Number of Servings 3

Calories	150
Protein	1 g
Carbohydrate	16 g
Fat	10 g
Cholesterol† ....(0 mg/100 g)	0 mg
Sodium	220 mg
Potassium	50 mg

Percentage of U.S. Recommended
Daily Allowances (U.S. RDA)

Protein	2
Vitamin A	*
Vitamin C	*
Thiamine	*
Riboflavin	*
Niacin	*
Calcium	2
Iron	*
Phosphorus	4
Magnesium	4

The Serving-Size Hoax

As you look at the label above, imagine a little bag of corn chips you buy at a delicatessen. This is an amount you would eat by yourself with your sub or sandwich. Let's look at the nutrition information.

FAT . . . . 10 g. The corn chips contain 10 × 9 or 90 calories of fat per serving. That's a lot of fat.

SERVING SIZE . . . . 1 oz. That makes it 90 calories of fat per ounce. Before you stick your hand into the bag to begin munching, take a look at the number of servings in the bag.

NUMBER OF SERVINGS 3. Three! 3 servings × 90 calories of fat = 270 calories of fat for the whole bag. Wow. And this is not a bag you would share. To put the fat calorie content of this bag of corn chips into perspective: 280 fat calories equals Nancy Goor's entire fat budget for the day.

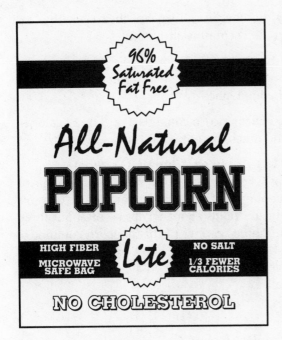

NUTRITIONAL INFORMATION
PER SERVING

Serving Size . . . . ½ oz.
  (Equals 1⅔ cups)
Servings Per Container 14
Calories 60
Protein. . . . . 1 gram
Carbohydrates. . . . . . 10 grams
Fat . . . . 3 grams
Cholesterol. 0**
Sodium . . . . 0 milligrams
Fiber . . . . 2000 milligrams

PERCENTAGE OF U.S.
RECOMMENDED DAILY
ALLOWANCES

Protein   *   Riboflavin 2
Vitamin A*   Niacin   *
Vitamin C*   Calcium   *
Thiamine *   Iron   *

Note: *Contains less than 2%
U.S. RDA of this nutrient.

**Information on cholesterol is provided for individuals who, on the advice of their physician, are modifying their dietary intake of cholesterol.

Our NATURAL popcorn contains one-third fewer calories than our regular buttered popcorn.

INGREDIENTS: Popped Corn, Canola Oil, Beta Carotene for Color.

Sifting through the Hype

The bag of popcorn above sports an amazing array of food claims.

1. LITE
   In color? in sodium content? in weight? in fat?
2. No cholesterol
   Popcorn is a vegetable product. So what else is new?
3. 96% Saturated Fat Free
   Saturated fat accounts for 4 percent of the weight. But what does this mean in terms of calories of saturated fat? You will notice that saturated fat content is not listed on the nutrition label.
4. No Salt

5. High Fiber

Popcorn is naturally high in fiber.

6. 1/3 Fewer Calories

Fewer than what? Fewer than air-popped popcorn? No, fewer than buttered popcorn.

7. All-Natural

"All-natural" does not necessarily mean "heart-healthy" or even healthy. After all, coconut is all-natural.

You may disregard all this promotion (unless you just want to be amused). To determine whether you have really purchased an ultra-healthy product, read the food label.

FAT . . . . 3 g. The popcorn contains 3 × 9 or 27 calories of fat per serving. Not too much fat, but what is the serving size?

SERVING SIZE . . . . ½ oz. (Equals 1⅔ cups)
One and two-thirds cups? Are they kidding? Who eats 1⅔ cups of popcorn? The smallest container of popcorn (about the size of a soft drink cup) at a movie theater holds about 5 cups — or about three servings of this popcorn. Three servings of this popcorn contain 81 fat calories (3 servings × 27 fat calories). You could easily eat half of this bag, or 7 servings. Seven servings contains 189 fat calories. Not so very LITE, after all.

Comparing Labels May Be Tricky

You can and should use the nutrient content information to make comparisons among products. But *be careful.* Be sure you are comparing equal portion sizes. As you have just seen, the manufacturers of some high-fat or high-calorie foods make their portion sizes small so the calorie, fat, sodium, or sugar content does not seem so high. If this is the case, adjust all nutrient content information to the same serving size so you can make meaningful comparisons.

For example, at first glance, a package of Promise Extra Light margarine and Land O Lakes Country margarine appear to be equally low in saturated fat — 9 calories per serving. But look more closely. You will see that the serving size of Promise Extra Light is 1 tablespoon, and the serving size of Land O Lakes Country margarine is 1 teaspoon. This is particularly misleading since the serving size of every other margarine is given in tablespoon amounts.

There are 3 teaspoons in a tablespoon, so the Land O Lakes Country margarine is actually 27 sat-fat calories per tablespoon — three times as high as you may have first assumed.

Oil Labels

Many food products list polyunsaturated oils (such as corn or soy oil) that have been hydrogenated or partially hydrogenated. This means that the oil has been treated by a chemical process that converts some or all of the polyunsaturated oil into trans fats. These trans fats act like saturated fat and raise LDL-cholesterol, thus increasing your risk of heart disease. (See the discussion of trans fats on page 80 in Chapter 7, "Where's the Fat?")

Products are often labeled as containing one or more oils; for example, corn, soybean, palm, or coconut oil. As you know from the food tables, there are large and important differences among these oils. Soybean is a predominantly polyunsaturated oil, while palm and especially coconut and palm kernel oils are predominantly saturated oils. In cases where a choice of oils is listed, the manufacturer uses whichever is cheapest at the moment. As you do not know which oil was used, the best course of action is to avoid the food altogether.

Consumer Beware

Know how to read labels and avoid being misled by the following kinds of advertising claims.

1. CLAIM: Cholesterol-free.
   TRUTH: The average consumer translates "cholesterol-free" to "heart-healthy." Hah! Of course, coconut, palm, and hydrogenated plant oils are cholesterol-free. Cholesterol is found only in animal products. Coconut and palm are plants. What the advertisers fail to say is the saturated fat in coconut, palm, and hydrogenated plant oils is much more heart-risky than cholesterol and should be avoided more assiduously.
2. CLAIM: Light, lower-fat, or lean.
   TRUTH: A food that is described as light, lower-fat, or lean may be lower in fat than other foods of the same type while still being a high-fat food. For example, some brands

of cream cheese are advertised as light, containing 50 percent less fat. While it is true that 5 grams of fat is half as much as 10 grams of fat, 5 × 9 calories per gram of fat or 45 calories of fat is still a lot of fat in one tablespoon of cream cheese.

3. CLAIM: LITE, light.

   TRUTH: Food producers bank on the fact that we associate the term *light* with low-fat. However, light may be used to describe color, texture, taste, size, sodium content, fat content, or amount of total calories. Dorman's Light Slim Jack cheese, for example, contains 7 grams or 63 calories of fat. Dorman's regular Monterey Jack cheese contains 8 grams or 72 calories of fat. A reduction of 9 calories of fat does not make this product light. Light, here, must refer to sodium content.

4. CLAIM: 2% milk is low-fat.

   TRUTH: 2% milk is lower in fat than whole milk but is hardly a low-fat food item. The percentages refer to the percent of the weight of the milk that is fat. Since most of the weight of the milk is water, the weight contributed by fat is small. However, 2% milk derives 34.6 percent of its calories from fat (45 calories of fat per cup). This is not what you would call a low-fat item. Expressing the fat content as a percentage of the weight trivializes the high-fat content.

5. CLAIM: Frankfurters contain no more than 30 percent fat.

   TRUTH: The Food and Drug Administration allows franks to contain up to 30 percent fat. This means at most 30 percent of the weight of the franks comes from fat. But about 80 percent of the calories of a frank come from fat. This amounts to 151 calories of fat in each beef frank. Expressing fat content in terms of weight grossly underestimates its contribution. You get a much better appreciation for the fat content when you express it in terms of calories.

6. CLAIM: 82% fat-free turkey bologna.

   TRUTH: White turkey breast meat is truly a low-fat food. To create 82 percent fat-free turkey bologna — which, according to the food label, has a whopping 45 fat calories per slice — the food manufacturer added turkey fat and skin. 82 percent fat-free, or 18 percent fat means that fat accounts for 18 percent of the weight of the product. Who cares? Actually, each slice of turkey bologna contains 45 fat calories and 60 total calories. Thus, fat accounts for 75 percent (45/60) of the total calories. Do you think the manufacturer could sell any of these cold cuts if the label read "25 percent fat-free!" or "75% fat!"?

<1 Gram: The New Math

If you read the food labels of many products, you might think that food manufacturers are responding to a more health-conscious public. Many food products contain less than 1 gram or 9 calories of fat or saturated fat. Some food labels list an asterisk (*) for fat or saturated fat to denote that the amount of fat or saturated fat is less than 1 gram. Are foods really becoming less fat-filled? Or are the serving sizes just becoming smaller?

You will notice on food labels that grams of fat, saturated fat, protein, and carbohydrate are always whole numbers, never fractions or decimals. This is because manufacturers are allowed to round the actual value to the nearest whole number. Thus, 2 grams may actually range from 1.5 grams to 2.49 grams.

If the amount of fat is 0.99 grams or less (8.9 calories of fat or less), the manufacturer is allowed to list it as <1 gram (less than 1 gram). Qualifying for a <1 gram listing can be accomplished by actually lowering the fat content of the product or by: 1. reducing the serving size without actually changing the product; 2. in the case of saturated fat, keeping the total fat the same but changing to a more unsaturated fat. Several examples will illustrate these points.

Let's look at Deli Thins turkey ham. According to the label, a slice contains less than 1 gram of fat and weighs 11 grams. A slice of regular turkey ham contains 1 gram of fat and weighs 28 grams. The slice of Deli Thins turkey ham contains 40 percent as much fat, but it is 40 percent as big as regular turkey ham. It is exactly the same product, but the manufacturer has cut one slice of regular turkey ham into two. If you put 3 ounces of either regular or Deli Thins turkey ham on a sandwich, you will be eating the same amount of fat.

Likewise, many cookie and cracker labels list their saturated fat content as <1 gram. Look at the Food Tables to see what manufacturers define as a typical serving size. We cookie and cracker lovers know that one cracker or cookie is not what we eat. In addition, by using hydrogenated or partially hydrogenated oils in place of more saturated fats (beef or pork fat, or coconut, palm, or palm kernel oils), manufacturers are able to reduce the saturated fat content listed on the nutrition label. The resulting sat-fat listing underrates the amount of heart-risky fat in the food because the amount of trans fat is not taken into account.

MODIFYING RECIPES

You will find many low-sat-fat recipes in this book. We have chosen only recipes that are low in saturated fat so that you can easily fit them into your daily sat-fat budget. To help you keep track of your saturated fat intake, sat-fat calories are listed at the end of each recipe along with total calories.

TOTAL FAT CALORIES OF RECIPES

For those of you who are reducing your total fat intake, a list of the total fat calories of the recipes begins on page 535.

And you can easily make a whole range of old and new favorites perfect for your new low-fat eating plan with a few simple adaptations.

Substituting Ingredients

Sour Cream Herb Bread can be modified easily without sacrificing taste or texture. Substitute 3 tablespoons of margarine for 3 tablespoons of butter, for a saving of 141 calories of saturated fat. Substitute ½ cup of buttermilk for ½ cup of sour cream for a saving of 135 calories of saturated fat. Buttermilk Herb Bread is just as delicious as Sour Cream Herb Bread and, with 276 fewer calories of saturated fat per loaf, it is much healthier.

Sour Cream Herb Bread	**Buttermilk Herb Bread**
1 tablespoon dry yeast	same
¼ cup very warm water	same
pinch of sugar	same
3 tablespoons **butter**	3 tablespoons **margarine**
3 cups flour	same
3 tablespoons sugar	2 tablespoons sugar
1 teaspoon salt	same
¼ teaspoon marjoram	same
¼ teaspoon oregano	same
¼ teaspoon thyme	same
½ cup **sour cream**	½ cup **buttermilk**
1 egg	same

	TOTAL CALORIES		SAT-FAT CALORIES	
	LOAF	SLICE	LOAF	SLICE
Sour Cream Herb Bread:	2145	126	351	21
Buttermilk Herb Bread:	1874	110	75	4

Silent Substitutions

These substitutions are termed silent because there is often little or no reduction in the quality (taste and texture) of the final product when ingredients rich in saturated fat are replaced by their low-fat counterparts.

When the recipe calls for:	**Use instead:**
Butter	Margarine
Lard or solid shortening	Liquid vegetable oil (olive oil is preferable) or margarine
Sour cream	Low-fat yogurt or buttermilk
Whole milk	Skim milk
1 tablespoon chocolate	3 tablespoons cocoa + 1 tablespoon margarine
3 egg yolks	1 egg yolk
2 whole eggs	1 egg + 1 egg white
Pork	Chicken, white meat
Chicken livers	Chicken, white meat
Veal cutlets	Turkey cutlets

COOKING TIPS

Here are some tips for cooking that will help you stay within your sat-fat budget:

- Steam vegetables. Purchase an inexpensive metal steamer that can be placed in any size saucepan. Buy fresh vegetables. Place about an inch of water in the saucepan. Spread out your steamer and place your vegetables on top. Cover the saucepan. Steam the vegetables until they are tender. Overcooking destroys taste, texture, and vitamins.
- Use a cast-iron griddle to cook turkey cutlets (pound and flour first) or chicken breasts. You will need to add little or no fat.
- Always remove skin *before* cooking chicken. The skin increases the saturated fat content by 2½ times. Bake, broil, or roast chicken. Sauté in a small amount of oil, preferably in a wok.
- Bake, broil, or poach fish. Fried vegetables or meats absorb fat that you do not need. Use a wok for sautéing.
- When cooking beef, trim off all visible fat. Broil or bake on a rack to drain the fat. Remove more fat from the cooked meat with paper towels. Avoid pan-frying.
- *Never* deep-fry foods.

Is Cooking the Low-Fat Way Expensive?

NO. NO. NO. Replacing foods high in saturated fat with vegetables, fruits, and whole grains will save you money as well as improve your health. Convenience foods that are highly processed and full of saturated fat are expensive. Beef is more expensive than chicken, turkey, and many fish. A rice dish with small amounts of chicken or even beef is much less expensive than a steak. Sour cream and sweet cream are costly, both in price and health. Get the picture? Popcorn (made with polyunsaturated oil or air-popped) is one of the healthiest and least expensive snack foods available. In contrast, commercial snack foods such as cookies, chips, and candies are highly saturated, heart-risky, and extremely expensive.

A NEW BEGINNING

You are making a dramatic change in your life. You have learned why it is so important for you to eat heart-healthy foods. In time you will find that a menu low in saturated fat and high in complex carbohydrates will be the most satisfying for you.

Making these changes may not be easy at first, but soon you will find that cooking and eating right is a normal part of your life. I can see you now, sitting in front of the fireplace with your great-great-great-grandchildren, sharing a bowl of air-popped popcorn.

Remember:

1. Take time to eat. Eating junk food from vending machines or at fast-food restaurants saves you time in the present but may cost you dearly in the future.
2. When eating out, *ask* what ingredients are in dishes. Choose broiled, baked, or roasted turkey or chicken without skin or fish. Choose dishes without butter or high-fat sauces. Ask for margarine instead of butter. Ask for dressings and toppings to be served on the side so you can regulate the amount you eat. Don't hesitate to send food back if it is not prepared the way you requested.
3. Learn to read labels carefully. Ingredients are listed in descending order according to weight. Pay particular attention to serving sizes when comparing foods or determining their contribution of saturated fat.
4. Consumer beware: All plant products are cholesterol-free. What they may not be is low in saturated fat. Foods advertised as light, lean, or lower-fat may be high in saturated fat. Some food labels list a choice of vegetable oils. If coconut, palm, palm kernel, or hydrogenated vegetable oils are among the choices, avoid the product.

11 ENSURING A BALANCED DIET

IN YOUR FERVOR to lower your sat-fat intake, don't forget to balance your diet with foods that will give you adequate amounts of vitamins, minerals, protein, and fiber. Eating a well-balanced diet should be no problem if you replace your excess sat-fat calories with a lot of fruits, vegetables, whole grains, and low-fat or nonfat dairy. You'll be amazed at how full and satisfied you'll feel.

The Eating Right Pyramid

More specifically, to maintain your health it is essential that you eat foods from each of the following food groups every day.

WHOLE-GRAIN BREADS, CEREALS, RICE, AND PASTA

For good health and weight control, you should consume 6 to 11 servings of whole-grain breads, cereals, rice, and pasta per day. (See Table 3 on page 141 for sizes of servings.)

The following whole-grain products are rich in starch, fiber, protein, thiamine, riboflavin, niacin, folic acid, vitamin E, iron, phosphorus, magnesium, zinc, and other trace minerals. Choose from:

brown rice	oatmeal	whole-wheat bread
buckwheat groats	pumpernickel	and rolls
bulgur	bread	whole-wheat pasta

The following enriched-grain products contain starch and protein, but thiamine, riboflavin, niacin, and iron have been added. Make

Figure 13: The Eating Right Pyramid *The Eating Right Pyramid proposed by the Department of Agriculture replaces the original four basic food groups wheel. Although both diagrams stress the importance of eating foods from all groups, the pyramid emphasizes the importance of eating more of some foods than others. You should consume whole-grain breads and cereals, rice, and pasta pictured in the base of the pyramid in greatest quantities, followed by vegetables and fruits. Milk products and meat should be eaten in smaller amounts, and fats, oils, and sweets (not even part of the four basic food groups) should be eaten sparingly. In general, Americans have turned this pyramid on its head and have, as a result, been totally out of balance for years.*

sure that saturated fat has not also been added. *Read the labels carefully!* Eat these foods less often. Whole-grain products are far more nutritious.

bagels	French bread	pasta
cereal (ready-to-eat)	noodles	rice

VEGETABLES

Vegetables contribute vital fiber, vitamins, and minerals to your diet. They should be varied and eaten in abundance, at least 3 to 5 servings a day.

The best way to prepare vegetables is to steam them for a short time so they are still crunchy (overcooking causes loss of vitamins and taste). In restaurants, beware of vegetables cooked in butter or drowned in high-fat sauces. To keep them delicious, healthy, and nonfattening, ask that vegetables be steamed with no fat and served with sauces on the side.

Dark green vegetables should be included several times a week. They are an excellent source of vitamins A and C, riboflavin, folic acid, iron, and magnesium. Choose from:

beet greens	endive	spinach
broccoli*	escarole	turnip greens
chard	kale	watercress
chicory	romaine lettuce	

Deep yellow vegetables are an excellent source of vitamin A. Choose from:

carrots	sweet potatoes
pumpkin	winter squash

Other vegetables also contribute varying amounts of vitamins and minerals. Choose from:

artichokes	chinese cabbage	okra
asparagus	cucumbers	onions
beets	eggplant	radishes
brussels sprouts*	green beans	summer squash
cabbage*	green peppers	tomatoes
cauliflower*	lettuce	turnips*
celery	mushrooms	zucchini

Starchy vegetables are rich in starch, fiber, vitamin B_6, folic acid, iron, magnesium, potassium, and phosphorus. Choose from:

corn	potatoes (white)
green peas	rutabaga*
lima beans	sweet potatoes (rich in vitamin A)

Dried beans and peas are excellent sources of protein, soluble fiber (known to reduce blood cholesterol levels), calcium, magnesium, phosphorus, potassium, iron, and zinc.

---

*These cruciferous vegetables may reduce your risk of colon cancer.

Choose from these dried beans and peas, which should be included as a starchy vegetable several times a week. Dried beans and peas are a healthy substitute for meat, poultry, fish, and eggs. They may be included in both the vegetable and meat food groups in the Eating Right Pyramid.

black beans	lentils	split peas
black-eyed peas	lima beans	other types of dried
chickpeas	navy beans	beans and peas
kidney beans	pinto beans	

FRUITS

Fruits contain vitamins, minerals, and fiber. Eat a variety — at least 2 to 4 servings of fruit daily. Have fruits available around the house instead of nuts, cookies, crackers, or candies. Bananas, oranges, pears, apples, strawberries, peaches, nectarines, cantaloupes . . . all fruits make sweet or crunchy treats. Take a bag of your favorite fruits to work: when hunger or boredom strikes, dip into the bag instead of heading for the vending machine and its high-fat temptations.

Citrus, melon, and berries are rich sources of vitamin C, other vitamins, folic acid, and minerals. Choose from:

blueberries	lemon	tangerine
cantaloupe	orange	watermelon
grapefruit	orange juice	other citrus fruits,
grapefruit juice	raspberries	melons, and
honeydew melon	strawberries	berries
kiwi fruit		

Other fruits are also a rich source of vitamins and minerals. Choose from:

apples	nectarines	prunes
apricots	peaches	raisins
bananas	pears	other fruit
cherries	pineapples	fruit juices
grapes	plums	

MILK, YOGURT, AND CHEESE

Milk products are rich in protein, calcium, riboflavin, vitamin B_{12}, magnesium, vitamin A, thiamine, and, if fortified, vitamin D. Milk products need not be high in saturated fat to contain high amounts of calcium. In fact, low-fat milk products contain more calcium than their high-fat counterparts. Do not skimp on low- or nonfat milk products. Even as an adult, you need all the nutrients they supply. Choose from these foods daily:

buttermilk   low- or nonfat yogurt
low-fat (1%) cottage cheese   skim milk

Calcium is also found in dark green vegetables.

Women need more calcium than men in order to avoid developing the bone-thinning disease osteoporosis.

MEAT, POULTRY, FISH, DRIED BEANS, EGGS, AND NUTS

Meats, poultry, fish, and eggs are good sources of protein, phosphorus, niacin, iron, zinc, and vitamins B_6 and B_{12}. However, Americans eat more meat than is necessary for good health. Limit your meat consumption to no more than 4 to 6 ounces a day.

Choose often from the following:

white meat chicken with no skin
white meat turkey with no skin
fish
shellfish

Choose less often (or not at all) from the following:

beef   lamb   veal
ham   pork   eggs

Eat organ meats such as liver, pancreas, and brain rarely, if at all. They are loaded with cholesterol. Pancreas and brain are also high in fat.

Cooked dried beans or peas, as well as nuts and seeds, may be substituted for meat, poultry, fish, and eggs. However, as these plant foods lack vitamin B_{12}, this vitamin must be supplied by other foods. Nuts and seeds are high in fat and should be eaten in moderation.

Here is a table that will make the recommendations easy to follow.

Table 3: Minimum Basic Nutritional Requirements

FOOD GROUP	RECOMMENDED	DAILY SERVINGS	SERVING SIZE
Fruits and Vegetables	All fruits* and	2–4	½ to 1 cup 1 fruit
	vegetables**	3–5	½ to 1 cup
Dairy		2–3 (adults) 3–4 (children)	
	1% low-fat cottage cheese		½ cup
	Dry-curd cottage cheese		½ cup
	Skim milk		1 cup
	1% low-fat milk		1 cup
	Nonfat yogurt		1 cup
Grain		6–11	
	Whole-grain bread		1 slice
	Bagels		1
	Rice		½ cup
	Bulgur		½ cup
	Whole-grain cereals		1 oz
	Pasta		½ cup
Meat		2	
Poultry	Chicken breast w/o skin**		(2–3 oz)
	Turkey breast w/o skin		
Fish	All fin fish**		(3–4 oz)
	Shellfish**		
	Tuna, water packed		
	Sardines (in fish oil)		
Meat alternatives	Dried beans, peas, lentils		½ cup

*Fresh preferred over canned.
**Not fried.

12 CHOLESTEROL GUIDELINES: FROM TOTS TO TEENS

HEART DISEASE has always been considered a disease of the old. Young people rarely die of heart attacks,* and when they do, it is considered an aberration. Heart disease was thought to be a natural consequence of aging. No more. In recent years, scientific research has shown that heart disease is a disease of lifestyle behaviors and may begin when you are a toddler. The heart attack that took your best buddy last year was not a result of something he did last year or even the year before. It was the accumulation of years of a lifestyle that began when he was just a boy. Do you remember him then — devouring hot dogs, chomping on potato chips?

How do we know heart disease begins when we are young? A variety of studies has shown that the atherosclerotic narrowing of the coronary arteries begins in childhood and is influenced by high blood cholesterol and diet.

EXPERT PANEL PROVIDES GUIDELINES

In 1987 the Adult Treatment Panel of the National Cholesterol Education Program of the National Institutes of Health provided guidelines to physicians and the public about diet and cholesterol in adults. Spurred on by the disturbing evidence that heart disease begins in childhood, a panel of experts was convened to study the problem and make recommendations for children. On April 7, 1991,

---

*About one child in a million has a rare genetic condition called homozygous familial hypercholesterolemia. Because they have no functional LDL receptors, these children have blood cholesterol levels around 700 mg/dL and develop severe atherosclerosis early in life. They suffer heart attacks during childhood, usually dying of heart disease before reaching adulthood.

the National Cholesterol Education Program issued the panel's report on blood cholesterol levels in children and adolescents (ages 2 to 19 years old).

The expert panel cited the following critical evidence to link diet, elevated blood cholesterol, and heart disease in children.

- Autopsies of American children and adolescents who died in accidents revealed fatty streaks in their coronary arteries. Fatty streaks, the earliest visible lesions of the atherosclerotic process, often develop into fibrous plaques, the lesions that narrow the arteries. Fibrous plaques appear in Americans as early as the second decade of life. Autopsies of young (average age: 22 years) American soldiers killed in Korea and Vietnam showed that almost 80 percent had gross evidence of coronary disease.
- High levels of total blood cholesterol and LDL-cholesterol and low levels of HDL-cholesterol have been shown to be directly related to the development of coronary-artery fatty streaks and fibrous plaques.
- As in adults, a diet high in saturated fat causes high blood cholesterol in children. An interesting international study has shown that in countries where the average saturated fat consumption is low, the cholesterol levels of children are also low. In Ghana the average saturated fat intake was 10.5 percent of total calories. The average cholesterol level was 128 mg/dL. The reverse is also true. In those countries where children eat a diet rich in saturated fat, they have higher levels of blood cholesterol. In Finland, where the saturated fat intake was 17.7 percent of total calories, the average cholesterol level was 190 mg/dL. As you might expect, Finland has the highest heart attack rate in the world.
- Children and adolescents in the United States have higher blood cholesterol levels and higher intakes of saturated fat and cholesterol than their counterparts in many other countries. Likewise, U.S. adults have higher blood cholesterol levels and higher rates of coronary heart disease and death than adults in these other countries.

The panel concluded that the fatty streaks and fibrous plaques that develop in the coronary arteries of many American children and adolescents are due largely to a diet high in saturated fat and cholesterol.

Who Is at Risk?

Studies have shown that children and adolescents with high blood cholesterol levels are more likely than the general population to have high levels as adults. Those at highest risk have elevated LDL levels, low HDL levels, a family history of premature heart disease, and the presence of other risk factors.

Are Your Children at Risk? The only way to find out if your children are at risk is to have their cholesterol tested. If you or a member of your family has elevated cholesterol, there is a good chance your children also have high cholesterol levels. Children with elevated blood cholesterol levels, especially those with high LDL levels, often come from families with high rates of coronary heart disease. Elevated blood cholesterol levels cluster in families as a result of both shared heredity and eating patterns.

What Can You Do about It? As we have stressed throughout *Eater's Choice,* a diet low in saturated fat is healthy, regardless of your cholesterol level. This is true for both children and adults alike. You don't have to limit your children to a diet of celery sticks and carrot juice. A low-sat-fat diet can be supremely delicious and satisfying. If you want your children to grow into healthy adults, you will have to put some thought into what you feed them. Before we offer some suggestions, you probably want to know whether to test your children's cholesterol, as well as what are the acceptable cholesterol levels in children.

Who Should Be Tested? In answer to the question, "Should all children have their blood cholesterol measured?" the panel responded "No." They rejected the recommendation of universal screening of children as too expensive. They advise screening only children who are at increased risk of having high blood cholesterol because:

- one parent or both have elevated cholesterol (≥240 mg/dL), **or**
- their parents or grandparents have a history of premature cardiovascular disease.*

---

*A person has premature cardiovascular disease if any of the following criteria is met before the age of 55:
- coronary atherosclerosis documented by coronary arteriography
- balloon angioplasty or coronary artery by-pass surgery
- a documented heart attack, angina pectoris, peripheral vascular disease, cerebrovascular disease, or sudden cardiac death

However, for children or adolescents whose parental or grandparental history is not known, cholesterol screening is advisable, particularly if the children have other risk factors, such as obesity, high blood pressure, or if they smoke. (See page 533 for a flowchart and explanation of recommendations for screening and treatment of children at risk.)

What Do Your Children's Cholesterol Numbers Mean?

The panel defined three categories of risk based on total cholesterol and/or LDL levels:

CHOLESTEROL LEVELS AND RISK FOR CHILDREN

CATEGORY	TOTAL CHOLESTEROL	LDL
Acceptable	<170 mg/dL	<110 mg/dL
Borderline*	170–199 mg/dL	110–129 mg/dL
High*	≥200 mg/dL	≥130 mg/dL

*Classification in the borderline and high categories is based on the average of two measurements and not on a single measurement.

All those with high LDL levels (≥130 mg/dL) should be evaluated for possible causes of elevated blood cholesterol other than a high-sat-fat diet. Some of the other factors commonly present in children and adolescents which raise blood cholesterol levels include:

• obesity
• oral contraceptive use
• isotretinoin (Accutane®)
• anabolic steroid use
• anorexia nervosa

Many of these other causes of high blood cholesterol are potentially reversible.

What Is the Recommended Treatment?

Category: Acceptable. If any of your children fit into the Acceptable category, the panel recommends that they have their cholesterol and/or LDL rechecked in five years and be taught and fed a healthy diet. If they have any of the following risk factors, they should be made aware of the ways to reduce them:

- elevated blood pressure
- low HDL (<35 mg/dL)
- severe obesity (≥30 percent overweight for height)
- diabetes mellitus
- smoking
- physical inactivity

Category: Borderline. If any of your children has cholesterol levels in the Borderline category, they should be eating less than 10 percent of their total calories from saturated fat — the Step 1 Diet (for more on the Step 1 Diet, see Table 4) — with a goal of lowering LDL-cholesterol to <110 mg/dL. They should also be told how to reduce any of the relevant risk factors for coronary heart disease. Children in the Borderline category should be reevaluated in one year.

Category: High Risk. If your child tests in the High category, get ready to gear up for a healthier regime. First, children in the High category should have a clinical evaluation and intensive clinical in-

Table 4: Features of Step 1 and Step 2 Diets

| NUTRIENT | RECOMMENDED INTAKE | |
	STEP 1 DIET	STEP 2 DIET
Total fat	Average of no more than 30% of total calories	Same as Step 1
Saturated fat	Less than 10% of total calories	Less than 7% of total calories
Polyunsaturated fat	Up to 10% of total calories	Same as Step 1
Monounsaturated fat	30% total calories minus (% saturated fat calories + % polyunsaturated fat calories)	Same as Step 1
Cholesterol	Less than 300 mg/day	Less than 200 mg/day
Carbohydrates	About 55% of total calories	Same as Step 1
Protein	About 15–20% of total calories	Same as Step 1
Total calories	To promote normal growth and development and to reach or maintain desirable body weight	Same as Step 1

tervention. They should start with a 10 percent sat-fat budget (see the Step 1 Diet, Table 4) and then move on to a sat-fat budget of less than 7 percent (see the Step 2 Diet, Table 4), with the goal of reducing their LDL-cholesterol to <130 mg/dL at a minimum and ideally to <110 mg/dL.

The expert panel recommends drug therapy for children ten years old and older if the following conditions remain after six months to a year of diet therapy:

• LDL ≥ 190 mg/dL or
• LDL ≥ 160 mg/dL *and* there is a positive family history of premature cardiovascular disease *or* the child or adolescent has two or more other cardiovascular risk factors that persist after energetic attempts to control them.

IMPORTANT!

With few exceptions, you can control your child's cholesterol through diet. Eating delicious food that is low in saturated fat can be a real treat. If you eat healthfully, your child will eat healthfully. Drugs are no panacea. They have side effects, they are expensive, and if diet is not changed, they must be taken forever. Diet also has side effects — weight control; lowering the risk of breast, colon, and prostate cancer; and regularity.

If your child tests High for cholesterol, you should make sure that all members of your family have their blood cholesterol measured.

The Balancing Act of the Pediatric Community

The dietary recommendations reflect the concern of the pediatric medical community that extreme changes in diet might compromise growth and development. The pediatric experts are reluctant to reduce total fat. Because fat has so many calories (9 calories per gram versus only 4 calories per gram for carbohydrates and protein), they fear that reducing total fat will overly reduce total calories, which children need to grow and develop.

Fat Habits Develop Early

On the other hand, children develop food tastes and food habits at a young age. If they eat a high-fat diet at age five, it is likely they will crave a high-fat diet at age thirty-five. And a high-fat diet is not healthy. The high-fat American diet increases the risks of obesity, diabetes, some common cancers, such as colon and breast cancer, and heart disease.

In fact, the total fat intake recommendations of the Step 1 and Step 2 diets may be too high for some children, especially if they are overweight. For such children, a total fat intake of 25 percent of total calories may be closer to the mark. Such a reduction should be made in consultation with your pediatrician, with close monitoring to ensure normal growth and development.

Don't Throw out the Baby with the Fat Calories. Eating too little fat is not an American problem. Our children eat anywhere from 35 to 50 percent of their calories as fat, and when they become adults they suffer the health consequences of such a high-fat diet. The opposite problem, undereating fat, is extremely rare, but occasionally one hears of fanatical parents who reduce their child's fat intake to almost nothing and the child fails to thrive. If you have a tendency toward overzealous behavior, be warned. Too little fat and total calories may cause long-term failure to thrive and seriously impair growth and development.

How Much Fat Do Kids Really Eat? To understand why so many American children are fat and have such high cholesterol levels, take a look at the percentage of fat in the current diets of American children and adolescents as compared to the recommended amounts:

Table 5: Comparison of Current and Recommended Diets of Children and Adolescents

NUTRIENT	CURRENT AVERAGE INTAKE	RECOMMENDED INTAKE	
		STEP 1	STEP 2
Saturated fat	14% of calories	<10%	<7%
Total fat	35–36% of calories	No more than 30%	Same
Cholesterol	193–296 mg/day	<300 mg/day	<200 mg/day

Remember Who's Boss. There is no reason why your children should eat so much fat and saturated fat. An average of 35 percent to 50 percent of calories is a tremendous amount of fat. You are in the fortunate position of being the parent or guardian and keeper of the keys to the kitchen. While your children are young, *you* determine what they eat. They may beg you for a cereal advertised on TV or insist on eating dinner at McDonald's. You are the parent and can just say no!

Good for Everyone

If one of your children has high cholesterol, chances are that you, your spouse, and/or your other children also have high cholesterol. And even if no one else in the family has elevated cholesterol, eating a diet low in saturated fat is healthy and delicious for everyone. Have you heard us say this before?! A diet low in fat and saturated fat is recommended by the American Heart Association for *everyone over 2 years old.*

Everyone in your family deserves the benefits of a low-fat diet. It is never too late for the older members to halt the atherosclerotic process and never too early for the younger members to develop good eating habits, which they can carry with them into old age. Eating healthfully when young will save them the difficulty of unlearning unhealthy eating habits later.

If everyone eats the same healthy diet, you avoid labeling the child who has a cholesterol problem. You do *not* want to single out a child who has high cholesterol by making him feel different and "sick." Why make special dishes just for one when the whole family will enjoy the same mouth-watering low-fat recipes?

IF YOUR CHILD HAS HIGH CHOLESTEROL: A PLAN OF ACTION

First, you have to make sure that *you* are eating a low-fat/high–complex carbohydrate diet. That's a snap now that you have read *Eater's Choice.* With no fanfare, gradually change the way you cook to include more low-sat-fat dishes. Look further on in the book to find almost 300 scrumptious recipes that are low in saturated fat. Try Bar-B-Que Chicken (page 242). It's similar to what your kids are used to. Kung Pao Chicken with Broccoli (page 232) is a dish they may have had in a Chinese restaurant. Try Tortilla Soup (page 206). They'll love the crunchy tortillas at the bottom of the bowl. Serve Divine Buttermilk Pound Cake (page 390) for dessert, and you'll convert the pickiest eater. Soon your family will be openminded about any dish you want to serve.

If your children are not willing to try a new soup or chicken dish, ask them to take just a bite. They'll change their tune after a taste. If they refuse to eat, don't force them, but don't feed them later. They won't starve. Be strong. Don't let food become the basis for a power struggle. Look at it this way. Not eating dinner one night won't kill them, but eating a diet of high-fat snacks may.

In the snack realm, replace chips, cookies, and crackers with fresh fruit, nonfat flavored yogurt, pretzels, homemade air-popped popcorn, cereal (be sure it's low-fat), nonfat frozen yogurt, and raw vegetables like carrot and celery sticks. Your children will soon look forward to a snack of sliced strawberries, half a grapefruit, or a banana. Or whip up a lot of fruit in your blender with ice or nonfat yogurt and create a Frothy Fruit Shake (page 348).

THE SNACK LAW

Never, never, never allow your children to snack — even healthy snacks — too close to dinnertime. You know what time that is. Be firm. If you must, serve dinner earlier or later so you are guaranteed a hungry audience. No matter how wonderful a low-sat-fat meal you prepare, if your children are not hungry, they will not eat it. Then, when they are hungry later, it will be easier to feed them something they won't refuse — high-fat junk. So never, never, never allow your children to snack — even healthy snacks — too close to mealtimes.

A Fly in the Ointment

If your spouse is not willing to cooperate ("I'm a steak and potatoes man. This food is for the birds" or "I can't be bothered changing my style of cooking just for one kid"), explain how vital family cooperation is to the health of your child. High cholesterol in children is a serious, life-threatening problem. Spouses should also read *Eat-*

er's Choice so they can understand the whole problem and see how a low-fat diet will benefit them personally, too.

Bringing Up the Problem

When your children are old enough, if they haven't already confronted you, you will want to tell them that they have high cholesterol. Explain it as a problem that lots and lots of people have. They are not strange or unique. They are lucky because it is a problem that can easily be controlled. Encourage them to read *Eater's Choice*. Treat them like adults. This is *their* problem and they need to make food choices to help them keep their cholesterol low. Being aware of the saturated fat in food will help them make better choices.

Handling the Problem

You might order an Eater's Choice Passbook (see the last page of the book) for them to keep track of their sat-fat calories. Looking up what they eat and recording the sat-fat calories can be extremely insightful. Some children will like the game of it. The adult angle will appeal to some because a Passbook is just like a checkbook. They don't have to keep track of their sat-fat intake forever, but keeping track for even a short period will make a tremendous impact on their future food choices.

IMPORTANT MESSAGE: DOWN WITH FAT — UP WITH COMPLEX CARBOHYDRATES

Eater's Choice emphasizes the reduction of saturated fat to lower blood cholesterol. But reducing fat is not enough. The sat-fat calories that your children eliminate must be replaced by calories of complex carbohydrates — vegetables and whole grains — as well as fruits and low- or nonfat dairy products. Your children need the vitamins, minerals, and fiber that these foods provide. Slip them an orange. Stick a carrot in their lunch. Add banana slices to their cereal. Make sure they are not just cutting out saturated fat. Make sure they are eating lots of vegetables, fruits, whole grains, and low- or nonfat dairy.

A Less Casual Approach

For most children, the changes you make to lower the saturated fat in the family diet will be adequate to lower their cholesterol. However, if your child is in the High category, or his cholesterol doesn't drop low enough with the changes you have made, you might want to try the following approach.

THE SAT-FAT BUDGET

You will notice that *Eater's Choice* has desirable weight tables to help you figure out your sat-fat budget. Such tables do not exist for children. To figure out your child's sat-fat budget:

1. Keep a food record for your child for 3 days. Read "The Nitty-Gritty of How to Keep a Food Record" (page 523) to find out exactly how to do it. (You may want to order a Passbook for keeping the food record. See the order form at the back of the book.) Be exact. Make sure your child's diet is typical of his normal daily food intake.
2. Add up the total calories for each day. Average the totals for the 3 days. Your child consumed an average of _____ total calories a day.
3. To determine the sat-fat budget, take 10 percent of the average total calories consumed a day. Here's how to do it:

$$10\% \times \underline{\hspace{2cm}} = \underline{\hspace{1.5cm}} \text{ sat-fat calories.}$$
$$\text{Total calories}$$

4. Add up the sat-fat calories for each day. Average the 3 totals. Your child consumed an average of _____ sat-fat calories a day.
5. Divide the average sat-fat calories a day by the average total calories consumed.

$$\frac{\text{Average sat-fat calories/day}}{\text{Average total calories/day}} \times 100\% = \underline{\hspace{1cm}} \begin{array}{l} \text{average \%} \\ \text{of calories as sat-fat} \end{array}$$

Your child consumed _____% of calories as saturated fat.

Here is an example to help you determine your child's sat-fat budget. Meet Billy.

1. Billy consumed 1800 total calories on Thursday, 2200 on Friday, and 2000 on Saturday.
2. 1800 + 2200 + 2000 = 6000 total calories.
   6000 total calories ÷ 3 days = 2000 total calories a day.
   Billy consumed an average of 2000 total calories a day.
3. 10% × 2000 = a sat-fat budget of 200 sat-fat calories.
4. Billy ate 400 sat-fat calories on Thursday, 500 on Friday, and 450 on Saturday. 400 + 500 + 450 = 1350 sat-fat calories.
   1350 ÷ 3 days = 450.
   Billy consumed an average of 450 sat-fat calories a day. Remember that his sat-fat budget is 200 sat-fat calories a day.
5. $\dfrac{450 \text{ average sat-fat calories}}{2000 \text{ average total calories}} = 22.5\%$ calories as saturated fat.

Billy consumed an average of 22.5 percent of his total calories as saturated fat and 250 sat-fat calories over his budget. The most important goal is to remove 250 sat-fat calories from Billy's daily diet.

If your child already consumes only 10 percent of total calories from saturated fat and has elevated cholesterol, you might want to reduce his sat-fat budget to 7 percent. But be sure to replace the fat removed with complex carbohydrates so that your child gets enough calories to grow and develop normally. Because complex carbohydrates have twice as much bulk as fat for a given number of calories, your child will be eating much more food. Don't be alarmed. Low-fat food is not fattening. If your child is overweight, consult your pediatrician to see if you should reduce his total calories, and if so, by how much.

EATING RIGHT

Knowing your child's sat-fat budget and the sat-fat calories in foods will help you make wise choices in buying and preparing foods. You do not want to make eating into a BIG THING. You want eating healthfully to be a natural part of your child's life.

When your children are young, you have almost complete control over their food choices. Include a variety of fresh fruits and vegetables, breads and cereals (not high-fat) and low- or nonfat dairy in their daily diet. The lure is great, but for the sake of your children's arteries avoid fast-food restaurants. The high-sat-fat temptations are overwhelming. If you must eat out, go to a sub shop instead and order turkey. You might even order a vegetarian pizza without cheese at a pizza parlor.

Cook (and have them help you) *Eater's Choice* or other low sat-fat recipes, and you will make everyone in the family happy.

It is disturbing to find that your child is at risk for heart disease. But consider how fortunate you are that you can easily prevent this risk. By controlling your child's cholesterol problem, you will be enriching the lives of your children, family, and yourself as well.

TWO WEEKS OF MEALS 13

THE FOLLOWING sample meal plans are provided as an example of how to use your sat-fat budget to plan meals and splurges. Here are two whole weeks of menus with a different breakfast, soup, main course, and dessert for each day to show you the variety of foods you can eat and still stay within your sat-fat budget. All the sample meal plans are based on a total consumption of 2000 calories per day. You can find the recipes for dishes printed in italics in the Cook's Choice section.

The first weekly meal plan provides menus that add up to approximately 200 sat-fat calories a day and thus conform to the *Eater's Choice* 10 Percent Plan. In addition, a 6 Percent Plan (120 sat-fat calories per day) is provided, which illustrates how you can modify your eating in the event the 10 Percent Plan does not lower your blood cholesterol sufficiently. Bold print highlights differences in foods or portion sizes between the 10 Percent and the 6 Percent eating plans.

The second weekly meal plan is based on the 6 Percent Plan. This meal plan illustrates how you can save up sat-fat calories to spend on a splurge later in the week. The saturated fat intake in the meals from Sunday through Friday is lower than allowed on the 6 Percent budget. Despite the fact that you will actually be eating more like a 5 Percent *Eater's Choice* Plan, you will have a most satisfying week. You will even have scrumptious desserts each day.

By eating below your sat-fat budget all week, you will be able to save up calories (in this plan, you will save 205 sat-fat calories) to spend at the end of the week. You can spend these calories any way you wish. Of course, since you ate so well all week, you might choose not to spend these calories at all. Eating less saturated fat than is in your sat-fat budget is always an option — a healthy option.

Armed with your own personal sat-fat budget and using the skills you have learned in this book, you can devise delicious and interesting meal plans based on your own food preferences.

MEAL PLANS — WEEK 1

FOOD	PORTION	10% PLAN TOTAL CALORIES	SAT-FAT CALORIES	PORTION	6% PLAN TOTAL CALORIES	SAT-FAT CALORIES
SUNDAY — WEEK 1						
Breakfast						
French Toast	2	212	16	2	212	16
Syrup	1 tbsp	61	0	1 tbsp	61	0
Orange juice	**6 fl oz**	83	0	**8 fl oz**	110	0
Coffee	1 cup	0	0	1 cup	0	0
2% milk	1 tbsp	8	2	1 tbsp	8	2
Breakfast subtotal		364	18		391	18
Lunch						
Potato Soup with Leeks and Broccoli	1 cup	107	3	1 cup	107	3
Oriental Chicken Salad	1 serving	325	20	1 serving	325	20
French Bread	**1 piece**	87	2	**2 pieces**	174	4
Coffee	1 cup	0	0	1 cup	0	0
2% milk	1 tbsp	8	2	1 tbsp	8	2
Apple				1 large	125	1
Lunch subtotal		527	27		739	30
Dinner						
Vegetable Soup Provençal	1½ cups	111	5	1½ cups	111	5
Calzone	1 serving	366	11	1 serving	366	11
2% milk	1 cup	121	27	1 cup	121	27
Mixed salad	1 serving	23	0	1 serving	23	0
Italian dressing	1 tbsp	69	9			
Low-cal Italian				1 tbsp	16	2
Ice cream	1 cup	269	80			
Ice milk				½ cup	92	16
Chocolate Cake with Chocolate Icing	1 slice	273	13	1 slice	273	13
Dinner subtotal		1232	145		1002	74
Daily total		2123	190		2132	122

MEAL PLANS — WEEK 1

FOOD	PORTION	10% PLAN TOTAL CALORIES	10% PLAN SAT-FAT CALORIES	PORTION	6% PLAN TOTAL CALORIES	6% PLAN SAT-FAT CALORIES
MONDAY — WEEK 1						
Breakfast						
Water bagel	1	200	3	1	200	3
Margarine	2 tsp	60	12			
Edam cheese	1 oz	101	45			
Peanut butter				1 tbsp	95	12
Jam				1 tbsp	55	0
Orange juice	6 oz	83	0	6 oz	83	0
Coffee	1 cup	0	0	1 cup	0	0
2% milk	1 tbsp	8	2	1 tbsp	8	2
Breakfast subtotal		452	62		441	17
Lunch						
Turkey sandwich						
White meat turkey w/o skin	3 oz	114	2	3 oz	114	2
Mayonnaise	1 tbsp	99	11			
Low-cal mayonnaise				1 tbsp	35	5
Whole-wheat bread	2 slices	140	8	2 slices	140	8
Tomato	¼ tomato	6	0	¼ tomato	6	0
Potato chips	1 oz	210	32			
Coffee	1 cup	0	0	1 cup	0	0
2% milk	1 tbsp	8	2	1 tbsp	8	2
Pear	1	100	0	1	100	0
Lunch subtotal		677	55		403	17
Dinner						
Carrot Soup	1½ cups	114	3	1½ cups	114	3
Chicken Kiev	1 serving	243	23	1 serving	243	23
Rice	½ cup	113	1	½ cup	113	1
Sesame Broccoli	1 serving	50	3	1 serving	50	3
Mixed salad	1 serving	23	0	1 serving	23	0
Thousand Island dressing	1 tbsp	59	8			
Low-cal Thousand Island				2 tbsp	48	4

MEAL PLANS — WEEK 1

FOOD	PORTION	10% PLAN		PORTION	6% PLAN	
		TOTAL CALORIES	SAT-FAT CALORIES		TOTAL CALORIES	SAT-FAT CALORIES
Coffee	1 cup	0	0	1 cup	0	0
2% milk	1 tbsp	8	2	1 tbsp	8	2
Ice milk	1 cup	184	32			
Applesauce Cake				1 slice	250	14
Dinner subtotal		794	72		849	50
Snack						
Mixed nuts				1½ oz	254	27
Daily total		1923	189		1947	111

TUESDAY — WEEK 1

Breakfast

FOOD	PORTION	TOTAL CALORIES	SAT-FAT CALORIES	PORTION	TOTAL CALORIES	SAT-FAT CALORIES
Cheerios	1 oz	110	3	1 oz	110	3
2% milk	1 cup	121	27			
Skim milk				1 cup	86	3
Whole-wheat bread	**2 slices**	140	8	**1 slice**	70	4
Margarine	**2 tsp**	60	12	**1 tsp**	30	6
Jelly	1 tbsp	50	0	1 tbsp	50	0
Coffee	1 cup	0	0	1 cup	0	0
2% milk	1 tbsp	8	2	1 tbsp	8	2
Orange juice	**6 fl oz**	83	0	**8 fl oz**	110	0
Breakfast subtotal		572	52		464	18

Lunch

FOOD	PORTION	TOTAL CALORIES	SAT-FAT CALORIES	PORTION	TOTAL CALORIES	SAT-FAT CALORIES
Arby's Junior roast beef sandwich	1	218	32	1	218	32
French fries	1 serving	220	33			
Apple juice				1 cup	115	0
Coffee	1 cup	0	0	1 cup	0	0
2% milk	1 tbsp	8	2	1 tbsp	8	2
Apple	**1 small**	80	1	**1 large**	125	1
Lunch subtotal		526	68		466	35

Dinner

FOOD	PORTION	TOTAL CALORIES	SAT-FAT CALORIES	PORTION	TOTAL CALORIES	SAT-FAT CALORIES
Zucchini Soup	1 cup	80	1	1 cup	80	1
Scallop Creole	1 serving	184	7	1 serving	184	7

MEAL PLANS — WEEK I

FOOD	10% PLAN			6% PLAN		
	PORTION	TOTAL CALORIES	SAT-FAT CALORIES	PORTION	TOTAL CALORIES	SAT-FAT CALORIES
White rice	½ cup	113	1	½ cup	113	1
Caraway Carrots	1 serving	40	2	1 serving	40	2
Mixed salad	1 serving	23	0	1 serving	23	0
Russian dressing	1 tbsp	76	10			
Low-cal French dressing				2 tbsp	44	2
Coffee	1 cup	0	0	1 cup	0	0
2% milk	1 tbsp	8	2	1 tbsp	8	2
Tante Nancy's Apple Crumb Cake	1 serving	225	15	1 serving	225	15
Dinner subtotal		749	38		717	30
Snack						
Swiss cheese	1 oz	107	45			
Wheat Thins	4	35	5			
Skim milk	1 cup	86	3			
Ice milk				1 cup	184	32
Daily total		2075	211		1831	115

WEDNESDAY — WEEK 1

Breakfast						
Whole-wheat toast	2 slices	140	8	2 slices	140	8
Peanut butter	1 tbsp	95	12	1 tbsp	95	12
Orange juice	**6 fl oz**	83	0	**8 fl oz**	110	0
Coffee	1 cup	0	0	1 cup	0	0
2% milk	1 tbsp	8	2	1 tbsp	8	2
Breakfast subtotal		326	22		353	22

Lunch						
Tuna sandwich						
White tuna (water packed)	3.25 oz	146	3	3.25 oz	146	3
Whole-wheat bread	2 slices	140	8	2 slices	140	8

MEAL PLANS — WEEK I

FOOD	10% PLAN PORTION	TOTAL CALORIES	SAT-FAT CALORIES	6% PLAN PORTION	TOTAL CALORIES	SAT-FAT CALORIES
Mayonnaise	1 tbsp	99	14			
Low-cal mayonnaise				1 tbsp	35	5
Apple	**1 small**	80	1	**1 large**	125	1
Coffee	1 cup	0	0	1 cup	0	0
2% milk	1 tbsp	8	2	1 tbsp	8	2
Lunch subtotal		473	28		454	19
Dinner						
Sirloin steak	**6 oz**	372	72	**4 oz**	248	48
Spinach, cooked	½ cup	20	0	½ cup	20	0
Baked potato w/skin, large	1	220	1	1	220	1
Margarine	**2 tsp**	60	12	**1 tbsp**	90	18
Mixed salad	1 serving	23	0	1 serving	23	0
French dressing, **regular**	2 tbsp	134	28			
low calorie				2 tbsp	44	2
Coffee	1 cup	0	0	1 cup	0	0
2% milk	1 tbsp	8	2	1 tbsp	8	2
Ice milk	½ cup	92	16			
Fruit cocktail				1 cup	185	0
Dinner subtotal		929	131		838	71
Snack						
Grapes				2 cups	194	2
Popcorn	**4 cups**	220	20	**2 cups**	110	10
Daily total		1948	201		1949	124

THURSDAY — WEEK 1

Breakfast

FOOD	PORTION	TOTAL CALORIES	SAT-FAT CALORIES	PORTION	TOTAL CALORIES	SAT-FAT CALORIES
Oat bran cereal	½ cup dry	165	2	½ cup dry	165	2
Raisins	1 tbsp	27	0	1 tbsp	27	0
Margarine	1 tsp	30	6	1 tsp	30	6
Orange juice	**6 fl oz**	83	0	**8 fl oz**	110	0
Coffee	1 cup	0	0	1 cup	0	0
2% milk	1 tbsp	8	2	1 tbsp	8	2
Breakfast subtotal		313	10		340	10

MEAL PLANS — WEEK I

| FOOD | 10% PLAN | | | 6% PLAN | | |
	PORTION	TOTAL CALORIES	SAT-FAT CALORIES	PORTION	TOTAL CALORIES	SAT-FAT CALORIES
Lunch						
Hamburger, lean broiled	**4 oz**	324	100	**3 oz**	243	75
Hamburger roll	1	115	5	1	115	5
Coleslaw	½ cup	42	2	½ cup	42	2
Coffee	1 cup	0	0	1 cup	0	0
2% milk	1 tbsp	8	2	1 tbsp	8	2
Grapes	1 cup	97	0			
Apple				1 large	125	1
Popcorn		___	___	2 cups	110	10
Lunch subtotal		586	109		643	95
Dinner						
Mushroom Soup	1 cup	95	5			
Minestrone				1½ cups	180	3
Turkey Scaloppine Limone	1 serving	246	14			
Turkey Mexique				1 serving	160	6
Steamed Zucchini Matchsticks	1 serving	17	0	1 serving	17	0
Whole-wheat bread	2 slices	140	8			
Rice	½ cup	113	1	½ cup	113	1
Cucumber Salad	1 serving	20	0	1 serving	20	0
Carrot Cake sans Oeufs	1 serving	122	5			
Apricots, canned				1 cup	215	0
2% milk	1 cup	121	27		___	___
Dinner subtotal		874	60		705	10
Snack						
Nonfat fruit yogurt	8 oz	200	0			
Anjou pear				1 pear	120	0
Skim milk		___	___	1 cup	86	3
Daily total		1973	179		1894	118

MEAL PLANS — WEEK 1

FOOD	PORTION	10% PLAN TOTAL CALORIES	SAT-FAT CALORIES	PORTION	6% PLAN TOTAL CALORIES	SAT-FAT CALORIES
FRIDAY — WEEK 1						
Breakfast						
Whole-wheat toast	**1 slice**	70	4	**2 slices**	140	8
Banana slices	**½ banana**	53	1	1 banana	105	2
1% cottage cheese	**¼ cup**	41	4	**½ cup**	82	7
Cantaloupe	½ melon	95	1	½ melon	95	1
Coffee	1 cup	0	0	1 cup	0	0
2% milk	1 tbsp	8	2	1 tbsp	8	2
Breakfast subtotal		267	12		430	20
Lunch						
Dijon Chicken Rice Salad	1 serving	285	12	1 serving	285	12
Apple Oat Bran Muffin	1 muffin	125	4	1 muffin	125	4
Orange	1 fruit	60	0	1 fruit	60	0
Coffee	1 cup	0	0	1 cup	0	0
2% milk	1 tbsp	8	2	1 tbsp	8	2
Pear				1 large	125	1
Lunch subtotal		478	18		603	19
Dinner						
Cucumber Soup	1 cup	78	0	1 cup	78	0
Rib chops	**2**	480	120	**1**	240	60
Potato Skins	1 serving	79	3	1 serving	79	3
Italian Mixed Vegetables	1 serving	35	2	1 serving	35	2
White wine	3½ fl oz	80	0	3½ fl oz	80	0
Coffee	1 cup	0	0	1 cup	0	0
2% milk	1 tbsp	8	2	1 tbsp	8	2
Cinnamon Sweet Cakes	2	296	16			
Apple				1 large	125	1
Dinner subtotal		1056	143		645	68

MEAL PLANS — WEEK I

	10% PLAN			6% PLAN		
FOOD	PORTION	TOTAL CALORIES	SAT-FAT CALORIES	PORTION	TOTAL CALORIES	SAT-FAT CALORIES
Snack						
Nonfat yogurt w/fruit	8 oz	200	0			
Grapes				1 cup	97	1
Skim milk		___	___	1 cup	86	3
Daily total		2001	173		1861	111

SATURDAY — WEEK 1

Breakfast

Buttermilk Waffles	1 square	158	5	1 square	158	5
Syrup	1 tbsp	61	0	1 tbsp	61	0
Grapefruit	1 fruit	95	0	1 fruit	95	0
Coffee	1 cup	0	0	1 cup	0	0
2% milk	1 tbsp	8	2	1 tbsp	8	2
Breakfast subtotal		322	7		322	7

Lunch

Pawtucket Chili	1½ cups	165	4	1½ cups	165	4
Anjou pear	1 fruit	120	0	1 fruit	120	0
Popcorn	4 cups	220	20	4 cups	220	20
Coffee	1 cup	0	0	1 cup	0	0
2% milk	1 tbsp	8	2	1 tbsp	8	2
Lunch subtotal		513	26		513	26

Dinner

Pesto on Spaghetti	1 serving	313	17	1 serving	313	17
Pink salmon steak	6 oz	246	12	6 oz	246	12
Cauliflower Sauté	1 serving	57	4	1 serving	57	4
Baked sweet potato	1	115	0	1	115	0
Margarine	1 tsp	30	6	1 tsp	30	6
Mixed salad	1 serving	23	0	1 serving	23	0
Blue cheese dressing	1 tbsp	77	14			
Low-cal Italian dressing				1 tbsp	16	2
Ice cream	½ cup	135	40			
Sherbet				½ cup	135	11

MEAL PLANS — WEEK 1

		10% PLAN			6% PLAN	
FOOD	PORTION	TOTAL CALORIES	SAT-FAT CALORIES	PORTION	TOTAL CALORIES	SAT-FAT CALORIES
Coffee	1 cup	0	0	1 cup	0	0
2% milk	1 tbsp	8	2	1 tbsp	8	2
Dinner subtotal		1004	95		943	54
Snack						
Blue cheese	1 oz	100	48			
Wheat Thins	8	70	10			
Oat Bran Muffin				1	160	6
Daily total		2009	186		1938	93

MEAL PLANS — WEEK 2

FOOD	PORTION	TOTAL CALORIES	SAT-FAT CALORIES
SUNDAY — WEEK 2			
Breakfast			
Buttermilk Pancakes	3	93	3
Syrup	3 tbsp	183	0
Orange sections	1 cup	85	0
Coffee, black	1 cup	0	0
Breakfast subtotal		361	3
Lunch			
Gazpacho I	1 cup	109	7
Scallop Curry	1 serving	187	7
Rice	¾ cup	170	2
Keema Eggplant	1 serving	100	4
Mixed salad	1 serving	23	0
Low-cal Russian dressing	1 tbsp	23	1
Banana Cake	1 slice	263	12
Lunch subtotal		875	33
Dinner			
Corn Chowder	1½ cups	288	12
Tomato Quiche	1 slice	220	21
Spinach with mushroom salad	1 cup	15	0
Dressing (oil, vinegar, Dijon mustard)	2 tbsp	119	16
Coffee, black	1 cup	0	0
Kiwifruit	1	45	0
Dinner subtotal		687	49
Daily total		1923	85
6% Plan sat-fat daily budget		120	
+ Carry-over		0	
Total		120	
− Day's expenditure		− 85	
New carry-over		35	

MEAL PLANS — WEEK 2

FOOD	PORTION	TOTAL CALORIES	SAT-FAT CALORIES
MONDAY — WEEK 2			
Breakfast			
Strawberries	1 cup	45	0
w/nonfat yogurt	½ cup	55	0
Oat Bran Muffins	2	320	12
Orange juice	6 fl oz	83	0
Coffee, black	1 cup	0	0
Breakfast subtotal		503	12
Lunch			
Tuna salad sandwich			
water-packed tuna	3¼ oz	146	3
whole-wheat toast	2 slices	140	8
low-cal salad dressing	1 tbsp	45	9
Orange	1	60	0
Marvelous Cookies	2	160	10
Skim milk	8 fl oz	86	3
Lunch subtotal		637	33
Dinner			
Watercress Soup	1 serving	82	7
Indonesian Chicken with Green Beans	1 serving	190	11
Rice	1 cup	226	1
Indian Vegetables	1 serving	86	2
Cucumber Salad	1 serving	20	0
Apple Cake	1 slice	220	13
Dinner subtotal		824	34
Daily total		1964	79

6% Plan sat-fat daily budget	120	
+ Carry-over	35	
Total	155	
− Day's expenditure	− 79	
New carry-over	76	

MEAL PLANS — WEEK 2

FOOD	PORTION	TOTAL CALORIES	SAT-FAT CALORIES
TUESDAY — WEEK 2			
Breakfast			
Cocoa	1 cup		
Cocoa	1 tsp	20	7
Sugar	2 tsp	30	0
Skim milk	8 fl oz	86	3
Low-fat cottage cheese	¼ cup	41	4
Honey Whole-Wheat Bread	1 slice	130	2
Orange juice	6 fl oz	83	0
Banana	1	105	2
Breakfast subtotal		495	18
Lunch			
Cold Ginger Carrot Soup	1 cup	60	2
Peppery Chicken	1 half breast	182	5
Whole-Wheat Bagels	2	230	2
Carrot sticks	1 carrot	30	0
Grapes	1 cup	97	1
Lunch subtotal		599	10
Dinner			
Lentil and Everything Soup	1 cup	94	2
Broiled Monkfish with Orange Sauce	1 serving	194	13
Rice Pilau with Apricots	½ cup	100	3
Cauliflower Sauté	1 serving	57	4
Mixed salad	1 serving	23	0
Dressing made with olive oil, vinegar, herbs	2 tbsp	179	24
Ice milk	¾ cup	138	24
Skim milk	8 fl oz	86	3
Dinner subtotal		871	73
Daily total		1965	101

6% Plan sat-fat daily budget	120	
+ Carry-over	76	
Total	196	
− Day's expenditure	− 101	
New carry-over	95	

MEAL PLANS — WEEK 2

FOOD	PORTION	TOTAL CALORIES	SAT-FAT CALORIES
WEDNESDAY — WEEK 2			
Breakfast			
Oat bran cereal	½ cup dry	165	2
Raisins	1 tbsp	14	0
Margarine	1 tsp	30	6
Orange	1	60	0
Breakfast subtotal		269	8
Lunch			
Fruit Salad with Cottage Cheese	1 serving	280	7
Honey Whole-Wheat Bread	1 slice	130	2
Margarine	1 tsp	30	6
Popcorn (sunflower oil)	4 cups	220	20
Lunch subtotal		660	35
Dinner			
Avgolemono Soup	1 cup	99	2
Chicken Kiev	1 serving	243	23
Sweet potato, baked	1	115	trace
Sliced tomato	1	23	0
Skim milk	8 fl oz	86	3
Cocoa Brownie	1 square	115	9
Dinner subtotal		681	37
Snack			
Focaccia	2½ pieces	351	9
Daily total		1961	89

6% Plan sat-fat daily budget	120
+ Carry-over	95
Total	215
− Day's expenditure	− 89
New carry-over	126

MEAL PLANS — WEEK 2

FOOD	PORTION	TOTAL CALORIES	SAT-FAT CALORIES
THURSDAY — WEEK 2			
Breakfast			
Nonfat yogurt w/fruit	8 fl oz	200	0
Whole-wheat toast	2 pieces	140	8
Jelly	1 tsp	15	0
Coffee, black	1 cup	0	0
Breakfast subtotal		355	8
Lunch			
Curried Tuna Salad w/Pears	1 serving	220	11
Apricot Oat Muffin	2	270	8
Fresh blueberries, cherries or grapefruit sections	1 cup	80	0
Skim milk	8 fl oz	86	3
Lunch subtotal		656	22
Dinner			
Apple Squash Soup	1 cup	148	5
Turkey Cutlets with Artichokes and Cream Sauce	1 serving	248	17
Rice	¾ cup	170	2
Acorn Squash	1 serving	55	3
Eastern Spinach Salad	1 serving	55	3
Mocha Cake with Mocha Frosting	1 square	174	13
Dinner subtotal		850	43
Daily total		1861	73
6% Plan sat-fat daily budget		120	
+ Carry-over		126	
Total		246	
− Day's expenditure		− 73	
New carry-over		173	

MEAL PLANS — WEEK 2

FOOD	PORTION	TOTAL CALORIES	SAT-FAT CALORIES
FRIDAY — WEEK 2			
Breakfast			
Cheerios	1 oz	110	3
Skim milk	½ cup	43	1
Banana, sliced	½	53	1
Orange juice	6 fl oz	83	0
Whole-wheat toast	1 piece	70	4
Margarine	1 tsp	30	6
Coffee, black	1 cup	0	0
Breakfast subtotal		389	15
Lunch			
Turkey submarine sandwich			
White meat turkey	3 oz	114	2
Low-cal mayonnaise	1 tbsp	45	9
Submarine roll	1	215	8
Bosc pear	1	100	0
Skim milk	8 fl oz	86	3
Lunch subtotal		560	22
Dinner			
Broccoli Soup	1 cup	116	4
Pizza	2 pieces	296	8
Mixed salad	1 serving	23	0
Low-cal Italian dressing	2 tbsp	32	4
Green Beans Basilico	1 serving	49	4
Deep-Dish Pear Pie	1 slice	236	11
Coffee, black	1 cup	0	0
Dinner subtotal		752	31
Snack			
Popcorn (sunflower oil)	4 cups	220	20
Daily total		1921	88

6% Plan sat-fat daily budget	120	
+ Carry-over	173	
Total	293	
− Day's expenditure	− 88	
New carry-over	205	

MEAL PLANS — WEEK 2

FOOD	PORTION	TOTAL CALORIES	SAT-FAT CALORIES
SATURDAY — WEEK 2 — Day to Splurge			
Breakfast			
Poached egg	1	79	15
Canadian bacon	2 slices	86	12
Buttermilk Waffles	2 squares	316	10
Orange juice	6 fl oz	83	0
Coffee, black	1 cup	0	0
Breakfast subtotal		564	37
Lunch			
Chili non Carne	1½ cups	190	4
with salad vegetables	¼ cup	15	0
Bran Muffin	1	116	4
Tangerine	1	35	0
Skim milk	8 fl oz	86	3
Lunch subtotal		442	11
Dinner			
Rib roast (lean, trimmed)	6 oz	420	102
Large baked potato	1	220	0
with sour cream	2 tbsps	52	28
Mixed salad	1 serving	23	0
Low-cal Italian dressing	1 tbsp	16	2
Cheese cake	1 slice	280	89
Coffee, black	1 cup	0	0
Dinner subtotal		1011	221
Daily total		2017	269

6% Plan sat-fat daily budget	120
+ Carry-over	205
Total	325
− Day's expenditure	− 269
New carry-over	56

TWO

COOK'S CHOICE

INTRODUCTION

COOK'S CHOICE is different and special. In the following pages, you will find only recipes that are *very low* in saturated fat. Not only are these recipes healthy, they make for delicious eating.

We wrote Cook's Choice to show you that low-sat-fat, heart-healthy foods can be just as tasty and satisfying as heart-risky foods. This is especially important for people who need to lower their blood cholesterol. It is also a must for those who want to lower their blood pressure or lose weight, and for diabetics.

But beyond any health considerations, this cookbook is for people who want to eat well. Dishes need not be filled with cream, sour cream, or cheese to taste good. Try Spinach Quiche (page 316), try Key Lime Pie (page 398), try Watercress Soup (page 192) — in fact, try any of the following recipes for a real taste treat.

Be advised: Because the Goor oven is not necessarily calibrated the same as your oven, and your chicken breasts or swordfish steaks may be thicker or thinner than ours, etc., consider the baking time in the recipes as an estimate. If the recipe tells you to bake a dish for 45 minutes, check your oven at 30. Your food may be ready.

A NOTE TO SODIUM WATCHERS

If you are monitoring your sodium intake, you may want to cut down on the amount of salt in some of these recipes.

A NOTE TO FAT WATCHERS

If you are monitoring your fat intake, check the fat calories for Eater's Choice recipes on pages 535–546.

Here are some tips for superior taste or nutritional benefits without excess effort or expense:

• In the recipes that call for pepper, use freshly ground black pepper. There really is a difference between the stale, tasteless pepper that comes in a can and the bright taste of pepper that has just been ground. It is definitely worth buying a peppermill (not necessarily expensive) and whole peppercorns (available in the spice section of your local grocery store).

• Grate a whole nutmeg (available in the spice section of your local grocery store) with a hand grater for a fresher, nuttier taste.

• Fresh garlic is available at grocery stores and is far superior to garlic powder or garlic salt. It will stay fresh for weeks in the refrigerator.

• Fresh ginger root is available at many grocery stores and is easily kept for months in the refrigerator in a jar filled with sherry. Slice off the outer covering and use ginger root with superior results in recipes that call for ginger.

• In any recipes that call for canned chicken broth, either strain the broth (we often skim the fat off the surface, then pour the broth through a fine tea strainer) or if the fat is hardened, lift it off the soup with a spoon, or use a gravy skimmer.

• Use *unbleached* white flour. When flour is bleached, it loses many of its important nutritional qualities.

NOTE: $\boxed{Q}$ indicates recipes that are quick and easy to prepare. But beware: some $\boxed{Q}$ recipes require marinating for several hours or overnight. Read recipes through before beginning!

STOCKING UP

For some of you, reducing your saturated fat will mean a big change in the foods you cook. You may wonder what foods will replace the cream in your refrigerator or the Twinkies in your cupboard. What foods should you have on hand to make cooking the following recipes a snap? Here is a list of foods and spices to keep in your cupboard, your freezer, and your refrigerator.

Foods to keep on your shelves:

almonds, slivered	apricots, dried
anchovies	apricot jelly

artichoke hearts in water
baking powder
baking soda
barley
beans, dried (black, pinto, etc.)
beans, kidney, canned
chicken broth
chickpeas
cocoa, unsweetened
cornstarch
flour, unbleached white
flour, whole-wheat
honey
lentils
molasses
oat bran
oatmeal (not quick)
oil, olive
oil, sunflower or safflower
olives, black and green
onions
pastas (spaghetti, noodles, etc.)

pineapple chunks, canned
peaches, canned
peanuts, unsalted
potatoes
prunes
raisins
salt
sesame paste (tahini)
sherry, dry
sugar, brown
sugar, white
sugar, confectioners'
tomatoes, canned
tomato juice
tomato paste (6 oz)
tomato sauce (8 oz)
vanilla
vermouth
vinegar
walnuts, shelled
yeast (if you plan to make
  bread)

Spices:

basil leaves
caraway seeds
cardamom, ground
cayenne pepper
chili powder, hot (if you like)
chili powder, mild
cinnamon, ground
cinnamon sticks
cloves, ground and whole
coriander
cream of tartar
cumin, ground and seeds
curry powder

dillweed
garam masala*
ginger, ground
mustard seed, black
nutmeg, whole
oregano
paprika
peppercorns, black
rosemary leaves
sesame seeds
tarragon
thyme leaves
turmeric

*Available in Indian groceries and specialty stores

Foods from the Oriental food store:

bamboo shoots, canned
bean sauce
black beans (fermented)
chili paste with garlic
hoisin sauce
mushrooms, dried black

sesame chili oil
sesame oil
soy sauce and double black
  soy sauce
water chestnuts, canned

Foods* to keep in your refrigerator:

buttermilk (for baking)
carrots
celery
garlic cloves
ginger root (store in jar with
  sherry)
lemons

limes
margarine
mayonnaise or salad dressing
mustard, Dijon
yogurt, nonfat plain

Foods to keep in your freezer:

boned and skinned chicken
  breasts
corn, frozen
margarine

peas, frozen
turkey cutlets
whole-wheat bread
whole-wheat pita bread

These all-season foods will enhance your meals — keep some on hand:

broccoli
carrots**
celery**
eggplant
mushrooms (always good in
  salads)
peppers, red or green

potatoes, white or sweet**
snow peas (Chinese peapods)
spinach
squash** (acorn, butternut,
  etc.)
tomatoes
zucchini

Buy fruits in season. Apples, oranges, and pears can usually be purchased year-round. Use for baking, cooking, and snacks.

---

*These foods will stay fresh at least several weeks.
**These vegetables will keep fresh at least a week or more.

SOUPS

14

SOUP! What a wonderful invention! Hot, cold, spicy, sweet, thick, thin, bland, tart — an unlimited source of goodness. Soup is the perfect way to start a meal. It is a delight to the senses and it is filling. In fact, a bowl of soup makes you feel so satisfied that by the time you get to the main course, your ravenous hunger is abated and you may eat less for the rest of the meal.

These are the major advantages of making your own soup:

- It will taste much better than anything you can buy.
- You have an enormous choice of great soups to make.
- You need not worry about whether the soup is too salty or fatty because you control the amount of salt and fat in your soup.
- You make the kind of soup you want when you want it: hot soup to warm you in the winter; cold soup to refresh you in the summer.
- You can make a large amount at one time and freeze it in small containers for use at a later time. Frozen soup is like money in the bank.

CHICKEN STOCK

Instead of using canned chicken broth, you can make your own chicken stock and freeze it in small amounts. It will be tastier, and it will have no fat or salt. There are many ways to make chicken stock; here is one example.

4 pounds chicken backs, or a
    4–5 pound stewing chicken,
    or 6–8 boneless chicken
    breasts
1 onion, sliced
2 carrots, cut into thirds

1 stalk celery, cut into thirds
1 bay leaf
2 sprigs parsley
¼ teaspoon thyme
1 can (10¾ oz) chicken broth,
    strained

In your largest kettle, combine all ingredients, cover with water, and bring to a boil. Reduce heat, cover, and simmer for 1½ hours.

Remove chicken and vegetables. (You may save both the chicken and the vegetables for another use.)

Refrigerate stock in kettle overnight.

Skim off fat.

Freeze in storage containers.

Q

AVGOLEMONO SOUP
(Greek Lemon Soup)

½ cup long-grain rice
2 quarts chicken stock, or 3 cans
    (10¾ oz each) chicken broth,
    strained, + 3 cans water
1 teaspoon salt (optional)

¾ cup spaghetti broken into
    ½-inch pieces
1 egg
1 egg white
Juice of 1½ lemons

In a soup pot, bring stock to a boil, reduce heat, and simmer with rice until tender (about 20 minutes).

Add salt and spaghetti pieces and simmer for 6 minutes more.

Just before serving, beat together egg and egg white.

Slowly add lemon juice to the eggs, beating constantly.

Take 1 cup of the broth from the soup pot and add it to the lemon-egg mixture, beating constantly.

Pour lemon-egg broth back into the soup pot, beating constantly. Bring to a boil and serve immediately.

Makes 9 one-cup servings
Per serving: 99 Total calories; 2 Sat-fat calories

Q   ## MATZO BALL SOUP

· Traditional matzo ball soup is made with chicken fat and several eggs. This low sat-fat version is as light as a feather and is equally tasty.

¼ cup water	¼ teaspoon salt (optional)
2 tablespoons margarine	6 cups chicken stock, or 2 cans
1 egg	(10¾ oz each) chicken broth,
1 egg white	strained, + 2½ cans water
½ cup matzo meal	

Combine water, margarine, egg, and egg white.
Blend in matzo meal and salt and refrigerate for 20 minutes.
Form chilled dough into balls.
Bring chicken stock to a full boil.
Add matzo balls and simmer, covered, for 20 minutes.

Makes 4 one-and-a-half cup servings (2 matzo balls each)
Per serving: 167 Total calories; 6 Sat-fat calories

Q   ## MUSHROOM SOUP

A must! In no more than ten minutes you can make this sophisticated and soothing soup and set it before your family or guests.

½ pound fresh mushrooms, sliced	Juice of 1 lemon (about ¼ cup)
1 tablespoon margarine	2 tablespoons dry vermouth
2 cans (10¾ oz each) chicken broth, strained	1 tablespoon dry sherry
	Dash of Tabasco sauce

In a medium saucepan, sauté mushrooms in margarine until just tender.
Gently mix in strained chicken broth.

Add lemon juice, vermouth, sherry, and Tabasco sauce, and heat until warm.

Makes 5 one-cup servings
Per serving: 95 Total calories; 5 Sat-fat calories

POTATO SOUP WITH LEEKS AND BROCCOLI

1 ½ tablespoons olive oil
1 ½ cups sliced leeks* (white part)
2 tablespoons unbleached white flour
3 ½ cups hot water
4 cups peeled and sliced potatoes

1 teaspoon salt (optional)
¼ teaspoon freshly ground black pepper
2 cups broccoli flowerets
1 ½ cups skim milk

In a soup pot, heat olive oil.
Mix in leeks, cover pot, and cook slowly until leeks are soft.
Blend in flour and cook for a few seconds. Remove pot from heat.
Add ½ cup of the hot water and blend thoroughly.
Add the remaining hot water, potatoes, salt, and pepper.
Bring to a boil, reduce heat, and simmer, partially covered, for about 40 minutes or until potatoes are tender.
While the potatoes are cooking, steam the broccoli until it is just tender. Set aside.
Pour the cooked potatoes and their liquid into a blender and purée until they are almost smooth (they should still have some texture).
Return soup to pot, add 1 cup of the skim milk, and blend well.
If the soup is too thick, slowly add more skim milk, ¼ cup at a time. Do not add so much skim milk that the soup becomes too thin. Soup should be *thick*.
Mix in broccoli, correct seasoning, and finish with several twists of your peppermill.

Makes 7 one-cup servings
Per serving: 122 Total calories; 3 Sat-fat calories

*If you have no leeks, you may use onions, but the special flavor of leeks enhances the soup.

☐ CARROT SOUP

Carrot soup is a great spur-of-the-moment soup because it is simple to make and you probably have the ingredients on hand. It is thick and tasty — wonderful to warm the soul and body on a nippy winter day.

1 medium onion, chopped
3 small cloves garlic, minced
2 teaspoons olive oil
1 teaspoon thyme
12 carrots, sliced (about 6 cups)
2 potatoes, peeled and sliced
 (about 2 cups)

1 bay leaf
Freshly ground black pepper to
 taste
2 cans (10¾ oz each) chicken
 broth, strained

In a soup pot or large casserole, sauté onion and garlic in olive oil until soft.
Stir in thyme.
Mix in carrots, potatoes, bay leaf, and pepper.
Add chicken broth and enough water to cover vegetables.
Bring soup to a boil. Reduce heat, cover, and simmer for 30 minutes.
Remove bay leaf and purée soup in blender.

Makes 11 one-cup servings
Per serving: 76 Total calories; 2 Sat-fat calories

☐ CARROT SOUP DES BASQUES

The fennel seeds and cumin combine with the carrots to give this soup a hearty robustness.

¼ teaspoon fennel seeds
2 green onions, sliced
1½ teaspoons olive oil
4 cups sliced carrots
3 cups sliced potatoes

1 small onion, minced
2 cans chicken broth (10¾ oz
 each) strained
¼ teaspoon marjoram
½ teaspoon cumin

Crush fennel seeds with the back of a spoon and set aside.
Sauté green onions in olive oil until soft.
Mix in carrots, potatoes, and onion.
Add chicken broth, plus enough water to cover vegetables.

Add fennel, marjoram, and cumin.

Bring to a boil, reduce heat, and simmer for 30 minutes or until vegetables are soft.

Coarsely purée in a blender.

Makes 7 one-cup servings
Per serving: 96 Total calories; 1 Sat-fat calorie

Q COLD GINGER-CARROT SOUP

This soup can be eaten either cold or warm. The lime and ginger give it an interesting flavor.

1 tablespoon minced ginger root
2 cloves garlic, minced
½ cup chopped onion
2 teaspoons olive oil
5 cups sliced carrots

2 cans (10¾ oz each) chicken broth, strained, + 1 can water
¼ cup fresh lime juice (approximately)
Nonfat yogurt, for garnish

In a soup pot or large casserole, sauté ginger, garlic, and onion in olive oil until tender.

Stir in carrots.

Add chicken broth and water and simmer until carrots are tender (about 20 minutes).

Add lime juice and purée soup in blender until smooth.

Chill or serve warm. Top each soup bowl with a large dollop of yogurt.

Makes 10 one-cup servings
Per serving: 60 Total calories; 2 Sat-fat calories

Q   # PEANUT BUTTER SOUP

A tasty soup that you can make easily in about 15 minutes.

1 cup chopped celery
½ cup chopped onion
1 tablespoon olive oil
¼ cup natural all-peanut peanut
    butter
1 can (10¾ oz) chicken broth,
    strained, + 1 can water

1 cup tomato juice
½ teaspoon coriander
Freshly ground black pepper to
    taste

In a soup pot or large casserole, sauté celery and onion in olive oil
until tender.
Stir in peanut butter.
Add chicken broth, water, tomato juice, coriander, and pepper.
Bring to a boil, reduce heat, and simmer for 10 minutes.

Makes 5 one-cup servings
Per serving: 136 Total calories; 13 Sat-fat calories

APPLE-SQUASH SOUP

Apple-Squash Soup is rich and delicious. Use acorn or butternut
squash or even yellow zucchini.

2 tablespoons olive oil
2 cups chopped onion
5 teaspoons curry powder
About 3 pounds squash, peeled,
    seeded, and cubed (about 6
    cups)
2 Granny Smith or other tart
    apples, peeled, cored, and
    cubed

3 cups chicken stock, or 1 can
    (10¾ oz) chicken broth,
    strained, + water to equal 3
    cups
1 teaspoon salt (optional)
1 cup apple cider or apple juice
Freshly ground pepper to taste
1–2 Granny Smith or other tart
    apples, for garnish

In a large soup pot, sauté onion in olive oil until tender.
Stir in curry powder.
Add squash, apples, chicken stock, and salt. Bring to a boil, reduce
heat, and simmer for 25 minutes or until squash and apples are
tender.

Remove 2 cups of liquid and set aside.

Purée remaining soup in blender and return to soup pot.

Stir cider into puréed soup.

Add liquid that you set aside, a bit at a time, making sure that soup remains thick, but not *too* thick.

If necessary, reheat soup until hot.

Pepper liberally.

Grate or chop apples into tiny pieces *just* before serving and garnish each bowl of soup.

Makes 9 one-cup servings
Per serving: 148 Total calories; 5 Sat-fat calories

Q GINGER SQUASH SOUP

½ cup chopped onion

2 tablespoons minced ginger root

2 teaspoons olive oil

6 cups butternut squash, peeled, seeded, and cut into thin slices

2 cans chicken broth (10¾ oz each), strained

1 cup water

½ teaspoon salt (optional)

4 cloves garlic

2–3 tablespoons fresh lime juice

Salt and freshly ground pepper to taste

In a large soup pot, sauté the onion and ginger root in olive oil until soft.

Mix in squash. Add broth, water, salt, and garlic, and bring to a boil.

Reduce heat and simmer, covered, until squash is tender, about 15 minutes.

Purée in blender or food processor.

Return to pot and stir in lime juice, salt, and pepper.

Makes 7 one-cup servings
Per serving: 63 Total calories; 2 Sat-fat calories

☑ TARRAGON SQUASH SOUP

A rich, creamy soup that uses no cream. Puréed bread is the secret ingredient.

2 pounds butternut squash, peeled, seeded, and coarsely chopped
2 cloves garlic, peeled
1 teaspoon salt (optional)
2 cans (10¾ oz each) chicken broth, strained, + ½ cup water

2 slices stale bread, crusts removed
¼ teaspoon freshly ground black pepper
1 teaspoon dried tarragon, or 1 tablespoon fresh tarragon, chopped

In a large pot, combine squash, garlic, salt, chicken broth, and water and bring to a boil. Reduce heat and simmer until squash is tender (about 20–25 minutes).

Tear bread into small pieces and add to squash. Simmer for 3 minutes more.

Purée in blender or food processor.

Just before serving, stir in pepper and tarragon.

Makes 6 one-cup servings
Per serving: 122 Total calories; 2 Sat-fat calories

☑ GREEN TOMATO SOUP

What does one do with all the green tomatoes left on the vine at the end of the summer growing season? Cook tangy, tasty Green Tomato Soup.

1 cup chopped green tomatoes
4 cups sliced green tomatoes
1 cup sliced onion
2 tablespoons olive oil

1 can (10¾ oz) chicken broth, strained, + 1 can water
2 cups shredded fresh spinach

Set aside the 1 cup chopped green tomatoes.

In a medium skillet, briefly sauté sliced green tomatoes and onion in olive oil. Cover and cook at low heat until tender.

Purée tomato-onion mixture in blender or food processor. Pour into casserole or soup pot.

Add chicken broth and water and heat through.

Five minutes before serving, add spinach and reserved chopped tomatoes.

Makes 7 one-cup servings
Per serving: 83 Total calories; 4 Sat-fat calories

⌷ SWEET CABBAGE SOUP

4 cups chopped cabbage
3 cups grated carrot
1 large can (28 oz) tomatoes
  with juice
1 teaspoon tarragon

1 teaspoon basil
1 teaspoon salt (optional)
Water
Juice of 1 lemon
¼ cup raisins

In a large pot, combine cabbage, carrots, tomatoes and their juice, tarragon, basil, and salt. Add water to cover.

Bring to a boil. Reduce heat, cover, and simmer until vegetables are tender.

Purée soup lightly in blender so it still has texture.

Add lemon juice and raisins.

Makes 9 one-cup servings
Per serving: 56 Total calories; 0 Sat-fat calories

⌷ CAULIFLOWER SOUP

Cauliflower Soup is a treasure. It is simple and quick to make and has a wonderful, delicate taste.

1 large head cauliflower
1 can chicken broth (10¾ oz),
  strained
2 stalks celery, diced
2 green onions, sliced

1 teaspoon olive oil
2 tablespoons unbleached white
  flour
1–2 cups water

Remove and discard cauliflower stem. Steam flowerets until tender. Reserve about ½ to 1½ cups and set aside. (You need about 4–5 cups cauliflower for the soup itself. Make sure you don't reserve too much!)

Purée cauliflower and chicken broth in blender. Set aside.

Sauté celery and green onions in oil until tender.

Reduce heat to medium and stir in flour.

Stir in cauliflower purée. Slowly mix in 1 cup of water, stirring constantly until soup thickens. If soup is too thick, stir in remaining water, ¼ cup at a time. Continue cooking until warmed through.

Cut reserved flowerets into bite-size pieces, add to soup, and serve.

Makes 6 one-cup servings (approximately)
Per serving: 47 Total calories; 1 Sat-fat calorie

Q BROCCOLI SOUP

1 cup chopped onion	⅛–¼ teaspoon cayenne pepper
½ cup chopped celery	½–1 teaspoon salt (optional)
1 tablespoon olive oil	6 cups broccoli flowerets (about
1 cup water	2 heads)
⅓ cup long-grain rice	3 cups skim milk

In a soup pot or large casserole, sauté onion and celery in olive oil until tender.

Stir in water, rice, cayenne pepper, and salt, and simmer, covered, for about 10 minutes.

Meanwhile, steam broccoli until just tender. Reserve 1 cup for garnish.

Stir remaining broccoli into soup and continue cooking for 10 minutes more or until rice is cooked and broccoli is soft.

Place in blender. Add skim milk and blend until smooth.

Reheat slowly. Add reserved broccoli and serve.

Makes 7 one-cup servings
Per serving: 116 Total calories; 4 Sat-fat calories

Q
CORN CHOWDER

2 tablespoons margarine
2 tablespoons flour
2 cups skim milk

2 cans creamed corn (16 oz
  each)
½ teaspoon salt (optional)
½ red pepper or green pepper,
  chopped

In a large pot, melt margarine.
Remove pot from heat and mix in flour until smooth.
Slowly stir in 1 cup of the skim milk.
Return pot to burner and heat slowly until milk thickens.
Stir creamed corn and salt into milk.
Slowly stir in the remaining 1 cup of skim milk. Heat but do not
boil.
Stir in peppers and serve.

Makes 6 one-cup servings
Per serving: 192 Total calories; 8 Sat-fat calories

Q
CUCUMBER SOUP

Cucumber soup gets a gold star for excellence. It is as refreshing
as a dip in a cool lake on a hot summer day. It is simple, quick, and
impressive.

2 cucumbers
2 cups nonfat yogurt
1 can (10¾ oz) chicken broth,
  strained

1 clove garlic, crushed
Walnuts, for garnish

Peel cucumbers and cut into bite-size cubes. Salt heavily and set
aside.
Spoon yogurt into a medium casserole and stir until smooth.
Stir in chicken broth.
Mix in garlic.
Rinse salt off cucumbers and add them to yogurt mixture. Add salt
to taste.

Chill in refrigerator for several hours. Garnish with chopped walnuts.

Makes 5 one-cup servings
Per serving: 78 Total calories; 0 Sat-fat calories
Per walnut half: 12 Total calories; 1 Sat-fat calorie

Q # ZUCCHINI SOUP

One of the greatest recipes known to mankind. Hot or cold, summer or winter, for family or company, zucchini soup is delicious — and easy. You can even prepare it 20 minutes before you eat. If you want to make more and freeze it, just add a few more zucchini and more broth. This recipe is very flexible. Add more or less of any ingredient, and it will still taste superb.

3 large or 4 medium zucchini
 (or more or less), sliced
½ cup chopped onion
¼ cup long-grain rice
Chicken stock to cover zucchini,
 or 2 cans (10¾ oz each)
 chicken broth, strained, +
 water to cover zucchini

1 teaspoon salt (optional)
1 teaspoon curry powder
 (approximately)
1 teaspoon Dijon mustard
 (approximately)
½–1 cup nonfat yogurt

In a large soup pot, combine zucchini, onion, rice, chicken stock, water, and salt (add more water, if necessary, to cover zucchini).
Simmer for 15 minutes or until zucchini are tender.
Purée in blender, adding curry powder, mustard, and yogurt to taste.
Eat warm or cool.
This soup freezes well. Reheat frozen soup for best results. Eat immediately or cool for later.

Makes 8 (approximately) one-cup servings
Per serving: 80 Total calories; 1 Sat-fat calorie

WATERCRESS SOUP

Watercress Soup is thick and creamy in texture but low in fat. It makes a refreshing first course in summer or winter.

1 tablespoon olive oil
1 cup chopped onion
2 bunches watercress, washed and stems removed
2 tablespoons unbleached white flour
5 cups chicken stock, or 2 cans (10¾ oz each) chicken broth, strained, + 2 cans water
1 teaspoon salt (optional)

½ teaspoon freshly ground black pepper
1 teaspoon tarragon
1 teaspoon dillweed
1 quart buttermilk
2 tablespoons fresh lemon juice
1 teaspoon Worcestershire sauce
½ teaspoon curry powder
10 sprigs watercress, for garnish

In a large soup pot, heat olive oil. Add onion and cook until soft. Stir in watercress.

Cover and cook slowly for 10 minutes or until watercress wilts. Sprinkle on flour and mix well.

Add chicken stock, salt, and pepper. Cover and simmer for 30 minutes. Add tarragon and dillweed at the last minute.

Cool slightly. Purée in blender or food processor.

Return soup to pot. Add buttermilk, lemon juice, and Worcestershire sauce and stir until smooth.

Add curry powder and heat through.

Cool and refrigerate.

Makes 10 one-cup servings
Per serving: 82 Total calories; 7 Sat-fat calories

Q GAZPACHO I

4 large tomatoes, quartered
1 medium onion, quartered
2 cloves garlic
1 green pepper, coarsely
  chopped
1 cucumber, peeled and coarsely
  chopped

2 tablespoons olive oil
¼ cup white vinegar
1 cup tomato juice
Salt to taste (optional)
Stale bread (1 or 2 slices, or
  bagel)

In a blender, roughly purée tomatoes, onion, garlic, green pepper, cucumber, olive oil, vinegar, tomato juice, and salt. Chill.

Before serving, make croutons by cutting bread (bagel, whole-wheat bread — whatever you have around) into cubes and toasting until crispy in toaster oven.

Garnish soup with croutons.

Makes 8 one-cup servings

Per serving:	Total calories	Sat-fat calories
Without croutons	85	6
With croutons	109	7

Q GAZPACHO II

If you hate wasting the juice from canned tomatoes, the following two recipes (Gazpacho II and Tomato-Rice Soup) will appeal to you. Each time you use canned tomatoes, accumulate their juice in a storage container in the freezer for future soups.

8 cups juice from canned
  tomatoes
2 green peppers, coarsely
  chopped
1 medium onion, coarsely
  chopped

2 cloves garlic, minced
1 cucumber, peeled and coarsely
  chopped
½ cup white vinegar
2 tablespoons olive oil
Salt and freshly ground black
  pepper to taste

Purée all ingredients in blender. Chill.
Add croutons as in Gazpacho I (page 193).

Makes 8 one-cup servings

Per serving:	Total calories	Sat-fat calories
Without croutons	83	4
With croutons	100	5

Q | # TOMATO-RICE SOUP

6 cups juice from canned tomatoes	½ cup long-grain rice
1 tablespoon grated onion	1 cup frozen peas
1 pinch ground cloves	1 cup frozen corn

Combine tomato juice, onion, cloves, and rice and bring to a boil.
Reduce heat and simmer for about 25 minutes.

Add peas and corn and cook about 5 minutes more.

Makes 8 one-cup servings
Per serving: 93 Total calories; 0 Sat-fat calories

Q | # ORIENTAL NOODLE SOUP

2 cans chicken broth (10¾ oz each), strained, + 2 cans water	¼ teaspoon white pepper
	1 cake tofu,* cubed
	1 green onion, sliced
2 ounces cellophane noodles*	10–15 snow peas
1 tablespoon soy sauce	

Bring broth and water to a boil in a soup pot. Add cellophane noodles.

Simmer about 10 minutes, until noodles are soft.

Add soy sauce and white pepper. Simmer a minute or two.

Add tofu, green onion, and snow peas and serve.

Makes 6 one-cup servings
Per serving: 64 Total calories; 1 Sat-fat calorie

HOT AND SOUR SOUP

The ingredients in Hot and Sour Soup seem exotic, but they are all available at Oriental food stores. This wonderful soup is worth an extra shopping trip. You may use the ingredients in many other recipes.

NOTE: This soup is spicy hot. Reduce chili oil and white pepper for a milder soup.

10 large dried black mushrooms*
½ cup tree ear fungi*
⅓ cup tiger lily stems (golden needles)*
2 tablespoons cornstarch
3 tablespoons water
¾ cup diced uncooked chicken breast
1 tablespoon olive oil
1 tablespoon soy sauce
1 can (8 oz) bamboo shoots,* sliced

6 cups chicken stock, or 3 cans (10¾ oz each) chicken broth, strained, + 2 cans water
3 tablespoons white vinegar
1 tablespoon double black soy sauce**
2 cakes tofu (fresh bean curd),* cubed
2 teaspoons chili oil*
½–1 teaspoon ground white pepper
2 egg whites, beaten
4 green onions, sliced

Place mushrooms, tree ears, and tiger lily stems in a small bowl and cover with boiling water. In about 15 minutes or when they are soft, drain off the water and chop off stems or any hard parts.

Slice mushrooms and tree ears and pull tiger lily stems into shreds. Set aside.

Combine cornstarch and water into a smooth paste. Set aside.

In a heated wok or skillet, sauté chicken in oil until chicken is cooked through.

Stir in regular soy sauce.

Stir in mushrooms, tree ears, tiger lily stems, and bamboo shoots.

Add chicken stock, vinegar, and double black soy sauce.

Stir cornstarch mixture into soup. Let thicken.

Add tofu and bring soup to a boil.

Stir in the chili oil and white pepper.

---

*Available at Oriental food stores and some supermarkets
**If double black soy sauce is not available, make your own by mixing 2 teaspoons regular soy sauce with 1 teaspoon molasses.

Turn off the heat for 1 minute and then slowly pour the egg whites into the soup, stirring constantly.

Garnish each bowl of soup with chopped green onions.

Makes 10 one-cup servings
Per serving: 105 Total calories; 5 Sat-fat calories

Q   MULLIGATAWNY SOUP

Customarily, Mulligatawny Soup is made with cream. Our Mulligatawny Soup dispenses with the cream (at 335 sat-fat calories a cup) or a cream substitute. The spicy flavors and interesting textures make this one of our favorite soups.

½ cup chopped onion
½ cup chopped carrot
½ cup chopped celery
1 tablespoon olive oil
1 ½ tablespoons flour
2 teaspoons curry powder
5 cups chicken stock, or 2 cans
   (10 oz each) chicken broth,
   strained, + 2 cans water

½ cup diced uncooked chicken
1 apple, peeled and diced
½ cup cooked long-grain rice
¼ teaspoon thyme
1 teaspoon salt (optional)
¼ teaspoon freshly ground
   black pepper

In a soup pot or large casserole, sauté onion, carrot, and celery in oil until vegetables are tender.

Stir in flour and curry powder and cook for about 1 minute.

Pour in chicken stock and bring to a boil.

Add chicken. Reduce heat, cover, and simmer for 15 minutes.

Add apple, rice, thyme, salt, and pepper and simmer for 15 minutes more.

Makes 6 one-cup servings
Per serving: 121 Total calories; 4 Sat-fat calories

⟨Q⟩ MONHEGAN ISLAND FISH CHOWDER

Eating Monhegan Island Fish Chowder will show you that fish chowders need not be made with cream to be delicious. This chowder uses one large can of evaporated skim milk, which has 3 calories of saturated fat. A comparable amount of cream has 335 calories of saturated fat.

3 large potatoes (about 4 cups)
1 cup chopped onion
1 tablespoon olive oil
2 cups water
1 teaspoon salt (optional)
1 teaspoon basil

¼ teaspoon freshly ground pepper
1 pound cod fillets
2 cups frozen corn kernels
1 large can (12 oz) evaporated skim milk

Scrub potatoes well and cut into bite-size pieces. *Do not peel.* Steam until just tender. Set aside.

In a large pot, sauté onion in olive oil until tender.

Add potatoes, water, salt, basil, and pepper and bring to a boil. Reduce heat, cover, and simmer for 15 minutes.

Gently place cod fillets on top of potatoes, cover, and simmer until fish flakes easily (about 10 minutes).

Carefully stir in corn and evaporated milk. Heat until corn and milk are hot and serve. Do not allow soup to boil.

Makes 9 one-cup servings
Per serving: 165 Total calories; 3 Sat-fat calories

MILD FISH CHOWDER

2 cans (10¾ oz each) chicken broth, strained, + 2 cans water
3 cups cubed potatoes
2 tablespoons long-grain rice
½ cup sliced carrot
1 teaspoon dillweed
1 tablespoon margarine
1 cup sliced leeks

2 green onions, sliced
1 tablespoon unbleached white flour
1 cup frozen corn
⅓ pound mild white fish (such as turbot)
½ can (6½ oz) solid white albacore tuna packed in water

In a large pot, combine chicken broth, water, potatoes, rice, carrots, and dillweed.

In a skillet, melt margarine. Sauté leeks and green onions until soft. Mix in flour until smooth and remove from heat.

Add leek-flour mixture to soup.

Simmer soup until potatoes are fully cooked (about 20 minutes).

Stir in corn, fish, tuna, and tuna liquid. Cook 5 minutes more or until fish is fully cooked.

Makes 7 one-cup servings
Per serving: 181 Total calories; 4 Sat-fat calories

Q   # MINESTRONE

Almost every Italian restaurant in Italy offers its own minestrone, or vegetable soup. Each one is slightly different and all are wonderful. Take whatever vegetables you have in the refrigerator, add some water or broth, pasta, rice and/or beans, to create your own minestrone.

½ onion, sliced	¼ cup long-grain rice
1 tablespoon olive oil	1 teaspoon basil
2 potatoes, diced	1 teaspoon oregano
4 carrots, sliced	½–1 teaspoon salt (optional)
2 celery stalks, sliced	1 can (15½ oz) kidney beans

In a soup pot or large casserole, sauté onion in olive oil until tender.

Mix in potatoes, carrots, and celery. Add water to cover.

Add rice, basil, oregano, salt, and kidney beans.

Bring to a boil. Reduce heat, cover, and simmer until rice is cooked and vegetables are tender (about 25 minutes).

Makes 8 one-cup servings
Per serving: 120 Total calories; 2 Sat-fat calories

VEGETABLE SOUP PROVENÇAL

A hearty Mediterranean soup with a distinctive taste. Use whatever vegetables you have on hand. The more the better! The secret ingredient is the pistou. Italy has its pesto and France has its pistou. Both sauces are combinations of basil, garlic, cheese (omitted here because it is so high in sat-fat), and olive oil, added to soups and pasta to enhance and enrich the flavor.

Make a lot of Vegetable Soup Provençal. It freezes well.
CAUTION: Reheat slowly.

1 large onion, chopped
3 cups sliced carrots
2–3 potatoes, diced
2½ quarts water
1 teaspoon salt (optional)
Any vegetables, such as:
   1 zucchini, sliced
   2 cups broccoli flowerets
   1 cup cauliflower flowerets
   2 cups green beans

2 slices stale bread, shredded
½ cup broken pieces of
   spaghetti

Pistou

8 cloves garlic, minced
⅓ cup chopped parsley
1 can (6 oz) tomato paste

3 tablespoons dried basil, or ½
   cup fresh basil
2 tablespoons olive oil

In a large soup pot, combine onion, carrot, and potato.

Add water and salt and heat to boiling. Reduce heat, cover, and simmer for 20 minutes.

Add zucchini, broccoli, cauliflower, green beans, any other vegetables of your choice, bread, and spaghetti and simmer, covered, for 15 minutes more.

Make pistou in food processor, blender, or with a fork by blending garlic, parsley, tomato paste, basil, and olive oil until smooth.
Stir the pistou into the soup, a little at a time.

Makes 15 one-cup servings
Per serving: 74 Total calories; 3 Sat-fat calories

Q VEGETABLE SOUP WITH SPINACH, POTATOES, RICE, AND CORN

2 cloves garlic, minced
2 teaspoons olive oil
5 ounces fresh spinach, torn into bite-size pieces
1 can chicken broth (10¾ oz), strained, + 2 cans water

½ teaspoon salt, optional
2 small potatoes, peeled and cubed
¼ cup long-grain rice
1 cup frozen corn

In soup pot, sauté garlic in oil until soft.
Stir in spinach and cook for about 1 minute.
Add broth, water, salt, potatoes, and rice, and bring to a boil.
Reduce to a simmer and cook for about 15 minutes or until potatoes are tender and rice is cooked.
Add corn and cook for about 1 minute.

Makes 5 one-cup servings
Per serving: 137 Total calories; 3 Sat-fat calories

GREEN PESTO SOUP

3 cups shredded spinach, washed, stems removed
6 green onions, sliced
1 tablespoon olive oil
1 cup shredded leaf lettuce
2 potatoes, peeled and diced (about 2 cups)

8 cups water
1 teaspoon salt (optional)
¼ teaspoon freshly ground black pepper
1 cup broken pieces of thin spaghetti

Pesto

2 cloves garlic
2 tablespoons olive oil
2 tablespoons basil
2 tablespoons chopped parsley

2 cups spinach, washed and
  stems removed
½ cup water

In a soup pot, sauté spinach and green onions in olive oil until tender.

Stir in lettuce, potatoes, water, salt, and pepper.

Cover pot and simmer until potatoes are tender (about 25 minutes).

Add spaghetti and bring soup to a boil. Reduce heat and simmer for 6 minutes.

Meanwhile, make pesto in a blender or food processor by blending garlic, olive oil, basil, parsley, spinach, and water until smooth.

Mix pesto into soup and serve.

Makes 11 one-cup servings
Per serving: 75 Total calories; 4 Sat-fat calories

Q
BARLEY-VEGETABLE SOUP

½ cup pearl barley, washed
2 quarts homemade chicken
  stock, or 3 cans (10¾ oz
  each) chicken broth, strained,
  + 3 cans water
1 small onion, cut into fourths
1 carrot, cut into thirds
1 stalk celery, cut into 1 inch
  slices

1 teaspoon thyme
1 bay leaf
Freshly ground pepper to taste
3–5 carrots, sliced
2 stalks celery, sliced
½ zucchini, sliced
½ cup onion, chopped
2 cups fresh spinach, chopped

Place barley, chicken stock, onion quarters, carrot thirds, celery slices, thyme, and bay leaf in a large soup pot and bring to a boil. Reduce heat, cover, and simmer for about 1 hour or until barley is tender.

Add sliced carrots, celery, zucchini, and chopped onion and cook until tender.

Add spinach a few minutes before serving.

Makes 9 one-cup servings
Per serving: 100 Total calories; Trace Sat-fat calories

Q LENTIL AND EVERYTHING BUT THE KITCHEN SINK SOUP

Lentils are legumes, which, besides tasting very good, are quite nutritious. They are rich in vitamin C, folic acid, and many minerals. They are a good source of soluble fiber, which has been found to lower blood cholesterol.

1 cup lentils
1 clove garlic, minced
2 stalks celery, sliced
½ cup chopped onion
1 tablespoon olive oil
1 cup grated carrot
1½–2 cups coarsely chopped potato

5 cups water
1 cup tomato juice
1 teaspoon salt (optional)
1 teaspoon thyme
1 tablespoon soy sauce
⅓ cup brown rice
1½ cups frozen corn

Place lentils in a bowl and cover with water.

In a large pot, sauté garlic, celery, and onion in olive oil until tender.

Stir in carrot and potatoes.

Drain water from lentils and add lentils to vegetables.

Add water, tomato juice, salt, thyme, soy sauce, and brown rice. Bring to a boil. Reduce heat, cover, and simmer until lentils and potatoes are tender (about 30 minutes).

Add corn and cook 10 to 20 minutes more.

If soup is too thick, add more water, ¼ cup at a time.

Makes 9 one-cup servings
Per serving: 94 Total calories; 2 Sat-fat calories

☒ LENTIL SOUP

½ pound lentils (1⅓ cups)
½ cup chopped onion
1 cup diced carrots
2 stalks celery, diced
1 green pepper, diced
2 teaspoons olive oil
1 small boiling potato, peeled
  and diced
1 teaspoon cumin
1 teaspoon chili powder

¾ teaspoon allspice
1 bay leaf
¼ cup chopped parsley
1 can chicken broth (10¾ oz),
  strained
4 cups water
½ teaspoon salt (optional)
Freshly ground black pepper
½ cup nonfat yogurt

Rinse off lentils and cover with water. Set aside.

In a large soup pot, sauté onion, carrots, celery, and green pepper in olive oil until onions are soft. After about 30 seconds, lower the heat to medium.

Mix in potato, cumin, chili powder, allspice, bay leaf, and parsley. Drain lentils and add to soup.

Add chicken broth, water, and salt and pepper.

Bring to boil, cover, and reduce to simmer for about an hour or until lentils are tender.

Remove bay leaf. If you wish, purée about ⅞ of the soup. Return purée to pot and mix into remaining soup.

Serve each bowl with a dollop of yogurt.

Makes 8 one-cup servings

Per serving:	*Total calories*	*Sat-fat calories*
Without yogurt	146	1
With yogurt	153	1

Even if you don't like beans, you'll love the following bean recipes: the secret to great bean soup is making a purée of most of the beans instead of leaving them whole. (Of course, you may prefer your beans not puréed at all.) See "Beans," page 291.

CUBAN BLACK BEAN SOUP

Beans are an excellent source of protein, soluble fiber, calcium, magnesium, phosphorus, potassium, iron, and zinc. Experiment with different types of beans to make this hearty, tasty soup. Spoon it over rice and top it with chopped onions.

½ pound dried black beans	1 teaspoon oregano
2 cloves garlic, minced	1 teaspoon salt, optional
1 large onion, chopped	1¼ cups cooked rice
1 green pepper, chopped	½ cup chopped onions, for
1 tablespoon olive oil	garnish
1 teaspoon cumin	2½ teaspoons vinegar

Cover black beans with cold water and soak overnight, or cover beans with boiling water and let soak for 4 hours.

Drain the beans and place in soup pot. Add water to cover. Simmer until tender (about 1–1½ hours).

In a medium skillet, sauté garlic, onions, and green pepper in olive oil until tender.

Stir in cumin, oregano, and salt. Add 1 tablespoon of water and simmer for one more minute to blend flavors.

Add vegetable mixture to beans. If you wish, purée ⅞ of the soup in blender and return purée to pot.

Place ¼ cup of rice in each soup bowl. Spoon soup over rice. Top with chopped onions and sprinkle with ½ teaspoon of vinegar.

Makes 5 one-cup servings
Per serving: 215 Total calories; 4 Sat-fat calories

BEAN SOUP WITH SPINACH, SQUASH, AND TOMATOES

2 cups dried red chili beans (or any other dried bean)
1 can chicken broth (10¾ oz), strained, + 1 can water
1 medium onion, minced
3 cloves garlic, minced
1 teaspoon minced ginger root
1 tablespoon olive oil
¾–1 teaspoon cumin
¾–1 teaspoon turmeric
½ teaspoon coriander
¼–½ teaspoon cayenne pepper
½–1 teaspoon salt (optional)
1 medium zucchini, quartered and sliced into ½-inch pieces
5 ounces fresh spinach, torn into bite-size pieces
1 can (16 oz) chopped tomatoes, with juice

Cover beans with boiling water and let soak for 4 hours. Drain. Add water to cover and cook 1 hour or until tender. Drain.

Remove about ⅞ of the beans and purée with chicken broth in blender. Add purée back to the whole beans.

In a large soup pot, sauté onion, garlic, and ginger root in olive oil until soft.

Mix in cumin, turmeric, coriander, cayenne, and salt.

Stir in bean mixture, zucchini, and spinach.

Add water and tomatoes. If mixture is too thick, slowly add more water, a few tablespoons at a time, until desired consistency is reached. Cook 5 minutes.

Makes 10 one-cup servings
Per serving: 162 Total calories; 2 Sat-fat calories

GREAT BLACK BEAN SOUP

1½ cups dried black beans
1 clove garlic, minced
½ cup chopped onion
4 carrots, chopped
2 teaspoons olive oil
1 tablespoon cumin
1 teaspoon coriander
¼–½ teaspoon cayenne
2 cans chicken broth (10¾ oz each), strained
½ cup long-grain rice
1 cup water
2 tablespoons nonfat yogurt per serving

Cover beans with boiling water. Let soak for 4 hours. Cook them for 1 hour–1 hour 15 minutes or until tender. Set aside.

In a large soup pot, sauté garlic, onion, and carrots in olive oil. After a minute, lower heat and cook until the carrots are tender.

Stir in cumin, coriander, and cayenne, and cook for about a minute.

Add chicken broth.

Drain beans and add them to the soup. Simmer for 5 minutes. Add rice and simmer, partially covered, for 15–20 minutes.

Purée ¾–⅞ of the soup in blender. Return purée to pot.

If soup is too thick, add water a little at a time until soup is a desirable consistancy — not too thick and not too watery.

Top with a dollop of yogurt (2 tablespoons) for each serving.

Makes 7 one-cup servings
Per serving: 233 Total calories; 2 Sat-fat calories

Q   TORTILLA SOUP

This instantaneous soup always gets rave reviews.

6 corn tortillas*	1 large can (28 oz) heavy
1 medium onion, diced	concentrated crushed
3 cloves garlic, minced	tomatoes
1 tablespoon olive oil	1 can (10¾ oz) chicken broth,
2 tablespoons chili powder	strained, + 1 can water
1 teaspoon oregano	1 green pepper, diced
	1 cup frozen corn
	Salt and pepper to taste

About 15 minutes before you serve soup, heat tortillas in a slow oven (325°F), until crisp.

In a soup pot, sauté onion and garlic in oil until soft.

Stir in chili powder and oregano.

Stir in tomatoes, chicken broth, and water.

Bring to a boil and simmer for a few minutes.

Add green pepper and corn.

Add salt and pepper to taste.

---

*Corn tortillas can be found in the refrigerator section of most supermarkets. Be sure they contain no lard or other saturated fat.

For each serving, break a tortilla into small pieces and place at the bottom of a soup bowl. Ladle soup over the tortilla and serve.

Makes 7 one-cup servings
Per serving: 155 Total calories; 4 Sat-fat calories

Q   CANTALOUPE SOUP

Cantaloupe is an excellent sources of vitamins A and C and fiber as well as being just plain delicious. Combined with ginger, orange juice, and buttermilk, cantaloupe makes a refreshing and unusual summer soup.

2 cantaloupes, chilled if possible	3 tablespoons sweet vermouth
¼ cup orange juice	½ cup buttermilk
1 teaspoon chopped ginger root	

Halve melons, discard seeds, scoop out meat, and place it in blender.
Add orange juice, ginger, vermouth, and buttermilk, and blend.
If cold, serve immediately. Otherwise, chill.

Makes 6 one-cup servings
Per serving: 80 Total calories; 1 Sat-fat calorie

Q   CHILLED STRAWBERRY SOUP

Ron says this soup should be in the dessert section. It is sweet and refreshing and easy to make.

2 oranges, peeled and thinly sliced	2 cups sliced strawberries*
	Dash of salt
1 cinnamon stick	1½ tablespoons cornstarch
2 cups water	1 tablespoon water
¼ cup sugar	

Simmer orange pieces and cinnamon stick in 2 cups of water for 5 minutes.

---

*Try peaches, cherries, apricots, or a combination of fruits.

Remove the cinnamon stick and set aside.

Add sugar, strawberries, and a dash of salt and bring to a boil. Turn heat to low.

Blend cornstarch with 1 tablespoon water and stir into soup until clear.

Chill with cinnamon stick.

Makes 5 one-cup servings
Per serving: 90 Total calories; 0 Sat-fat calories

Q   ## BLUEBERRY SOUP

This is a wonderful, sweet, refreshing soup that couldn't be easier to make. I have made it with blueberries and with strawberries — each makes an elegant and scrumptious soup. To make more or less soup than the recipe calls for, use the same ingredients, just keep the proportions the same.

3 cups blueberries (or other fruit, such as strawberries, raspberries)	½ cup sugar
	1 cinnamon stick
2¼ cups water	1½ cups nonfat yogurt

Combine fruit, water, sugar, and cinnamon stick in a saucepan.

Bring to a boil and remove from heat. Pour into blender and let cool. (If soup is too hot, it will curdle the yogurt.)

Remove cinnamon stick (but do not discard it) and blend. Add yogurt and blend.

Chill with cinnamon stick. Refrigerate until cold.

Makes 7 one-cup servings
Per serving: 104 Total calories; 0 Sat-fat calories

Q   # SOUR CHERRY SOUP

Sour Cherry Soup is a sweet soup. It is ideal for a luncheon or dinner party and *very* simple to make. It has no fat but does have quite a lot of sugar.

2 cans (1 lb each) undrained   2 tablespoons unbleached white
  sour cherries packed in water   flour
¾ cup sugar   6 tablespoons cold water
1 stick cinnamon   2 cups water

Remove about 12 cherries from one can and put aside for garnish. (Or buy another whole can of cherries.)

In a medium saucepan, cook cherries with their juice, sugar, and cinnamon stick for 10 to 15 minutes.

In a small bowl, mix flour and 3 tablespoons of the cold water until smooth. Blend in remaining 3 tablespoons cold water.

Remove cinnamon stick from cooked cherries and set aside.

Pour cherry mixture into blender. Add flour mixture and blend until soup is smooth.

Return soup to saucepan, add 2 cups water, and heat just to boiling.

Return cinnamon stick to soup and chill.

Garnish each bowl of soup with a few cherries before serving.

Makes 6 one-cup servings
Per serving: 165 Total calories; trace Sat-fat calories

15 CHICKEN

CHICKEN IS ONE of the most versatile meats. You can sauté it, bake it, broil it, boil it, roast it, or make it into chicken salad, chicken pot pie, or chicken brochettes. You can cook it with fruit, vegetables, grains, wine, herbs, or spices and it will be different and delicious each time.

Almost all of the following recipes use chicken breasts without skin. Chicken breast without skin is the preferred chicken choice for anyone concerned about saturated fat intake. Both thighs and drumsticks without skin are low in saturated fat (2.6 calories of sat-fat per ounce for a thigh, which amounts to about 6 sat-fat calories per thigh or 12 sat-fat calories for 2 thighs. There are 2 calories of saturated fat per ounce for a drumstick, which amounts to 5 sat-fat calories per drumstick or 10 sat-fat calories for 2). However, chicken breasts without skin are even lower (about 0.8 calories of sat-fat per ounce, which amounts to about 3.5 sat-fat calories per breast) and more versatile. If you do substitute chicken thighs or drumsticks in any of the recipes, make sure you adjust the total sat-fat values to reflect that change.

Chicken breasts may be purchased with bones or already boned. You may have avoided buying *boneless* chicken breasts without skin because of their expense. However, the skin and bones of a chicken breast account for half their weight. You are paying much more for chicken breasts with skin and bones than you think. Look for boned chicken breasts without skin on sale for a real bargain.

If chicken breast tenderloins are available in your supermarket, we recommend them highly. They are wonderfully tender. Substitute about 4 tenderloins for 1 chicken breast. Be sure to pull out the tendon.

210

COOKING FOR ONE OR TWO

In case you find that one of our recipes makes more servings than you need, just divide all the ingredients proportionately. For example, if the recipe calls for 8 chicken breasts, use 4 or 2, and instead of ½ cup of lime juice, use ¼ cup or 2 tablespoons; instead of 1 teaspoon of ginger, use ½ teaspoon, or ¼ teaspoon, etc. You may also want to make the full or half recipe and eat one half and freeze the rest. If you have a big dinner party, you can double or triple all the ingredients. The recipes are quite flexible, so just relax and adapt them to your needs.

NOTE: It is easier to slice chicken when it is slightly frozen. If you do not mind unusual-looking chicken pieces, the following advice will save you time. Slice slightly frozen (but not rock-hard frozen) boneless chicken breasts without skin lengthwise into 1½-inch-wide chunks. Feed into food processor using the thickest slicer you have. Sauté the chicken in oil and freeze for later use.

If you use canned chicken broth in any of these recipes, either strain the broth (pour it through a fine tea strainer) or, if the fat is hardened, lift it off the surface of the broth with a spoon. You can also use a gravy skimmer to skim off the fat.

▣ INDONESIAN CHICKEN WITH GREEN BEANS

A beautiful dish — green beans set against ochre-colored sauce — and very tasty. This is one of our all-time favorites. To save fat and sat-fat calories, read the "Lower-Fat Approach" at the end of the recipe.

6 boned and skinned chicken breast halves, cut into bite-size pieces
4 tablespoons olive oil
10 cloves garlic, minced
1 tablespoon minced ginger root
1 small onion, chopped
1 pound green beans, washed and cut into bite-size pieces

Juice of 1 lime (preferred) or lemon
1 tablespoon double black soy sauce*
2 teaspoons brown sugar
2 teaspoons turmeric
1 teaspoon salt
½ cup water

Sauté chicken in 2 tablespoons of the olive oil until chicken turns white and is cooked through. Set aside.

Heat the remaining 2 tablespoons olive oil and sauté garlic, ginger, and onion until soft.

Add green beans. Stir until green beans turn bright green.

Add lime juice, soy sauce, brown sugar, turmeric, salt, and ¼ cup of the water.

Slowly add remaining water, if necessary, but sauce should not be watery.

Add chicken pieces and stir until completely covered with sauce.

Serve over rice.

Lower-Fat Approach:

To make this recipe even lower in fat and saturated fat, while you sauté the chicken, cook the beans in a large pot of boiling water for about 5–10 minutes. Boil until they are tender but still crisp and a bright green. Drain and pour cool water over them to stop the cooking process. Set them aside and add when called for in the directions

---

*Double black soy sauce is available at Oriental food stores and some supermarkets. You can make your own by mixing 2 teaspoons soy sauce with 1 teaspoon dark molasses.

above. Sauté the garlic, ginger, and onion in only 1 tablespoon of olive oil, rather than 2 as originally suggested.

8 servings

Per serving:	Total calories	Sat-fat calories
Original recipe	190	11
Lower-fat recipe	175	9

Q   # LEMON CHICKEN

A delicate blending of tart and sweet, Lemon Chicken can't help but become one of your most popular family or company dishes.

4 boned and skinned chicken breast halves
Juice of 2 lemons
½ cup unbleached white flour
¼ teaspoon freshly ground black pepper
½ teaspoon salt (optional)

¼ teaspoon paprika
1 tablespoon grated lemon peel
2 tablespoons brown sugar
1 tablespoon lemon juice
1 tablespoon water
1 lemon, sliced thin

Place chicken in a bowl or casserole. Pour lemon juice over breasts and marinate in refrigerator for several hours or overnight, turning chicken periodically.

Preheat oven to 350°F.

Combine flour, pepper, salt, and paprika in plastic bag.

Remove chicken breasts from marinade and coat each with flour by shaking it in the plastic bag.

Place chicken in a baking pan in a single layer.

Either peel the yellow (zest) from a lemon and chop it fine in your food processor (a mini food chopper makes a perfect grater), or grate the zest with a hand grater. Mix 1 tablespoon of the grated peel with the brown sugar.

Sprinkle the lemon zest–sugar mixture evenly over the chicken breasts. Combine 1 tablespoon lemon juice and water and sprinkle evenly over chicken.

Put 1 lemon slice on each chicken breast and bake chicken for 35–40 minutes or until cooked through.

4 servings
Per serving: 176 Total calories; 4 Sat-fat calories

LIME-PEANUT-GINGER CHICKEN

Don't be put off by our ho-hum name for this chicken recipe. Although it contains these three ingredients (actually peanut butter), the flavors combine to produce a unique and simply delectable taste.

6 boned and skinned chicken
   breast halves
½ cup fresh lime juice
1 clove garlic
1 tablespoon sliced ginger root
1 teaspoon whole peppercorns
1 teaspoon dried basil
1 tablespoon soy sauce
1 tablespoon white vinegar
1 teaspoon honey
1 tablespoon water

1 tablespoon grated lemon peel
3 tablespoons olive oil
1 tablespoon sesame oil
1 tablespoon natural all-peanut
   peanut butter
2–3 cups sliced mushrooms
1 tablespoon cornstarch diluted
   in 2 tablespoons water
¼–½ cup sliced green onions

Cut chicken into bite-size pieces and marinate in lime juice for at least 2 hours in refrigerator.

Make a dressing by chopping garlic, ginger, and peppercorns in food processor or blender until pepper is no longer whole. (It will probably be impossible to break up all peppercorns.)

Blend in basil, soy sauce, vinegar, honey, water, and grated lemon peel.

Pour 1 tablespoon of the olive oil into the processor or blender and process until smooth. Set dressing aside.

Remove chicken from marinade and sauté it in sesame oil and the remaining 2 tablespoons of olive oil until it turns white.

Add dressing and stir until chicken is well coated and sauce is warm.

Mix in peanut butter. Stir in mushrooms. Add cornstarch mixture to thicken sauce.

Sprinkle green onions on top and serve over rice.

8 servings
Per serving: 190 Total calories; 13 Sat-fat calories

Q

CHICKEN KIEV

This recipe is a gem: it uses ingredients you probably have on hand; it takes no time to make; and the resulting dish is so special you can proudly serve it to the most discriminating of guests.

2 cloves garlic, finely chopped
1 teaspoon basil
1 teaspoon oregano
½ teaspoon salt (optional)
2 cups fine bread crumbs made from 3–4 slices of white bread or challah*

½ cup margarine
8 boned and skinned chicken breast halves
¼ cup dry white wine or vermouth
¼ cup sliced green onions

Preheat oven to 375°F.

Mix garlic, basil, oregano, and salt with bread crumbs and place on a large plate. (You can mince the garlic in a food processor, add bread slices and process until they become crumbs, then add spices and process again.)

Melt ¼ cup of the margarine. Dip each chicken breast in the melted margarine, roll it in bread crumbs, and place it in a shallow baking pan.

Bake near center of oven for 30–45 minutes or until fully cooked.

Melt the remaining ¼ cup margarine. Mix in wine and green onions.

Pour sauce over chicken.

Return chicken to oven for 3–5 minutes or until sauce is hot. Serve over rice.

8 servings
Per serving: 243 Total calories; 23 Sat-fat calories

*Avoid commercial bread crumbs. They are high in total calories (390 per cup) and high in saturated fat calories (14 per cup). Use your food processor or blender to make your own bread crumbs from a few slices of bread (about 65 total calories and 2 sat-fat calories per slice).

⊡ INDONESIAN PEANUT CHICKEN

Peanuts are a major ingredient in Indonesian cooking. The spicy peanut sauce that covers this chicken dish is called a satay. The satay may also be used as a dip for vegetables or slices of cold chicken.

6 boned and skinned chicken breast halves

2 tablespoons olive oil

Satay sauce

1 clove garlic
1 small onion
1-inch piece ginger root
1 cup shelled roasted peanuts, unsalted
1 tablespoon soy sauce

1 teaspoon turmeric
Juice of 1 lime or lemon
1–3 hot chili peppers
1 cup water
1 large onion, sliced
1 tablespoon olive oil

Cut chicken into bite-size pieces. (Cutting the chicken into small pieces takes a few minutes, but everything else is quick and easy. You may also keep the chicken pieces whole and bake them covered with the satay sauce.)

Sauté chicken in olive oil until white and cooked through. Set aside.

Blend garlic, onion, ginger, peanuts, soy sauce, turmeric, lime or lemon juice, chili peppers, and water in blender or food processor until smooth.

Place sauce in top of double boiler and heat water to boiling. Cover pot and cook sauce for 10–20 minutes or until thick.

Sauté onion rings in olive oil until soft.

Pour satay sauce over chicken and stir until chicken is well coated. Stir in onion rings and serve over rice.

8 servings
Per serving: 218 Total calories; 18 Sat-fat calories

Ⓠ TANDOORI CHICKEN

1 clove garlic, minced
½ tablespoon sliced ginger root
2 tablespoons chopped onion
½ teaspoon Dijon mustard
⅛ teaspoon cardamom
⅛ teaspoon coriander
¼ teaspoon salt (optional)

¼ teaspoon freshly ground
  black pepper
1½ tablespoons fresh lemon
  juice
¾ cup nonfat yogurt
4 skinned chicken breast halves

Combine all ingredients except chicken (may be done in food processor, mincing garlic and ginger first) and pour over chicken breasts.

Marinate in refrigerator for at least 24 hours.

Place chicken with marinade in a shallow baking pan.

Bake at 375°F for 30–45 minutes or until chicken is fully cooked.

4 servings
Per serving: 152 Total calories; 4 Sat-fat calories

Ⓠ CHICKEN WITH APPLES AND ONIONS

6 skinned chicken breast halves
1 cup sliced onion
1 tablespoon olive oil
2 cups sliced tart apples

1 tablespoon margarine
1½ cups apple juice
2 tablespoons honey
½–1 teaspoon salt (optional)

Preheat oven to 350°F.

Place chicken breasts in a shallow baking pan.

In a skillet, sauté onions in olive oil until tender. Add apples and sauté for 1 more minute.

Pour onions and apples over chicken.

Melt margarine in a small saucepan. Combine apple juice, honey, salt, and margarine and pour over chicken and vegetables.

Bake for 30–45 minutes or until chicken is cooked through.

6 servings
Per serving: 245 Total calories; 10 Sat-fat calories

Q CHICKEN SMOTHERED IN VEGETABLES

8 boned and skinned chicken
  breast halves
½ cup unbleached white flour
1 teaspoon salt (optional)
¼ teaspoon freshly ground
  black pepper
2 tablespoons olive oil

2 cloves garlic, minced
1½ cups sliced onion
1 green pepper, sliced
2 cups sliced mushrooms
2 teaspoons oregano
10 cherry tomatoes or 3 whole
  tomatoes, sliced

Preheat oven to 375°F. Grease a shallow baking pan with margarine.

Cut each chicken breast into four pieces.

Coat chicken by shaking in a plastic bag with flour, salt, and pepper.

Place chicken in baking pan and grind additional pepper over it.

In a large skillet, sauté garlic and onion in oil until soft.

Stir in green pepper, mushrooms, and oregano and cook for 1 minute.

Add tomatoes.

Pour vegetables over chicken and bake for 30–45 minutes or until chicken is fully cooked.

8 servings
Per serving: 199 Total calories; 8 Sat-fat calories

Q PEPPERY CHICKEN

A very peppery chicken that tastes good grilled or roasted in the oven.

4 skinned chicken breast halves
1 teaspoon olive oil
2 tablespoons soy sauce
2 tablespoons honey
½ teaspoon thyme
½ teaspoon paprika

¼ teaspoon cayenne pepper
1 tablespoon white vinegar
½ teaspoon allspice
1 teaspoon freshly ground
  pepper
1 cup sliced mushrooms

Place chicken in a shallow casserole.

Combine olive oil, soy sauce, honey, thyme, paprika, cayenne pepper, vinegar, allspice, and pepper and pour over chicken. Marinate in refrigerator for about 1 hour.

Preheat oven to 375°F.

Bake chicken for 30–45 minutes or until cooked through.

Surround chicken with sliced mushrooms, spoon the sauce over them, and bake 1 minute more.

For grilling: remove breasts from marinade and grill until cooked through, basting periodically with marinade.

Add mushrooms to the marinade and simmer for 1 minute. Spoon over grilled chicken breasts.

4 servings
Per serving: 182 Total calories; 5 Sat-fat calories

Q   MA-PO BEAN CURD

This dish may be used as an entree although it barely has any meat (chicken) in it. It is extremely tasty.

1½ tablespoons olive oil
1 tablespoon minced ginger root
2 boned and skinned chicken breast halves, ground (can be ground in food processor)
3 cakes (each about 3 × 3 × 1¼ inches) tofu (fresh bean curd),* cubed
½ cup water
1½–3 tablespoons soy sauce

½ teaspoon sugar
1–3 teaspoons chili paste with garlic*
1 tablespoon fermented black beans*
1 tablespoon cornstarch mixed with 2 tablespoons water
½ tablespoon sesame oil*
2 tablespoons sliced green onion

*Available at Oriental food stores and some supermarkets

Heat a wok or large skillet to hot. Add olive oil and sauté ginger until fragrant (about 10 seconds).

Add chicken and stir until it turns white.

Stir in tofu, water, 1½ tablespoons of the soy sauce, and sugar. Reduce heat, cover, and simmer for 5–10 minutes.

Uncover and stir in chili paste with garlic and fermented black beans.

Raise heat and stir in cornstarch mixture and sesame oil until sauce thickens. Taste. Add remaining soy sauce, a teaspoon at a time, if needed for flavor.

Stir in green onion and serve over rice.

6 servings
Per serving: 136 Total calories; 10 Sat-fat calories

CHICKEN COUSCOUS

Couscous is the national dish of the Maghreb region of Morocco, Algeria, and Tunisia. The grain, made from semolina, is eaten as a cereal, as a main dish with meat and vegetables, and as a dessert with fruit and nuts. Our Chicken Couscous combines interesting textures and exotic tastes to create a complete meal in one dish.

3 boned and skinned chicken breast halves, cut into bite-size pieces
½ cup sliced carrot
¼ cup sliced celery
1 small turnip, quartered
½ cup dry white wine or vermouth
½ teaspoon thyme
¼ teaspoon rosemary
¼ teaspoon salt (optional)

¼ teaspoon paprika
1 tablespoon slivered almonds
1 cup sliced onion
1 tablespoon olive oil
½ teaspoon coriander
2 tablespoons raisins
¾ cup chopped tomatoes
½ teaspoon cinnamon
1 cup quick-cooking couscous
1 teaspoon margarine

In a large casserole, combine chicken, carrot, celery, turnip, wine, thyme, rosemary, salt, and paprika, with water to cover.

Bring to a boil, reduce heat, and simmer, covered, until chicken is cooked (about 10–20 minutes).

Meanwhile, in a medium skillet, toast almonds over low heat until golden. Remove almonds and set aside.

In same skillet, cook onion in olive oil over low heat, covered, until soft, stirring often.

Mix in coriander and raisins and cook slowly for 5 minutes more. Set aside.

When chicken is finished cooking, pour out all but about ½ cup of the liquid.

Add tomatoes and cinnamon to the chicken mixture and mix well. Cook, covered, for 5 minutes more.

Make couscous according to package directions. It takes about 5 minutes. (Add 1 teaspoon margarine instead of any amount of butter they suggest.)

Reheat onion-raisin mixture and sprinkle almonds over it.

Place couscous on a large platter. Cover with onions. Top with chicken and vegetables. Spoon on remaining sauce from casserole.

5 servings
Per serving: 291 Total calories; 10 Sat-fat calories

Q APRICOT CHICKEN DIVINE

One-half cup of nonfat yogurt (0 sat-fat calories, 55 total calories) replaces ½ cup of sour cream (135 sat-fat calories, 247 total calories) to create this divine chicken.

8 skinned chicken breast halves	⅓–½ cup apricot preserves
½ cup unbleached white flour	1 tablespoon Dijon mustard
1 teaspoon salt (optional)	½ cup nonfat yogurt
	2 tablespoons slivered almonds

Preheat oven to 375°F.

Shake chicken in a plastic bag filled with flour and salt until chicken is coated.

Place chicken in a single layer in a shallow baking pan and bake for 25 minutes.

Combine apricot preserves, mustard, and yogurt.

Spread apricot mixture on chicken and bake for 10–15 minutes more or until done.

Just before serving, brown almonds lightly in toaster oven.

Sprinkle almonds over chicken and serve over rice.

8 servings
Per serving: 215 Total calories; 5 Sat-fat calories

Q GRILLED APRICOT-GINGER CHICKEN

¾ cup dried apricots
Juice of ½ lemon
1 clove garlic, minced
½ teaspoon minced ginger root
¼–½ teaspoon cardamom

⅛–¼ teaspoon cayenne pepper
¼–½ teaspoon salt (optional)
2 teaspoons olive oil
5 skinned chicken breast halves

Place apricots in a small saucepan and add water to cover. Add lemon juice, bring to a boil, reduce heat, and simmer until tender.

In a blender or food processor, purée apricots and liquid with garlic, ginger, cardamom, cayenne pepper, salt, and olive oil. Add more water if too thick. Score the chicken breasts several times on each side. Cover with the apricot mixture and marinate in refrigerator for several hours or overnight.

Remove chicken from marinade and reserve marinade.

Preheat oven to broil or prepare grill.

Broil or grill chicken until cooked through.

Heat marinade and spoon over chicken.

Serve over rice.

5 servings
Per serving: 191 Total calories; 6 Sat-fat calories

☑ SESAME CHICKEN BROCHETTES

6 boned and skinned chicken
  breast halves
¼ cup soy sauce
½ cup dry white wine or
  vermouth

1 clove garlic, minced
1 tablespoon sesame seeds,
  lightly toasted

Cut chicken breasts into 1-inch cubes and place in a bowl or casserole.

Combine soy sauce, wine, and garlic and pour over chicken. Marinate in refrigerator for at least 30 minutes.

Preheat oven to broil or prepare grill.

Remove chicken from marinade and reserve marinade.

Skewer chicken and broil or grill until cooked through, basting occasionally with marinade.

Roll chicken in sesame seeds and serve over rice.

Heat marinade and spoon over chicken and rice.

6 servings
Per serving: 160 Total calories; 5 Sat-fat calories

☑ CHICKEN WITH RICE, TOMATOES, AND ARTICHOKES

4 boned and skinned chicken
  breast halves
2 cloves garlic, minced
½ cup chopped onion
2 teaspoons olive oil
1 large can (28 oz) tomatoes,
  chopped
2 cups water

½ teaspoon thyme
½ teaspoon oregano
1 teaspoon salt (optional)
¼ teaspoon freshly ground
  pepper
1 bay leaf
2 cups uncooked long-grain rice
1 jar (11½ oz) artichoke hearts,
  packed in water

Cut chicken into bite-size pieces and set aside.

In a large casserole, sauté garlic and onion in olive oil until soft.

Stir in tomatoes and their liquid, water, thyme, oregano, salt, pepper, and bay leaf and bring to a boil.

Add chicken and rice, cover casserole, and reduce heat to low.

Cook for 25 minutes or until rice is tender, most liquid is absorbed, and chicken is cooked through.

Stir in artichokes and serve.

8 servings
Per serving: 289 Total calories; 5 Sat-fat calories

BAGHDAD CHICKEN

¾ cup chopped onion
2 teaspoons garam masala*
1 tablespoon olive oil
⅓ cup uncooked long-grain rice
⅔ cup water
3 tablespoons raisins
3 tablespoons chopped peanuts

¼ cup nonfat yogurt
8 boned and skinned chicken
　breast halves
Salt and freshly ground pepper
　to taste
4 cups cooked long-grain rice
　(optional)

Preheat oven to 375°F.

Sauté onion in garam masala and olive oil until soft. Stir in rice.

Add water, cover saucepan, and cook over low heat until liquid is absorbed (about 20 minutes).

Remove from heat. Stir in raisins, peanuts, and yogurt. Let cool.

Flatten chicken breasts between two sheets of wax paper. Salt and pepper chicken.

Put a portion of the rice mixture in the center of each breast.

Bring together the sides of the breast to enclose the rice.

Place the breast seam-side down in a shallow casserole.

Bake until chicken is cooked through (about 30–45 minutes).

Combine any rice mixture you have remaining with plain rice and serve on the side.

8 servings
Per serving: 210 Total calories; 8 Sat-fat calories

---

*Available at specialty food stores. Or make your own by combining ½ teaspoon ground cloves, ¾ teaspoon ground cardamom, and ¾ teaspoon cinnamon.

Q CHINESE CHICKEN

¼ cup + 2 tablespoons soy
   sauce (approximately)
¼ cup dry sherry
1 clove garlic
3 or 4 shakes ground ginger or 1
   thin slice ginger root
½ cup + 1 tablespoon sugar
   (approximately)

5–6 star anise*
2 cups water (approximately)
10 boned and skinned chicken
   breast halves**
2 tablespoons soy sauce
1 tablespoon sugar

Place ¼ cup soy sauce, sherry, garlic, ginger, ½ cup sugar, star anise, and 1 cup of the water in an electric frying pan (or large frying pan). Add chicken in one layer and cook over medium heat for 20 minutes. Sauce will be thick.

Turn chicken. Add remaining 1 cup water, 2 tablespoons soy sauce, and 1 tablespoon sugar.

Taste. If too salty, add more sugar. If too sweet, add more soy sauce.

Cook for 10–30 minutes more or until chicken is cooked through. Keep adding water when sauce gets too thick. Periodically turn chicken. Keep tasting sauce and add soy sauce or sugar if necessary.

Chicken should be a deep brown.

10 servings

	Total calories	Sat-fat calories
1 breast	183	3
1 drumstick	130	5
1 thigh	134	5

---

*Available at Oriental food stores and some supermarkets
**You may substitute chicken thighs or drumsticks without skin for some of the chicken breasts.

PHYLLO-WRAPPED CHICKEN WITH RICE, ARTICHOKES, AND CREAM SAUCE

What a wonderful combination of tastes and textures! This very elegant chicken can be made a day ahead and refrigerated. (We recommend that you do make this chicken dish ahead because it involves many steps. To cook it along with all the other dishes that comprise a dinner will make you a nervous wreck and frazzled host.)

Phyllo dough that has been stored in the freezer has to be thawed in the refrigerator for 8 hours or overnight and then set out at room temperature for 2–4 hours before using. Take this into account when planning to cook this dish.

Chicken

10 boned and skinned chicken breast halves
1 cup dry white wine or vermouth

1 teaspoon salt (optional)
1½ teaspoons thyme
½ teaspoon rosemary
1 bay leaf

Rice

3 tablespoons margarine
2 cloves garlic, minced
½ cup chopped onion

½ pound sliced mushrooms
¾ cup long-grain rice

Cream Sauce

3 tablespoons margarine
¼ cup unbleached white flour

½ cup skim milk

Assembly

1 package (9 oz) frozen artichoke hearts, thawed, or 1 jar (11½ oz) artichoke hearts, packed in water and drained

3 tablespoons margarine
16 sheets phyllo dough,* thawed (usually comes in 16-oz package)

*Available at Greek or Mideast food stores or in the freezer section of many supermarkets.

The Chicken and Broth

In a large pot, combine chicken, wine, salt, thyme, rosemary, bay leaf, and water to cover. Bring to a boil. Reduce heat, cover, and simmer for 25 minutes or until chicken is cooked through.

Remove chicken and cut into bite-size pieces. Set aside.

Boil chicken broth gently, uncovered, until it is reduced to about 3½ cups.

Set aside and make the rice.

The Rice

In a large saucepan, melt margarine.

Add garlic, onion, and mushrooms and cook until tender.

Stir in rice.

Add 1½ cups of the reduced chicken broth. Simmer, covered, until liquid is absorbed (about 20 minutes).

While rice is cooking, make the cream sauce.

The Cream Sauce

Melt margarine over low heat.

Stir in the flour and cook until bubbly.

Remove from heat and slowly stir in remaining 2 cups of broth.

Gradually add skim milk. Return to low heat and stir until thick.

Back to the Rice and Chicken

When the rice is cooked, stir in the artichoke hearts and 1 cup of the cream sauce. Set aside.

Stir remaining cream sauce into chicken pieces. Set aside.

Putting It All Together

Preheat oven to 350°F.

Grease a 13 × 9-inch baking pan with margarine.

Melt the 3 tablespoons margarine.

Unfold phyllo leaves. Cover with plastic or damp towel.

Place 1 phyllo sheet into bottom of pan. Brush lightly with melted margarine.

Repeat procedure with 6 more sheets of phyllo.

Spread half of the rice mixture over phyllo dough.

Spread chicken over rice mixture.

Spread remaining rice mixture over chicken.

Cover with 6 sheets of phyllo, brushing with margarine between each sheet.

Tuck in edges of last sheet and brush the top with margarine.

Cut lightly through 3 or 4 layers of phyllo dough to indicate pieces to be cut later.

Bake chicken for 30–45 minutes or until golden brown and bubbly. Or refrigerate it for up to 24 hours and bake later for 60 minutes.

12 servings
Per serving: 292 Total calories; 18 Sat-fat calories

CUBAN CHICKEN

2 potatoes, peeled and cubed
6 boned and skinned chicken
    breast halves, cut into thirds
½ cup unbleached white flour
⅓ cup water
1 large can (28 oz) tomatoes
    with juice
1 large green pepper, chopped

¾ cup chopped onion
2 cloves garlic, minced
¾ teaspoon oregano
¾ teaspoon cumin
½ teaspoon salt (optional)
¼ cup raisins
½ cup stuffed green olives

Preheat oven to 425°F.

Place potatoes in a saucepan, cover with water, and boil for 10 minutes.

Shake chicken breasts, one at a time, in a plastic bag filled with flour until breast is completely coated.

Arrange floured chicken in a shallow baking pan in one layer. Add water. Place potatoes evenly over chicken.

Reduce heat to 375°F and bake chicken for 20 minutes.

Meanwhile, chop tomatoes either in food processor or by hand and place them with juice in a large bowl.

Add green pepper, onion, garlic, oregano, cumin, salt, raisins, and olives.

Spread tomato mixture over chicken and bake for 10–20 minutes more or until chicken is fully cooked.

Serve over rice.

6 servings
Per serving: 252 Total calories; 7 Sat-fat calories

Ⓠ LEMON-MUSTARD CHICKEN

6 skinned chicken breast halves	3 tablespoons fresh lemon juice
¼ cup margarine	1 teaspoon tarragon
3 tablespoons Dijon mustard	½ teaspoon salt (optional)

Preheat oven to 375°F.

Place chicken in a shallow baking pan.

In a small saucepan, melt margarine. Stir in mustard, lemon juice, tarragon, and salt. Pour over chicken.

Bake chicken for 30–45 minutes or until cooked through.

Spoon sauce from pan over chicken.

6 servings
Per serving: 191 Total calories; 16 Sat-fat calories

COQ AU VIN

2 whole frying chickens	1 teaspoon salt (optional)
¼ cup olive oil	1 bay leaf
¼ cup cognac or brandy	½ teaspoon thyme
2 cups full-bodied red wine (*not* Hearty Burgundy)	12 small white onions, peeled
	½–1 pound mushrooms
1 can (10¾ oz) chicken broth, strained	4 tablespoons margarine
	3 tablespoons unbleached white flour
2 cloves garlic, minced	

Cut chickens into parts and remove skin. If you cannot remove the skin from a part (such as the wings) do not use that part.

In a large casserole, brown chicken on all sides in olive oil.

Pour cognac over chicken and ignite it. Shake pan while cognac is burning.

When flame subsides, add wine, chicken broth, garlic, salt, bay leaf, thyme, and onions and simmer, covered, until chicken is tender (about 25 minutes).

Remove chicken from casserole and cover to keep warm.

Boil liquid in casserole until it is reduced to about 3 cups (about 10 minutes). Remove from heat.

Sauté mushrooms in 2 tablespoons of the margarine for about 1 minute and set aside.

Make a paste of the remaining 2 tablespoons margarine and the flour.

Mix the paste into the reduced liquid in the casserole. Reheat slowly until liquid is thickened.

Return chicken and mushrooms to casserole and heat through.

Serve over noodles (shells, rotini, etc.).

10 servings

	Total calories	Sat-fat calories
1 chicken breast half	217	10
1 drumstick	162	12
1 thigh	166	12

Q ## PINEAPPLE CHICKEN

1 cup unbleached white flour
1 teaspoon salt (optional)
1 teaspoon paprika
¼ teaspoon freshly ground
   black pepper
8 skinned chicken breast halves

1 can (20 oz) pineapple chunks
   in heavy syrup
½ cup sliced green pepper
2 green onions, sliced
1 tablespoon brown sugar
¼ cup dry sherry

Preheat oven to 425°F.

Combine flour, salt, paprika, and pepper in a plastic bag.

Piece by piece, coat chicken by shaking it in the bag with the seasoned flour.

Arrange floured chicken in a shallow baking pan in one layer. Bake at 425°F for 20 minutes. Turn chicken.

Combine pineapple, green pepper, green onions, brown sugar, and sherry and pour over chicken.

Lower heat to 375°F and bake until chicken is golden brown and sauce is thick (about 15–30 minutes).

8 servings
Per serving: 210 Total calories; 4 Sat-fat calories

CREAMY CHICKEN PIE

Creamy Chicken Pie is so rich and creamy you will think you are eating something that is clogging your arteries. Not so! Low-fat cottage cheese is the secret ingredient. This recipe is great for using up leftover turkey or chicken.

Partially baked nonsweet pie crust (page 396)

2 tablespoons margarine

½ cup chopped onion

3 cups sliced mushrooms

3 tablespoons unbleached white flour

1 cup low-fat (1%) cottage cheese

2 cups diced cooked chicken or turkey breast

⅓ cup chopped parsley

¼ teaspoon freshly ground pepper

¼ teaspoon rosemary

Prepare partially cooked nonsweet pastry for pie bottom crust but use 1¾ cups flour, and ⅓ cup margarine. Refrigerate remaining dough.

Preheat oven to 375°F.

In a large skillet, melt margarine over medium heat.

Cook onion and mushrooms until most liquid has evaporated.

Stir in flour and cook until bubbly. Remove skillet from heat.

Stir in cottage cheese, chicken, parsley, pepper, and rosemary.

Spoon chicken mixture into partially baked pie shell.

Roll out extra dough and cut it into strips. Place over chicken, making a lattice top.

Bake for 45 minutes or until crust is golden brown.

7 servings
Per serving: 300 Total calories; 23 Sat-fat calories

KUNG PAO CHICKEN WITH BROCCOLI

You can easily make Chinese cooking low-fat and low-sat-fat by limiting the amount of oil you use. Vegetables or rice are mixed with small amounts of poultry or other meats to create tantalizing combinations of textures and tastes. This recipe calls for some exotic ingredients, which are available at Oriental food stores and may be stored forever (almost) in the refrigerator or pantry.

6 boned and skinned chicken breast halves

2 tablespoons cornstarch

2 tablespoons water + 1 cup water

2 tablespoons + 2 teaspoons bean sauce*

1 tablespoon + 1 teaspoon hoisin sauce*

1–2 teaspoons chili paste with garlic*

¾ teaspoon sugar

1 tablespoon + 1 teaspoon dry sherry

1 tablespoon + 1 teaspoon white vinegar

2 cloves garlic, peeled and flattened

1 head broccoli, stem trimmed, cut into flowerets

2 tablespoons olive oil

¼ cup unsalted roasted peanuts, shelled

2–4 dried hot red peppers

Cut chicken into bite-size pieces. Set aside.

Combine cornstarch with 2 tablespoons water. Stir in remaining cup of water. Set aside.

Combine bean sauce, hoisin sauce, chili paste with garlic, sugar, sherry, vinegar, and garlic and set aside.

Steam broccoli in wok or saucepan until tender. Set aside.

Sauté chicken in olive oil in wok or large frying pan until cooked through.

Add sauce. Stir until chicken is well coated. Add cornstarch mixture.

When sauce thickens, stir in peanuts and red peppers. Add broccoli and mix until well coated with sauce.

Serve over rice.

10 servings
Per serving: 191 Total calories; 10 Sat-fat calories

---

*Available at Oriental food stores and some supermarkets

Q

CHICKEN MARRAKESH

4 boned and skinned chicken
  breast halves
3 tablespoons fresh lemon juice
1 tablespoon grated lemon peel
1 clove garlic, minced
2–3 teaspoons thyme

½ teaspoon salt (optional)
½ teaspoon freshly ground
  pepper
1 lemon, thinly sliced

Place chicken in a bowl or casserole.

Mix together lemon juice, lemon peel, garlic, thyme, salt, and pepper and pour over chicken. Marinate chicken in refrigerator for at least 3 hours.

Preheat oven to 350°F.

Remove chicken from marinade and place in shallow baking dish.

Pour marinade over chicken and bake chicken for 30–45 minutes or until cooked through.

Garnish with lemon slices.

4 servings
Per serving: 132 Total calories; 4 Sat-fat calories

CHICKEN PAPRIKASH

Paprikash dishes typically use sour cream. Nonfat yogurt has been substituted here without affecting the taste. Half a cup of nonfat yogurt contains 0 sat-fat calories. Half a cup of sour cream contains about 135 sat-fat calories.

½ cup unbleached white flour
½–1 teaspoon salt (optional)
¼ teaspoon freshly ground
  black pepper
6 boned and skinned chicken
  breast halves
3 tablespoons water
1½ tablespoons cornstarch
½ cup chopped onion
2–3 cups sliced mushrooms

1 tablespoon olive oil
1½ teaspoons paprika
½ teaspoon dillweed
½ teaspoon salt
¼ teaspoon freshly ground
  black pepper
1 cup chicken broth, strained
½ cup nonfat yogurt
½–1 cup water

Preheat oven to 375°F.

Place flour, ½–1 teaspoon salt, and ¼ teaspoon pepper in a plastic bag. Piece by piece, coat chicken by shaking it in the bag with the seasoned flour.

Arrange floured chicken in one layer in a shallow baking pan and bake for 30–40 minutes or until chicken is cooked through.

In a small bowl, add water to cornstarch and mix until smooth. Set aside.

Meanwhile, in a large skillet, sauté onion and mushrooms in oil until tender.

Stir in paprika, dillweed, ½ teaspoon salt, ¼ teaspoon pepper, and chicken broth.

Add cornstarch mixture and bring to a boil, stirring constantly. Lower heat to medium.

Cut chicken into bite-size pieces and add to sauce. Stir until chicken is heated.

Remove from heat and stir in yogurt. Add water, ¼ cup at a time, if sauce is too thick.

Serve over rice or noodles.

8 servings
Per serving: 157 Total calories; 5 Sat-fat calories

Q CHICKEN WITH APRICOTS, SWEET POTATOES, AND PRUNES

This dish is colorful to look at and a pleasure to eat. What's more, it is quick and easy and can be prepared ahead of time.

6 boned and skinned chicken
  breast halves
¾ cup dried prunes
½ cup dried apricots
1 tablespoon olive oil
3 tablespoons white vinegar

½ cup dry vermouth
2 cloves garlic, minced
1½ tablespoons brown sugar
1 tablespoon oregano
2 cups sweet potatoes, peeled
  and cut into ½-inch cubes

Place chicken breasts in a medium-large bowl or casserole.

Combine prunes, apricots, olive oil, vinegar, vermouth, garlic, brown sugar, and oregano and pour over chicken. Cover and marinate in refrigerator for several hours or overnight.

When you are ready to bake the chicken, place sweet potato cubes in saucepan with water to cover. Bring to a boil and boil gently for 3 minutes. Drain and set aside.

Remove chicken from marinade. Arrange in shallow baking pan.

Spread marinade over chicken, cover with sweet potatoes, and bake for 30–45 minutes until chicken is fully cooked.

6 servings
Per serving: 301 Total calories; 7 Sat-fat calories

SINGAPORE CHICKEN

Singapore Chicken includes salad greens, but it is more like a main dish than a salad. You can eat it warm or chilled. It tastes even better the second day.

4 boned and skinned chicken breast halves
½ teaspoon minced garlic
½ teaspoon minced ginger root
1 tablespoon soy sauce
1 tablespoon hoisin sauce*
½ tablespoon white vinegar
½ teaspoon five-spice powder**
½ teaspoon Dijon mustard
1 teaspoon sugar
¼ cup white vinegar

1 teaspoon soy sauce
1½ tablespoons olive oil
½ Chinese celery cabbage, or ½ head lettuce, chopped (about 3 cups)
2 green onions, thinly sliced
1½ tablespoons slivered almonds, toasted
½ tablespoon sesame seeds, toasted

Place chicken breasts in a bowl or small casserole.

Combine garlic, ginger, 1 tablespoon soy sauce, hoisin sauce, ½ tablespoon vinegar, and five-spice powder and pour over chicken. Cover bowl and marinate chicken in refrigerator overnight.

Preheat oven to 350°F.

---

*Available at Oriental food stores and some supermarkets
**Five-spice powder is available at Oriental food stores, or you can make your own by pulverizing the following in a blender: 30 peppercorns, 2 whole star anise (optional), 1 teaspoon fennel seeds, 2 one-inch pieces cinnamon stick, ¼ teaspoon cloves. Store excess in covered jar.

Bake chicken in marinade for 30–45 minutes or until cooked through.

Meanwhile, prepare dressing by combining mustard, sugar, ¼ cup vinegar, 1 teaspoon soy sauce, and olive oil in a jar and shaking well.

Slice chicken into narrow strips and combine with celery cabbage and green onions.

Pour dressing over all and mix until well coated.

Top with almonds and sesame seeds.

Serve or refrigerate overnight.

5 servings
Per serving: 176 Total calories; 10 Sat-fat calories

TORTILLAS CON POLLO

Chicken, yogurt, and rice make this tortilla unusual, low-fat, and, of course, delicious.

Tomato Sauce

1 clove garlic, minced
⅓ cup chopped onion
1 tablespoon olive oil
1 large can (28 oz) tomatoes,
    drained and chopped

¼ cup chopped green pepper
½ teaspoon cumin seed
½ teaspoon oregano

Filling

3 cups cooked long-grain rice
1½ cups diced cooked chicken
½–1 teaspoon chili powder

½ teaspoon ground cumin
½ cup nonfat yogurt

8 tortillas*

At least 30 minutes before serving, prepare the tomato sauce: Cook garlic and onion in olive oil until soft. Add tomatoes, green pepper, cumin seed, and oregano and cook until thick (about 30 minutes).

---

*Read the label. Packaged tortillas should contain only corn (perhaps some lime) and should *not* contain any of the following: shortening, fat, salt, or preservatives.

Preheat oven to 350°F. Grease a shallow baking dish with margarine.

Combine rice, chicken, chili powder, cumin, and yogurt.

Place ½ cup rice mixture in center of each tortilla and roll.

Place seam-side down in baking dish.

When all eight tortillas have been placed in baking dish, cover with tomato sauce and bake for 25 minutes.

8 servings
Per serving: 217 Total calories; 4 Sat-fat calories

[Q] # CHICKEN CURRY

6 boned and skinned chicken breast halves, cut into bite-size pieces
2 tablespoons olive oil
2 cloves garlic, minced
¾ cup chopped onion
½ cup chopped green pepper

1 tablespoon olive oil
1–2 teaspoons curry powder
½ teaspoon thyme
½ teaspoon salt (optional)
2 cups cherry tomato halves (or whole tomatoes or drained canned tomatoes, chopped)

In a large skillet or wok, sauté chicken in 2 tablespoons olive oil until chicken is cooked through.

Remove chicken and set aside.

Sauté garlic, onion, and green pepper in the remaining 1 tablespoon olive oil until soft.

Blend in curry powder, thyme, and salt.

Add chicken and stir until well coated with sauce. Stir in tomatoes.

6 servings
Per serving: 210 Total calories; 13 Sat-fat calories

Q

KEEMA MATAR

Traditionally, Keema Matar is made with ground lamb or beef. It tastes equally good with ground chicken, and instead of spending 111 sat-fat calories on ground lean beef, you spend a mere 17.

5 boned and skinned chicken breast halves
3 tablespoons olive oil
1 tablespoon minced garlic (about 4–5 cloves)

2–3 tablespoons curry powder
1 cinnamon stick
½ teaspoon salt (optional)
1 cup frozen peas

Grind chicken breasts in a food processor or a meat grinder. If you are using a food processor, first cut the cold (but not frozen) chicken breasts into 1-inch cubes. Place the cubes in the work bowl. Press the Pulse/Off button until chicken is ground (not puréed!). In a large skillet, sauté ground chicken in olive oil, stirring constantly, until it is cooked through.

Mix in garlic, curry powder, cinnamon stick, and salt.

Add peas and stir until heated through.

Serve over Indian Rice (page 331).

4 servings
Per serving: 279 Total calories; 17 Sat-fat calories

MONGOLIAN HOT POT

Making this dish is a group activity that allows each person to be his own cook. It works like a fondue. Everyone skewers a piece of meat or vegetable and dips it into simmering broth in a large Oriental "hot pot" or in an electric frying pan or wok. When the meat is finished cooking, the enriched broth becomes an after-dinner soup.

6 boned and skinned chicken breast halves

Marinade

2 cloves garlic, minced
1 teaspoon olive oil
1 tablespoon white vinegar

2 tablespoons honey
¼ cup soy sauce
1 teaspoon sherry

Sauce

½ cup soy sauce
½ cup dry sherry
5 tablespoons honey

2 tablespoons minced ginger
  root
2 cloves garlic, minced

The Rest

4 ounces cellophane noodles*
4 cakes fresh tofu (bean curd),*
  cubed
½ pound snow peas
1 zucchini, cut into ¼-inch
  slices

½ head celery cabbage, coarsely
  chopped
1 pound bay scallops

Broth

10 cups chicken stock, or 2 cans
  (10¾ oz each) chicken broth,
  strained, + 6 cans water

3 green onions, sliced
1½ teaspoons sliced ginger root
2 cloves garlic, minced

4 cups hot cooked rice

Slice chicken breasts into slender, bite-size pieces. Marinate in garlic, olive oil, vinegar, honey, soy sauce, and sherry in refrigerator for several hours or overnight.

Mix all sauce ingredients together and set aside.

Pour boiling water over cellophane noodles and let stand for 5–10 minutes or until soft. Drain and set aside.

Remove chicken from marinade and arrange artistically on a plate.

Arrange another plate with tofu, snow peas, zucchini slices, and celery cabbage. Set aside.

Arrange bay scallops on another plate.

Pour chicken broth and water in a hot pot, chafing dish, or electric wok or frying pan set in the center of the table. Heat to a slow boil.

Mix in green onions, ginger, and garlic.

Give each person a bowl of rice, a plate, and a small custard dish for the sauce. Pass around the trays of chicken, scallops, and vegetables so people may take what they wish. Each person should also

---

*Available at Oriental food stores and some supermarkets

have a fondue fork, skewer, or sharp implement to dip chicken, scallops, and vegetables in broth until cooked.

When food is all devoured or everyone is almost full, add noodles and celery cabbage to the broth and cook for 2–3 minutes.

Serve resulting soup in bowls.

8 servings

Per serving:	Total calories	Sat-fat calories
2 tablespoons sauce	69	0
Meat and vegetables	199	7
Broth	184	1
Total	452	8

Q

SATE AJAM
(BROILED CHICKEN ON SKEWERS)

4 boned and skinned chicken
  breast halves
12 medium mushrooms
1 teaspoon olive oil
2 tablespoons fresh lime juice

⅛ teaspoon freshly ground
  black pepper
1 teaspoon cumin
1 teaspoon minced garlic

Cut chicken into 1-inch pieces and cut stems off mushrooms.

Alternate pieces of chicken with mushrooms on skewers. (Push skewers through the *tops* of the mushrooms so the mushrooms will not split.)

Place skewered chicken in a shallow casserole.

Combine olive oil, lime juice, pepper, cumin, and garlic and pour over chicken.

Turn skewers to coat chicken and mushrooms with oil mixture.

Refrigerate for at least 30 minutes.

Preheat broiler.

Place skewers on broiler pan and broil 6 inches from heat for about 10 minutes or until cooked through. Turn and baste several times.

Serve over rice and spoon warm marinade over chicken pieces.

4 servings
Per serving: 151 Total calories; 5 Sat-fat calories

Q CAJUN CHICKEN

8 boned and skinned chicken
breast halves

½ cup unbleached white flour
½ teaspoon salt, optional

Seasoning Mix (Use more or less of the peppers for a hotter or milder taste.)

¾ teaspoon oregano
½ teaspoon thyme
½ teaspoon basil
½ teaspoon salt

½ teaspoon paprika
¼ teaspoon freshly ground
black pepper
½ teaspoon cayenne pepper
¼ teaspoon white pepper

3 cloves garlic, minced
¾ cup chopped onion
2 stalks celery, diced
½ cup chopped green pepper
1 tomato, coarsely chopped

1½ tablespoons olive oil
1 can (10¾ oz) chicken broth,
strained
1 small can (8 oz) tomato sauce
1 potato, peeled and diced
2 bay leaves

Preheat oven to 350°F.

Shake chicken in a plastic bag filled with flour and salt until chicken is coated.

Place chicken in a single layer in a shallow baking pan and bake for 25–30 minutes until almost cooked through.

While chicken is baking, combine oregano, thyme, basil, salt, paprika, and peppers, and set aside.

In a large frying pan, sauté garlic, onion, celery, green pepper, and tomato in oil until soft.

Mix in seasoning mixture and let simmer for about a minute.

Mix in broth and tomato sauce. Bring to a boil, then simmer for 5 minutes.

Lower heat and add chicken breasts, potato, and bay leaves. Cook until potatoes are soft and chicken is done.

NOTE: If you find the finished dish too "hot" for your taste, dilute with an additional can of tomato sauce.

8 servings
Per serving: 204 Total calories; 3 Sat-fat calories

☒ BAR-B-QUE CHICKEN

Bar-B-Que Chicken is a popular main dish with food lovers of all ages. It also makes a great sandwich. Place the barbecued chicken on a slice of bread, top with sauce, a slice of tomato, a few slices of onion, and another slice of bread.

2 tablespoons Dijon mustard
¼ cup vinegar
¼ cup molasses
½ cup ketchup
½ teaspoon Worcestershire
   sauce

2 cloves garlic, minced
Dash of Tabasco sauce
8 skinned chicken breast halves
   or thighs*

In a large bowl, mix together Dijon mustard, vinegar, molasses, ketchup, Worcestershire sauce, garlic, and Tabasco for marinade.

Pour about half of the marinade over the chicken and refrigerate the rest to use later.

Marinate chicken for an hour (or less, if you haven't planned ahead).

Remove chicken and reserve marinade.

Barbecue, broil, or use a cast-iron pancake griddle to grill chicken for 10 minutes or until fully cooked.

Turn and coat chicken with marinade and continue cooking until done.

Combine reserved marinade with the marinade you refrigerated. Heat to boiling and simmer for 2 minutes. Spoon over chicken before serving.

8 servings

	Total calories	Sat-fat calories
1 breast	173	4
1 thigh	126	6

---

*For a barbecue, you may want greater quantities of chicken. Just double, triple, quadruple, etc., the recipe.

Q GINGER CHICKEN WITH GREEN ONIONS

5 boned and skinned chicken
  breast halves
1 teaspoon ground ginger
2 tablespoons cornstarch
1¼ cups water
3 tablespoons soy sauce

2 tablespoons olive oil
2 cloves garlic, minced
2 teaspoons minced ginger root
2 dried red peppers, crushed, or
  1 teaspoon dried red pepper
  flakes
1½ cups green onions cut into
  1-inch pieces

Cut chicken into bite-size pieces, sprinkle with ground ginger, and set aside for 15 minutes.

Make a smooth paste of the cornstarch and 2 tablespoons of the water. Stir in 2 more tablespoons of water and soy sauce. Set aside.

Sauté chicken in oil until cooked through.

Stir in garlic, ginger root, and red pepper flakes.

Mix in soy sauce mixture and heat until the sauce thickens.

If sauce is too thick, add remaining water, ¼ cup at a time, until desired consistency is achieved.

Stir in green onions and serve over rice.

6 servings
Per serving: 172 Total calories; 9 Sat-fat calories

Q ORANGE-SOY CHICKEN

4 boned and skinned chicken
  breast halves
2 tablespoons soy sauce
1½ tablespoons cornstarch
½ tablespoon hoisin sauce*
3 tablespoons dry sherry
⅓ cup water
1 clove garlic, minced

1 teaspoon minced ginger root
2 tablespoons orange peel slivers
1 tablespoon olive oil
1 teaspoon marmalade
½–1 teaspoon red pepper flakes
1 orange, peeled and cut into
  bite-size pieces
10–20 snow peas

Place chicken between two pieces of wax paper and pound with a meat mallet to flatten. Then steam in a vegetable steamer or on a steamer tray in a wok until cooked through. Pull or slice them into thin strips about 2–3 inches long.

*Available at Oriental food stores and some supermarkets

Mix soy sauce into cornstarch, a tablespoon at a time, creating a smooth paste.

Mix in hoisin sauce, sherry, and water, and set aside.

Sauté garlic, ginger, and orange peel slivers in oil until soft.

Stir in cooked chicken pieces.

Stir in cornstarch mixture and cook until it thickens. Add more water if too dry.

Mix in marmalade, red pepper, orange pieces, and snow peas, and serve over rice.

6 servings
Per serving: 136 Total calories; 5 Sat-fat calories

Q | ## CHICKEN VERDE

16 spears asparagus
4 boned and skinned chicken
   breast halves
1 clove garlic, minced
1 teaspoon basil

6 anchovies
2 tablespoons olive oil
2 tablespoons fresh lemon juice
1 teaspoon water

Preheat oven to 375°F.

Snap off bottoms of asparagus.

Pound breasts between two sheets of wax paper with a meat mallet, until flat. This is important, as they must be thin to cook quickly.

Combine garlic, basil, anchovies, olive oil, and lemon juice into a sauce in blender or food processor, or mash and mix by hand.

In a small rectangular glass casserole, place four asparagus spears closely together and wrap a chicken breast around them. Repeat this process for the rest of the breasts.

Spread sauce over chicken.

Sprinkle teaspoon of water over exposed asparagus.

Cover casserole tightly with aluminum foil.

Bake for 20–30 minutes, or until chicken is cooked through.

DO NOT OVERCOOK. If you cook asparagus too long, it becomes soggy and the sauce becomes watery.

4 servings
Per serving: 217 Total calories; 14 Sat-fat calories

VEGETABLES, CHICKEN, AND CELLOPHANE NOODLES

2 ounces cellophane noodles*
2 boned and skinned chicken
   breast halves
8 mushrooms (approximately)
2 carrots
1 zucchini
4 green onions
4 leaves Chinese cabbage*

3 cloves garlic, minced
1 tablespoon olive oil
1 tablespoon sesame oil*
3 tablespoons soy sauce
½ teaspoon sugar
½ teaspoon salt, optional

Cover cellophane noodles with warm water and set aside.

Steam chicken breasts in a vegetable steamer. When cooked through (about 10 minutes), cut them into bite-size pieces and set aside.

Cut mushrooms into thin slices. Cut carrot and zucchini into julienne strips. Cut green onions into 1-inch pieces. Set aside.

Remove the green leaf from the cabbage. Cut into bite-size pieces. Julienne the white part of the leaf. Set aside.

Drain water from cellophane noodles.

Sauté garlic in both oils.

Add vegetables and stir-fry until tender but crisp.

Stir in chicken.

Stir in soy sauce, sugar, salt, and cellophane noodles. Mix to distribute sauce evenly. Serve over rice.

6 servings
Per serving: 111 Total calories; 7 Sat-fat calories

Q CHICKEN NUGGETS CHEZ GOOR

The chicken nuggets that you get at fast-food chains are deep-fried in highly saturated oils. Instead of devouring 46 calories of saturated fat per serving, try Chicken Nuggets Chez Goor, marinated in olive oil and garlic and baked in the oven. A mere 5 sat-fat calories per serving.

---

*Available at Oriental food stores and some supermarkets

4 boned and skinned chicken
  breast halves
1 tablespoon olive oil
2 cloves garlic, minced
¼ teaspoon freshly ground
  pepper

1 cup finely ground bread
  crumbs, made from 2–3 slices
  French or other bread
¼ teaspoon cayenne pepper
2½ teaspoons honey
2 tablespoons Dijon mustard

Preheat oven to 475°F.

Cut each chicken breast half into 8 pieces.

Mix oil, garlic, and pepper with chicken pieces and marinate about 30 minutes.

Combine bread crumbs and cayenne and place on plate.

Roll chicken pieces in bread crumbs and place on large cookie sheet in a single layer.

Bake for about 15 minutes until browned and cooked through. For extra browning, broil for a few more minutes.

Combine honey and mustard. Dip nuggets into honey-mustard sauce.

4 servings

	Total calories	*Sat-fat calories*
Per serving	191	5
With honey-mustard sauce	211	5

SHEPHERD'S CHICKEN CHILI PIE

1½–2 pounds potatoes, peeled
  and cut into chunks
4 boned and skinned chicken
  breast halves, cubed
1 can (16 oz) whole tomatoes,
  with juice
1 large onion, sliced
3 cloves garlic, minced
1 tablespoon olive oil

1½ tablespoons chili powder
½ teaspoon oregano
1 teaspoon cumin
2 tablespoons water
1 tablespoon tomato paste
1 teaspoon margarine
Salt and pepper to taste
1 tablespoon skim milk

Place potatoes in a saucepan with water to cover, bring to a boil, and simmer for about 10–15 minutes, until tender.

Steam chicken pieces in a vegetable steamer or on a steamer tray in a wok until cooked through, about 10 minutes.

Drain tomatoes. Reserve liquid.

Preheat oven to 350°F.

In a large skillet, sauté onion and garlic in olive oil until soft.

Mix in chili powder, oregano, and cumin.

Add water, tomato paste, and tomatoes. Cook until sauce is thick. If sauce becomes *too* thick, add a few tablespoons of the reserved tomato juice.

Mix chicken cubes into sauce.

Drain potatoes and whip them. Add margarine, salt, and pepper. Add skim milk and mix until potatoes are smooth. Add more milk if necessary.

Place chicken mixture in a shallow casserole. Spread potatoes on top. Bake for about 30 minutes.

6 servings
Per serving: 218 Total calories; 7 Sat-fat calories

▣ BLACKENED CHICKEN

Ron is in seventh heaven when he bites into a chunk of chicken and the chicken bites back. The spicier it is, the better he likes it. He likes Blackened Chicken a lot.

Spice Mix

1 teaspoon thyme
1 teaspoon basil
½ teaspoon onion powder
¼ teaspoon salt (optional)
½ teaspoon cayenne pepper

½ teaspoon paprika
½ teaspoon white pepper
¼ teaspoon freshly ground
   black pepper

1 tablespoon olive oil
1 large clove garlic, minced

5 skinned chicken breast halves

Combine seasonings in a small bowl and set aside.

Combine olive oil and garlic in a small bowl.

Spread garlic-oil mixture over both sides of chicken breasts.

Sprinkle seasoning mix over each chicken breast and rub spices into both sides. (For a milder chicken, use less seasoning on each breast.)

Either grill on a cast-iron pancake griddle or barbecue grill, broil, or bake chicken until cooked through. Don't overcook.

NOTE: If you are using a cast-iron griddle, don't let it get too hot or it will char the chicken. You may need to turn on your exhaust fan to clear the hot spices from the air.

5 servings
Per serving: 154 Total calories; 7 Sat-fat calories

▣ CHICKEN WITH DRIED FRUIT AND LEMON

4 boned and skinned chicken
   breast halves
¼ cup chopped onion
1 tablespoon brown sugar
½ teaspoon ground ginger
¼–½ teaspoon salt (optional)
10 pitted prunes

2 tablespoons raisins
1 lemon, thinly sliced
¼ cup canned beef broth
¼ cup water
1 tablespoon soy sauce
1 tablespoon cornstarch

If you have a clay cooker, soak it in water for 15 minutes. Preheat oven to 450°F.

Place chicken in clay cooker or shallow baking pan.

Distribute onion evenly over chicken.

Combine sugar, ginger, and salt and spread half of the mixture over chicken.

Distribute prunes and raisins evenly over chicken.

Cover with lemon slices.

Sprinkle remaining sugar mixture over lemon.

Combine beef broth, water, and soy sauce and pour over chicken.

Cover clay cooker with top or cover baking pan tightly with aluminum foil.

Cook for 30–45 minutes or until chicken is cooked through.

Remove chicken to plate and cover with foil to keep warm.

Pour remaining liquid and fruit into small saucepan.

Mix cornstarch with about 2 tablespoons of liquid until smooth and add to saucepan. Heat until sauce thickens.

Serve chicken with fruited sauce.

4 servings
Per serving: 226 Total calories; 4 Sat-fat calories

Q SZECHUAN CHICKEN WITH SWEET RED PEPPER AND PINEAPPLE

The Chinese typically cook chicken by cutting it into small pieces and sautéing it in oil. To save fat calories, the chicken in this sweet-spicy and delectable dish is baked first with no fat, then cut into bite-size pieces and thrown into the sauce.

NOTE: For a different taste, try this recipe with a sliced green pepper and no pineapple.

⅓ cup unbleached white flour
Salt to taste (optional)
¼ teaspoon freshly ground
   black pepper
5 boned and skinned chicken
   breast halves
2 tablespoons soy sauce
2 tablespoons dry sherry
1–2 teaspoons chili paste with
   garlic*

1½ tablespoons tomato paste
¼ teaspoon sugar
2 tablespoons cornstarch
1 cup water + 2 tablespoons
1–2 teaspoons chopped ginger
   root
2 green onions, sliced
1 teaspoon olive oil
1 sweet red pepper, sliced
1½ cups pineapple chunks
¼ cup water

Preheat oven to 375°F.

Place flour, salt, and pepper in a plastic bag. Piece by piece, coat chicken by shaking it in the bag with the seasoned flour.

Arrange floured chicken in one layer in a shallow baking pan and bake for 20–40 minutes or until chicken is cooked through.

Meanwhile, combine soy sauce, sherry, chili paste, tomato paste, and sugar. Set aside.

Combine cornstarch with 2 tablespoons water. Then stir in remaining cup of water. Set aside.

When chicken is cooked through, cut into bite-size pieces and set aside.

In a large skillet or wok, sauté ginger and green onions in olive oil for a few seconds.

Remove skillet from heat and mix in soy sauce mixture. Stir in cornstarch-water mixture and return skillet to high heat.

---

*Available at Oriental food stores and some supermarkets

When sauce begins to thicken, add the chicken, red pepper, and pineapple and stir until well coated. If sauce is too thick, add more water, 1 tablespoon at a time.

5 servings
Per serving: 203 Total calories; 5 Sat-fat calories

Q **HUNAN CHICKEN WITH ONIONS AND PEPPERS**

2 tablespoons cornstarch
3 tablespoons soy sauce
1 tablespoon dry sherry
4 boned and skinned chicken breast halves, cut into bite-size pieces
1 can (8 oz) water chestnuts
3 tablespoons white vinegar
¾ cup water
2½ tablespoons olive oil

1 clove garlic, minced
2 medium onions, sliced (about 1½ cups)
1 red pepper and 1 green pepper (or 2 green peppers), seeded and cut into strips
2–3 whole dried chili peppers, crumbled*
¼–½ teaspoon salt (optional)

Combine 1 tablespoon cornstarch, 1 tablespoon soy sauce, and the sherry until smooth, and stir in chicken pieces.

Drain water chestnuts and roughly chop in half.

Combine remaining cornstarch with soy sauce and vinegar and mix with water. Set aside.

Heat 1 tablespoon olive oil in large skillet or wok. Sauté garlic, onions, red and green peppers, and water chestnuts on high heat for 1 minute. Lower to medium and cook until soft but not limp. Add chili peppers. Remove vegetables and set aside.

Sauté chicken in remaining olive oil until cooked through. (You may have to remove the chicken and clean the skillet before you proceed.)

Mix in vegetables and sauce and stir until sauce thickens.

6 servings
Per serving: 192 Total calories; 9 Sat-fat calories

---

*Do not crumble with bare fingers or you may burn your skin.

☐ BALSAMIC CHICKEN WITH POTATOES AND ONIONS

4 tablespoons balsamic or other
flavored vinegar
4 boned and skinned chicken
breast halves
2 medium-large potatoes
¾ cup sliced onion

2 teaspoons olive oil
¼–½ teaspoon thyme
Salt to taste (optional)
Freshly ground black pepper to
taste

Pour 3 tablespoons of vinegar over chicken and marinate for several hours or overnight.

Preheat oven to 350°F.

Wash potatoes thoroughly and cut into ¼-inch slices. (You should have about 2 cups.) Steam in a vegetable steamer for ten minutes (until almost tender).

Meanwhile, in a small skillet sauté onion in olive oil on medium heat until soft.

Mix in remaining tablespoon vinegar.

Mix in potatoes.

Pour the potato mixture into a shallow casserole large enough to accommodate a layer of potatoes covered by chicken breasts. Sprinkle potatoes with about ¼ teaspoon thyme.

Remove chicken from marinade and place on top of potatoes. Season with salt and pepper to taste and sprinkle with remaining thyme.

Bake for 30–45 minutes or until chicken is cooked through.

Makes 4 servings
Per serving: 203 Total calories; 6 Sat-fat calories

☐ THAI CHICKEN WITH ASPARAGUS

1 pound asparagus
2 tablespoons cornstarch
2 tablespoons water
1 pound boned and skinned
chicken breasts
1 tablespoon olive oil
¼–½ teaspoon red pepper
flakes
½ teaspoon caraway seeds

½ teaspoon coriander
½ teaspoon salt (optional)
¼ teaspoon freshly ground
black pepper
1 tablespoon minced shallot
1 clove garlic, minced
1 can chicken broth (10¾ oz),
strained

Snap off and discard the bottoms of asparagus. Cut spears into 1½-inch pieces.

Bring a pot of water to a boil and cook asparagus 3–5 minutes, until tender. Drain, run cool water over asparagus, and set aside.

Mix cornstarch with water until smooth and set aside.

Cut chicken breasts into bite-size pieces and sauté in oil until cooked through.

While chicken is cooking, combine the seasonings, shallot, and garlic (this step is easy to do in a food processor or mini food processor) and mix them together with chicken broth. Add cornstarch mixture. When chicken is cooked through, add seasoned broth. Bring to a boil and let sauce thicken. Lower heat and add asparagus.

4 servings
Per serving: 201 Total calories; 8 Sat-fat calories

Q   # CHICKEN FAJITAS

4 boned and skinned chicken
    breast halves

Marinade

2 cloves garlic, minced   ½ teaspoon salt (optional)
1½ teaspoons cumin   3 tablespoons fresh lime juice

Tomato Salsa

1 pound tomatoes, chopped   1 fresh chili pepper, sliced thin
1 small onion, minced   1 tablespoon fresh lime juice

Vegetable Mélange

1 large onion, sliced   1 red or yellow sweet pepper,
1 clove garlic, minced   sliced
1 green pepper, sliced   1 tablespoon olive oil

6 large flour tortillas

Place chicken breasts in a bowl, combine marinade ingredients, and pour over chicken. Marinate in refrigerator at least 30 minutes.

Combine tomato salsa ingredients and refrigerate until ready to use.

Sauté onion, garlic, and peppers in olive oil until soft. Set aside.

Grill** or broil chicken breasts until cooked through. Slice into strips.

Warm the tortillas as directed on the package. They should be soft. (Don't bake them too long or you will have 6 very large crackers.)

To assemble each tortilla, lay pepper mixture across half, cover with chicken, and top with tomato salsa. Fold over top and serve.

Makes 6 tortillas
Per serving: 212 Total calories; 6 Sat-fat calories

Q ALEX'S CHINESE CHICKEN WITH ONIONS, MUSHROOMS, AND ZUCCHINI

1 medium zucchini
1–1½ pounds boned and
    skinned chicken breast halves
    (or tenderloins), cut into bite-
    size pieces
2 tablespoons olive oil
3 tablespoons soy sauce
3 tablespoons white vinegar
1–1½ tablespoons chili paste
    with garlic

¼–1 teaspoon red pepper flakes
    (optional)
2 tablespoons + 1 cup water
2 tablespoons cornstarch
2 large onions, sliced
1 tablespoon olive oil
3 cups mushrooms, sliced

Quarter zucchini into 4 long sections. Cut these into ½-inch pieces. Steam zucchini 1–3 minutes until tender. Set aside.

Sauté chicken in 2 tablespoons olive oil until cooked through. Set aside.

Combine soy sauce, vinegar, chili paste, and red pepper flakes and set aside.

---

*You may find tortillas in your grocery store in a refrigerated case. Look for tortillas with the least amount of fat. Do not use tortillas made with lard.
**Cast-iron griddles make great indoor grills.

Add 2 tablespoons of water to cornstarch and mix until smooth. Add remaining water to cornstarch and set aside.

Sauté onions in the remaining 1 tablespoon olive oil until soft. Add mushrooms and cook for a minute. Stir in chicken.

Add soy sauce and cornstarch mixtures and stir until vegetables and chicken are covered.

Stir in zucchini.

Serve over rice.

6 generous servings
Per serving: 232 Total calories; 11 Sat-fat calories

FIFTIES CHICKEN

¼ cup unbleached white flour
1 clove garlic, crushed
4 boned and skinned chicken
  breasts
½ cup chopped onion

½ cup chopped green pepper
2 teaspoons olive oil
¾ cup orange juice
½ cup chili sauce
1 tablespoon Dijon mustard
1 tablespoon soy sauce

Preheat oven to 350°F.

Combine flour and garlic and place on a plate. Roll chicken pieces into flour, covering both sides. Place in shallow baking pan just large enough to hold chicken pieces in one layer. Set aside.

Sauté onion and green pepper in olive oil until tender. Mix in orange juice, chili sauce, Dijon mustard, and soy sauce. Use half the sauce to cover chicken. Reserve the other half in the refrigerator.

Bake chicken for 30–45 minutes or until cooked through. Heat reserved sauce and spoon over chicken.

4 servings
Per serving: 200 Total calories; 7 Sat-fat calories

TURKEY 16

TURKEY IS the heart of any Thanksgiving dinner, but it makes delicious eating throughout the rest of the year. Turkey can be stuffed and roasted and the leftovers made into numerous interesting dishes. Turkey cutlets can replace veal cutlets with no one being the wiser (but everyone being the healthier).

White meat turkey breast is a must for everyone who wants to consume less saturated fat and who also enjoys eating. One ounce of turkey breast has only ½ calorie of saturated fat!

NOTE: Turkey contains so much protein and so little fat, it tends to cook quickly. Be careful. Overcooking makes turkey tough.

BASIC TURKEY CUTLET

Turkey cutlets provide a quick and extremely elegant meal. In addition, they are low in fat (even lower than chicken), they are inexpensive, and they can be substituted for exorbitantly expensive veal scaloppine. Turkey cutlets can usually be found in the poultry section of your grocery store.

1 pound turkey cutlets
½ cup unbleached white flour
1 tablespoon olive oil*

1 tablespoon margarine*
Salt and freshly ground black
   pepper to taste

Here are two methods to prepare turkey cutlets for any veal scaloppine recipe:

With fat: Place cutlets between two pieces of wax paper and pound with meat mallet or rolling pin until thin.

---

*No fat is used in the second cooking method.

Place flour on a plate. Dip each cutlet in flour, coating it on both sides, and place it on a large plate. When the plate is completely covered with one layer of cutlets, cover them with a sheet of wax paper to hold the next layer.

Heat olive oil and margarine in a large frying pan or wok.

When very hot (margarine should bubble) place cutlets in frying pan. Do not crowd cutlets.

When the edges turn white, turn the cutlets and cook them until they become light brown and are no longer pink inside. Cutlets cook very quickly. Turn again. Do not overcook or cutlets will be tough.

Remove cutlets to a plate and salt and pepper them liberally.

Do not clean skillet. Now you are ready for any number of scaloppine recipes.

With no fat added: If you wish to reduce the total fat content of turkey cutlets (the sat-fat content is already low), instead of sautéing after you pound and flour them, place them on a cast-iron pancake griddle and cook them with no fat. You will find this method works particularly well in the Turkey with Capers recipe.

4 servings

	Total calories	Sat-fat calories
Per serving	211	12
With no added fat	158	4

Q TURKEY SCALOPPINE LIMONE

1 pound turkey cutlets	⅓ cup chopped parsley
1 teaspoon margarine	½ pound mushrooms, sliced
½ cup fresh lemon juice	(optional)
1 teaspoon unbleached white flour	1 lemon, thinly sliced

Prepare turkey cutlets as in master recipe (page 255).

Melt margarine in skillet. Add lemon juice.

Sprinkle on flour and blend into mixture. Add cutlets. Stir and turn cutlets until they are covered with sauce but do not overcook them.

Add parsley and mushrooms, stirring until mushrooms are covered with sauce.

Garnish with lemon slices and serve immediately.

4 servings

	Total calories	Sat-fat calories
Per serving	246	14
With no added fat	194	6

Ⓠ TURKEY SCALOPPINE MARSALA

1 pound turkey cutlets	2 teaspoons unbleached white
½–¾ cup Marsala	flour
1 teaspoon margarine	½ pound mushrooms, sliced

Prepare turkey cutlets as in master recipe (page 255).

Add Marsala to pan over high heat. When it begins to boil, add margarine and reduce heat to medium.

Sprinkle on flour and blend.

Add cutlets and stir and turn until covered with sauce.

Add mushrooms and stir until covered with sauce.

Serve immediately.

4 servings

	Total calories	Sat-fat calories
Per serving	268	14
With no added fat	216	6

Q

TURKEY WITH CAPERS

You may sauté turkey cutlets as in the first method for preparing turkey cutlets (page 255), but this takes a lot of fat. Flouring turkey cutlets, then grilling them on a cast-iron pancake griddle with no added fat, as in the second method (page 256), produces cutlets that are also tender but have almost no fat calories.

1 pound turkey breast cutlets	3 tablespoons red wine vinegar
2 teaspoons olive oil	2 tablespoons Dijon mustard
1 clove garlic, minced	1 cup chicken broth, strained
¼ cup chopped onion	2 tablespoons tomato paste
3 tablespoons capers, drained	⅓ cup chopped parsley

Prepare turkey cutlets as in master recipe (pages 255–256). Set aside.

In a large skillet, sauté garlic and onion in 2 teaspoons olive oil until soft.

Stir in capers, vinegar, Dijon mustard, chicken broth, and tomato paste. Add parsley.

Add turkey cutlets and mix until they are covered with sauce.

4 servings

	Total calories	Sat-fat calories
Per serving	237	13
With no added fat	184	5

Q

TURKEY NIÇOISE

1 pound turkey breast cutlets	1 tablespoon capers
¾ cup chopped onion	8 large black olives, halved
3 cloves garlic, minced	¼–½ teaspoon red pepper
1 tablespoon olive oil	flakes
1½ pounds fresh tomatoes, chopped	¼ teaspoon thyme
6 flat anchovies, chopped	¼ teaspoon basil
½ cup dry vermouth	¼ teaspoon oregano
	Salt to taste (optional)

Prepare turkey cutlets as in master recipe (pages 255–256).

In a large skillet, sauté onion and garlic in 1 tablespoon olive oil until soft.

Add tomatoes and anchovies and cook for 10–20 minutes until tomato sauce thickens.

Add vermouth, capers, olives, red pepper flakes, thyme, basil, oregano, and salt to taste, and cook for about 5 minutes until sauce thickens.

Mix turkey cutlets into the sauce and serve.

6 servings

	Total calories	Sat-fat calories
Per serving	219	13
With no added fat	184	7

TURKEY WITH SWEET RED PEPPER SAUCE

The sauce takes about an hour to cook but no time to prepare. You may make this tasty dish in advance and refrigerate it.

Sweet Red Pepper Sauce

2 red peppers, chopped (about 2 cups)
1½ cups sliced tomatoes
1 can chicken broth (10¾ oz), strained
1 cup dry vermouth

Juice of ½ lemon
¼–½ teaspoon red pepper flakes
Salt to taste (optional)
Freshly ground black pepper to taste

½ cup chopped parsley
Peel of ½ lemon

4 cloves garlic

1 pound turkey cutlets

In a medium (about 8-inch) skillet, combine red peppers, tomatoes, chicken broth, vermouth, lemon juice, red pepper flakes, salt, and black pepper.

Bring to a boil, lower heat to medium, and cook until liquid is reduced and sauce is thick, about 50–60 minutes.

Meanwhile, in a food processor or by hand, chop or mince parsley, together with the lemon peel and garlic. Set aside.

Prepare the turkey cutlets as in master recipe (pages 255–256).

Heat red pepper sauce.

Sprinkle parsley mixture over cutlets and cover with sauce.

Q ## TURKEY CUTLETS WITH ARTICHOKE-CREAM SAUCE

This turkey dish is so creamy, you would swear it was a no-no! With only 21 sat-fat calories per serving, it is a good choice for keeping your family healthy and impressing your company.

1 pound turkey cutlets
2 tablespoons margarine
3 tablespoons unbleached white flour

1 cup skim milk
1 jar (11½ oz) artichoke hearts, packed in water

Prepare cutlets as in master recipe (page 255).

In a medium saucepan, melt margarine. Remove from heat and stir in flour to make a smooth paste.

Slowly stir in skim milk and liquid from artichokes. Heat until thick.

Mix in artichoke hearts.

Pour sauce over cutlets and serve.

5 servings

	Total calories	Sat-fat calories
Per serving	248	17
With no added fat	206	11

TURKEY VÉRONIQUE

6 turkey cutlets (about 1 pound)
½ cup unbleached white flour
1 teaspoon tarragon
¼ teaspoon salt (optional)
¼ teaspoon freshly ground
  black pepper
1 tablespoon margarine

2 tablespoons olive oil
½ cup minced onion
1 cup sliced mushrooms
⅔ cup dry white wine or
  vermouth
2 cups seedless grapes

Preheat oven to 375°F.

Flatten turkey cutlets between two sheets of waxed paper.

Combine flour, tarragon, salt, and pepper on a plate.

Dredge cutlets in flour, coating evenly.

Melt margarine and 1 tablespoon olive oil in a large skillet. Brown cutlets (they brown quickly).

Remove cutlets with a slotted spoon and place in a shallow baking pan.

Add onions and mushrooms to the skillet and sauté in the remaining tablespoon olive oil until tender.

Add wine and heat to boiling. Pour over cutlets.

Cover with foil, place in oven, and bake for 5 minutes.

Add grapes and bake for 5 minutes more.

6 servings
Per serving: 234 Total calories; 12 Sat-fat calories

TURKEY ROLL-UPS FIRENZE

Avoid commercial bread crumbs. They are high in fat calories (45 per cup) and high in saturated fat calories (14 per cup). Use your food processor or blender to make your own from a few slices of bread (about 9 fat calories and 2 sat-fat calories per slice).

If you forget to thaw the spinach, cook it first until it is no longer frozen.

2 cups bread crumbs made from 3–4 slices bread
2 cloves garlic, minced
1 teaspoon thyme
1 teaspoon oregano
6 turkey cutlets (about 1 pound)
1 package frozen spinach, thawed, or 10 ounces fresh spinach

¼ cup low-fat (1%) cottage cheese
¼ cup chopped mushrooms
¼ cup chopped onion
2 tablespoons margarine, melted

Preheat oven to 400°F.

Combine bread crumbs, garlic, thyme, and oregano. Or chop garlic in food processor, then add bread slices and spices.

Pound cutlets between two sheets of wax paper until thin.

Squeeze liquid out of spinach.

Combine spinach, cottage cheese, mushrooms, and onions.

Place ⅙ spinach mixture on one side of each cutlet.

Roll up cutlets. Dip in melted margarine. Roll in bread crumbs.

Place rolled cutlets in a shallow casserole greased with margarine.

Bake for 10–20 minutes or until cooked through.

6 servings
Per serving: 176 Total calories; 10 Sat-fat calories

Q
BREADED TURKEY CUTLET

2 tablespoons margarine
1 pound turkey cutlets
¼ teaspoon salt (optional)
½ teaspoon basil or oregano

1 cup bread crumbs made from
  2 slices of bread
2 tablespoons olive oil

Melt margarine and set aside.

Pound turkey cutlets between two sheets of wax paper until thin.

Combine salt, herbs, and bread crumbs on a plate.

Dip cutlet into melted margarine, then coat on both sides with bread crumbs and shake off excess.

Heat olive oil in large skillet until bubbly.

Cook cutlets a few at a time until golden brown on each side.

Place on paper towels to absorb excess fat and serve immediately.

4 servings
Per serving: 273 Total calories; 22 Sat-fat calories

Q
TURKEY MEXIQUE

A great dish with a chili taste.

1 cup chopped onion
2 teaspoons minced garlic
1 tablespoon olive oil
1–2 tablespoons chili powder
1 tablespoon cumin seed
½ teaspoon salt (optional)
1 tablespoon unbleached white
  flour

1½ cups chicken broth, strained
3 tablespoons tomato paste
3 cups diced turkey breast, raw
  or cooked
1 green pepper, diced
¼ cup stuffed green olives,
  sliced

In a large skillet, sauté onion and garlic in olive oil until soft.

Stir in chili powder, cumin seed, salt, and flour.

Add chicken broth and tomato paste and blend well.

Cook for 5 minutes over low heat.

Stir in turkey, green pepper, and olives and heat through. (If turkey is raw, cook until turkey turns white and is fully cooked.)

Serve over rice.

6 servings
Per serving: 160 Total calories; 6 Sat-fat calories

Ⓠ TURKEY SAUTÉED WITH ONIONS AND ALMONDS

3 tablespoons slivered almonds
2 cups thinly sliced onion
1 tablespoon olive oil
¼ teaspoon cardamom
½ teaspoon coriander

1 teaspoon salt (optional)
⅓ cup dry sherry
¼ cup raisins
3 cups diced cooked turkey
  breast
¼ cup chopped parsley

Brown almond slivers in a toaster oven and set aside. Watch them carefully — they burn quickly.

In a large skillet or wok, sauté onion in olive oil until tender.

Stir in cardamom, coriander, salt, sherry, and raisins. Cook until all excess liquid evaporates.

Stir in turkey, parsley, and almonds and heat through.

6 servings
Per serving: 200 Total calories; 8 Sat-fat calories

Ⓠ BROCCOLI BAKED TURKEY

1 head broccoli
2 tablespoons margarine
3 tablespoons unbleached white
  flour
1 can (10¾ oz) chicken broth,
  strained

½ teaspoon salt (optional)
½ pound mushrooms, sliced
2 cups diced cooked turkey
  breast

Trim stems and leaves off broccoli and separate flowerets.

Steam flowerets until just tender. Set aside.

In a medium saucepan, melt margarine.

Remove from heat and stir flour into margarine to make a smooth paste.

Return to low heat and blend in chicken broth, stirring constantly until sauce is thick and smooth.

Stir salt and mushrooms into sauce.

Preheat oven to 375°F. Grease a shallow baking pan with margarine.

Place broccoli in baking pan, cover with turkey, and pour mushroom sauce over both.

Bake, uncovered, 15–25 minutes.

6 servings
Per serving: 145 Total calories; 19 Sat-fat calories

CREAMY TURKEY CASSEROLE

2 egg whites
2 tablespoons margarine
3 tablespoons unbleached white flour
1 can (10¾ oz) chicken broth, strained
1 cup diced celery
2 tablespoons minced green onion
½ cup (2 oz) chopped pecans
½ teaspoon salt (optional)
¼ teaspoon Worcestershire sauce
1 egg yolk
1 tablespoon fresh lemon juice
¼ cup reduced-calorie mayonnaise
3 cups diced cooked turkey breast

Preheat oven to 400°F. Grease a casserole with margarine.

Whip egg whites until stiff but not dry and set aside.

In a medium saucepan, melt margarine. Remove from heat and stir in flour to make a paste. Gradually blend in chicken broth over low heat. Stir constantly until sauce is thick and smooth.

Stir celery, green onion, pecans, salt, Worcestershire sauce, egg yolk, and lemon juice into sauce.

Fold in egg whites.

Mix mayonnaise with turkey so that turkey is well coated.

Add turkey mixture to sauce and pour into casserole. Bake for 20 minutes.

6 servings
Per serving: 255 Total calories; 22 Sat-fat calories

TURKEY WITH SNOW PEAS

1 pound turkey tenderloin
2 tablespoons white vinegar
2 tablespoons soy sauce
1 tablespoon brown sugar
2 slices ginger root
2 tablespoons dry sherry

1 tablespoon cornstarch
¼ cup water
3 ounces (about 1 cup) snow
  peas
10 water chestnuts, thinly sliced

Place turkey in a casserole.

Combine vinegar, soy sauce, brown sugar, ginger, and sherry and pour over turkey.

Simmer for about 20 minutes or until tender. *Do not overcook.*

Remove turkey from casserole and slice into bite-size pieces.

Return sliced turkey to casserole and refrigerate in marinade for several hours or overnight.

Place turkey in a large skillet or wok.

Combine cornstarch and water into a smooth paste. Stir into remaining marinade.

Heat turkey. Pour marinade over turkey and stir until well coated. Stir in snow peas and water chestnuts.

5 servings
Per serving: 190 Total calories; 9 Sat-fat calories

FISH AND SHELLFISH 17

ISH IS AN excellent choice for heart-healthy eating. It is a fine source of complete protein. The quality of this protein is about the same as that of red meat. Fish also contains important vitamins and minerals. And, in addition to all this good nutrition, fish contains much less fat than red meat. While 6 ounces of trimmed sirloin steak contains 150 calories of saturated fat, 6 ounces of haddock or flounder contain 6 calories of saturated fat. Fish oils are polyunsaturated and have an unusually potent effect in lowering blood triglyceride levels.

Fish cooks quickly — within minutes — and may be prepared in a multitude of tasty ways: broiled, baked, poached, oven-fried. Fish may be used as the base for soups, salads, pastas, and stews. Even when prepared most simply to enhance its delicacy, fish is delicious. The key is freshness.

Q BROILED MONKFISH WITH ORANGE SAUCE

Very special and delicious. Skim milk makes a great cream sauce. (And look at the difference in sat-fat calories per cup: 3 for a cup of skim milk versus 335 for a cup of cream.)

2 tablespoons margarine
2 tablespoons unbleached white
  flour
¼ cup orange juice
¾ cup skim milk
Grated peel of 1 orange
1 green onion, sliced
¼ teaspoon salt (optional)

¼ cup flour
½ teaspoon salt (optional)
¼ teaspoon freshly ground
  black pepper
1½ pounds monkfish fillets (or
  any whitefish fillets)
2 teaspoons margarine

Preheat broiler and grease broiler pan with oil.

Melt margarine in a small saucepan. Remove from heat and mix in 2 tablespoons flour to make a smooth paste.

Mix in orange juice and skim milk, stirring until smooth.

Cook over medium heat until sauce thickens, stirring constantly.

Stir in 2 tablespoons grated orange rind, green onion, and salt and set aside.

Combine ¼ cup flour, salt, and pepper and place on large plate.

Dredge fillets in flour so both sides are coated.

Lay fillets on broiler pan and dot them with 2 teaspoons margarine.

Sprinkle remaining orange rind on fillets (grate more if needed).

Broil for 5–15 minutes, depending on the thickness of the fish, or until fish flakes easily.

Reheat orange sauce and spoon 1 tablespoon over each serving.

6 servings
Per serving: 194 Total calories; 13 Sat-fat calories

Q MARINATED FISH STEAKS

1½ pounds fish steaks
   (swordfish, monkfish, halibut,
   etc.)
2 tablespoons ketchup
1 tablespoon fresh lemon juice
1 clove garlic, minced

1 teaspoon oregano
½ teaspoon salt (optional)
1 tablespoon olive oil
¼ cup orange juice
¼ cup dry vermouth
¼ cup chopped parsley

Place steaks in a shallow casserole.

Combine ketchup, lemon juice, garlic, oregano, salt, olive oil, orange juice, vermouth, and parsley and pour over fish. Marinate several hours or overnight in refrigerator.

Preheat broiler and grease broiler pan with oil.

Broil fish for 5–15 minutes or until it flakes easily.

Heat marinade and spoon over fish.

4 servings
Per serving: 297 Total calories; 16 Sat-fat calories

Q

FISH BAKED IN OLIVE, CHILI PEPPER, AND TOMATO SAUCE

¾ cup chopped onion
2 cloves garlic, minced
1 tablespoon olive oil
1 tablespoon cornstarch
1 can (16 oz) tomatoes, chopped, juice reserved
⅓ cup sliced stuffed green olives

1 teaspoon chopped red or green chili pepper
1½ pounds flounder fillets (or other mild fish)
Salt to taste (optional)
1 tablespoon fresh lemon juice

Preheat oven to 375°F.

In a medium skillet, sauté onion and garlic in olive oil until soft. Mix in cornstarch.

Add tomatoes and their juice and mix until well blended.

Cook over medium-high heat until sauce thickens.

Stir in olives and chili pepper.

Spoon half the sauce into a baking pan large enough to hold the fillets in one layer. Place fillets over sauce.

Salt fillets and sprinkle them with lemon juice.

Cover fillets with remaining sauce and bake for 10 minutes or until they flake easily.

6 servings
Per serving: 163 Total calories; 8 Sat-fat calories

Q ## SALMON WITH CUCUMBER-GRAPE SAUCE

½ cup nonfat yogurt
3 tablespoons reduced-calorie mayonnaise
1 tablespoon fresh lemon juice
⅓ cup grated cucumber

1 cup seedless grapes
6 salmon steaks* (6 oz each)
3 tablespoons margarine
¼ cup fresh lemon juice

Preheat broiler and grease broiler pan.

Combine yogurt, mayonnaise, lemon juice, cucumber, and grapes. Set aside.

Place salmon steaks on broiler pan.

---

*Salmon varies greatly in total calories and sat-fat calories depending on the species. This will affect the total calories per serving.

Melt margarine and combine it with lemon juice.
Baste salmon with lemon-margarine sauce.
Broil 3–5 minutes, turn salmon, and baste again.
Broil 3–5 minutes more or until fish flakes easily.
Spoon cucumber-grape sauce over salmon steaks and serve.

6 servings

Per serving:	Total calories	Sat-fat calories
Atlantic	528	30
Chinook	540	60
Pink	330	24
Sockeye (red)	365	42

⧠ BROILED GINGER FISH

1 cup flour
1 teaspoon salt (optional)
½ teaspoon freshly ground
   black pepper
4 six-ounce fish fillets
   (monkfish, haddock, etc.)

4 teaspoons margarine
4 teaspoons diced ginger root
Lemon slices to cover fillets

Set oven to broil and grease broiler pan with oil.
Combine flour, salt, and pepper on a large plate.
Dredge fillets in flour, covering both sides.
Dot fillets with margarine, sprinkle them with ginger, and cover
with lemon slices.
Broil for 5–15 minutes or until fish flakes easily.

4 servings
Per serving: 209 Total calories; 6 Sat-fat calories

Q

CURRY FISH

A simple but impressive dish, which tastes as good as it looks. Fun for company.

2 pounds any white fish fillets	Raisins
2 teaspoons margarine	Peanuts
Salt to taste	Crushed pineapple
¼ cup margarine	Scallions
1–2 tablespoons curry powder	Chutney
5 cups cooked long-grain rice	
3–4 hard-boiled egg whites, chopped	

Preheat oven to 425°F. Grease a baking dish with margarine.

Place fillets in baking dish, dot with 2 teaspoons margarine, salt lightly, and bake for 20 minutes.

Flake the fish. (If you wish to serve it later, you can refrigerate the fish now.)

Melt ¼ cup margarine in a large skillet and mix in curry powder.

Add fish and stir until it is covered with curry sauce.

Mix cooked rice and fish together gently.

Place egg whites, raisins, peanuts, crushed pineapple, scallions, and chutney in small dishes and pass with main dish.

10 servings

Per serving:	Total calories	Sat-fat calories
Without condiments	251	12
With teaspoon of each	317	18

Q

DILL FISH

1½ pounds fish fillets (flounder, sole, turbot, etc.)	1 clove garlic, minced
¼ cup fresh lime juice	Salt and freshly ground black pepper to taste
1 teaspoon dillweed	

Preheat oven to 350°F.

Squeeze lime juice over fillets and marinate for at least 30 minutes in refrigerator.

Grease a shallow baking pan with margarine.

Place fillets in baking pan and sprinkle with dill, garlic, salt, and pepper.

Bake for 5–10 minutes or until fish flakes easily.

6 servings
Per serving: 115 Total calories; 4 Sat-fat calories

FLOUNDER FILLETS STUFFED
WITH FENNEL RICE

Raw fennel, or *finocchio,* as the Italians call it, tastes of licorice or anise. The taste of cooked fennel is more subtle and sweet. Cook sliced fennel bulb with margarine and water to cover for a delicious vegetable dish. You may substitute celery in this recipe, but try to find fennel at your grocery store or an Italian market for a more unusual dish. Despite its lack of cream or whole milk, this dish is quite creamy.

⅓ cup sliced fennel stalks
⅓ cup sliced mushrooms
1 teaspoon fennel seeds
1 tablespoon margarine

1½ cups cooked long-grain rice
2 tablespoons margarine
3 tablespoons fresh lemon juice
8 flounder fillets

Preheat oven to 375°F. Grease a shallow baking pan with margarine.

In a medium skillet, sauté fennel and mushrooms in 1 tablespoon margarine until just tender.

Add fennel seeds and cooked rice. Stir for a minute and set aside.

Melt 2 tablespoons margarine in a small saucepan. Add lemon juice and set aside.

Lay out fillets on waxed paper.

Place several tablespoons of rice mixture in the middle of each fillet.

Roll up the fillets and place them seam-side down in the baking dish. (The sides may barely reach each other, but that is okay.)

Pour margarine-lemon mixture over fish and bake for about 20 minutes or until fish flake easily. (Measure thickness of rolled fish and allow 10 minutes per inch.)

If you have any rice mixture left over, reheat and serve with the fish.

8 servings
Per serving: 140 Total calories; 10 Sat-fat calories

PHYLLO-WRAPPED FISH AND MUSHROOM SAUCE

Fish wrapped in phyllo dough is an elegant company dish. If you want a simpler (as in less work) dish, just ignore the phyllo part of the recipe. The fish with the mushroom sauce is still luscious.

NOTE: If you are using phyllo dough, the directions on the box usually recommend that you thaw it in the refrigerator overnight and 2–3 hours at room temperature before you use it.

Fish

8 fillets (6 oz each) pollack,
   monkfish, or other white fish
Salt and freshly ground pepper

1 pound phyllo leaves
¼ cup melted margarine

Mushroom Sauce

2 tablespoons margarine
¼ cup unbleached white flour
3 cups sliced mushrooms
3 tablespoons margarine
¼ cup dry sherry

1½ cups skim milk
¼ teaspoon salt
⅛ teaspoon freshly ground
   pepper
Grated nutmeg to taste

The Fish

Preheat oven to 350°F. Grease a baking sheet with margarine.
Check fillets for small bones and remove them.

Lightly salt and pepper fish.

Unroll phyllo dough and cover it with plastic wrap or a towel to keep it from drying out and becoming brittle.

Place one sheet of phyllo dough on the counter with a narrow end toward you. Brush phyllo with melted margarine. Cover with a second sheet of phyllo and brush it with melted margarine. Repeat process for third sheet.

Place fillet on the phyllo edge nearest you. (If fillet is long and narrow, you may have to fold the fillet in half.) Fold left side, then right side of phyllo over fillet and roll it up.

Place seam-side down on baking sheet.

Wrap each fillet in phyllo dough and place on baking sheet.

Bake for 20 minutes. Make a small slit in phyllo to see if fish is done. Bake until fish flakes easily and is opaque.

While fish is baking, make mushroom sauce.

The Mushroom Sauce

In a medium saucepan, melt margarine.

Lower heat and mix in flour.

In a medium skillet, sauté mushrooms in 3 tablespoons of margarine until tender.

Add sherry to mushrooms and boil until alcohol is evaporated.

Add skim milk to mushrooms and heat until steaming but *not boiling*.

Slowly pour milk mixture into flour mixture, blending until sauce is smooth.

Return saucepan to burner and slowly heat sauce to boiling.

Add salt, pepper, and nutmeg to thickened sauce.

Serve over phyllo-wrapped fish.

8 servings

Per serving:	Total calories	Sat-fat calories
With mushroom sauce	431	22
Without mushroom sauce	342	10

▣ FISH WITH MUSHROOM SAUCE

8 fillets (6 oz each) pollack,   1 tablespoon margarine
    monkfish, or other white fish

Make mushroom sauce (see page 274).

Preheat oven to 350°F. Grease a shallow baking pan with margarine.

Place fish in baking pan and dot with margarine.

Bake for 5–10 minutes or until fish flakes easily and is opaque.

Spoon mushroom sauce over fish and serve.

8 servings
Per serving: 302 Total calories; 14 Sat-fat calories

▣ ORIENTAL FISH KEBABS

1¼ pounds swordfish steaks
½ cup fresh lime juice
1 tablespoon soy sauce
1 tablespoon brown sugar
2 cloves garlic, minced
2 tablespoons sliced green onion

1 medium onion, cut into
    eighths
1 green pepper, cut into 1½-
    inch pieces
8 cherry tomatoes

Cut fish into 1½-inch cubes.

Combine lime juice, soy sauce, brown sugar, garlic, and green onion and pour over fish. Marinate for at least 2 hours in refrigerator.

Arrange fish, onion chunks, green pepper, and tomatoes on skewers. Rotate skewers in marinade to cover vegetables and let sit for several minutes so the vegetables can absorb the flavor.

Broil for 10 minutes per inch of thickness of fish or until it flakes easily.

Heat remaining marinade and spoon over fish.

4 servings
Per serving: 243 Total calories; 10 Sat-fat calories

Q

SHANGHAI FISH

1½ pounds white fish fillets 　 2 tablespoons dry sherry
2 tablespoons soy sauce 　 3 green onions, sliced
1 clove garlic, minced 　 1 tablespoon hoisin sauce*

Marinate fish in soy sauce, garlic, sherry, green onions, and hoisin sauce for several hours in refrigerator.

Broil for 5–10 minutes or until fish flakes easily and is opaque.

Heat marinade to boiling and serve over fish.

6 servings
Per serving: 117 Total calories; 4 Sat-fat calories

Q

FISH WITH PEPPERCORNS, THYME, AND MUSTARD

¼–½ teaspoon black 　 2 tablespoons vermouth
　 peppercorns 　 ½ teaspoon olive oil
4 teaspoons Dijon mustard 　 1 pound fish fillets (sole,
1 teaspoon thyme 　 　 flounder, etc.)

Preheat oven to 450°F. With margarine, grease shallow glass casserole or baking pan large enough to hold fish.

Crush peppercorns coarsely in food processor or mortar and pestle.

Combine and mix with mustard, thyme, vermouth.

Make several diagonal slashes across the fillets.

Place fish in baking pan and spread mustard mixture over it.

Bake for 5–20 minutes, until fish flakes easily.

3 servings
Per serving: 70 Total calories; 5 Sat-fat calories

---

*Available at Oriental food stores and some supermarkets

SALMON SOUFFLÉ

1 can (8 oz) salmon
1 cup skim milk
1 cup fine bread crumbs made
    from 2 slices whole-wheat
    bread

3 egg whites

Preheat oven to 350°F. Grease a small casserole with margarine.

Prepare salmon by carefully rinsing it with water and removing any bones. Set aside.

Heat skim milk and bread crumbs slowly in a double boiler until thick.

Meanwhile, whip egg whites until stiff but not dry. Set aside.

Flake salmon with a fork and add it to the thickened milk mixture. Remove from heat.

Fold salmon mixture into egg whites.

Pour into casserole and bake for 30 minutes.

4 servings
Per serving: 149 Total calories; 9 Sat-fat calories

CAJUN FISH

This spicy fish will wake up your taste buds.

Seasoning Mix

1 teaspoon paprika
¼ teaspoon white pepper
¼ teaspoon cayenne pepper
½ teaspoon freshly ground
    black pepper

½ teaspoon oregano
½ teaspoon thyme
½ teaspoon basil
½ teaspoon salt (optional)

1 clove garlic, minced
2 teaspoons olive oil

1¼ pound skinned fish fillets,
    such as swordfish, grouper, or
    other thick fish

Preheat broiler.

Combine seasonings and set aside.

Combine garlic and oil in a small bowl.

Spread garlic-oil mixture over both sides of fillets.

Sprinkle herb mixture over fillets and rub it into each side. (For a milder version, use seasonings more sparingly.)

Broil fillets until cooked through (5–20 minutes depending on thickness of fish).

4 servings
Per serving: 188 Total calories; 9 Sat-fat calories

Q FENNEL FISH

Quick and *delicious* are words that aptly describe Fennel Fish. The fennel seeds add an exotic-tasting crunch.

1¼ pound thick fish fillets, such as grouper	3 tablespoons fennel seed
	2 tablespoons water
1 tablespoon olive oil	

Cut fish crosswise into ½-inch-thick slices. Set aside.

Pour oil into a skillet large enough to hold the fish pieces in one layer. Add fennel and sauté for a few seconds.

Add fish. Let cook for about 2 minutes on medium heat.

Add 1 tablespoon of the water and cover skillet. In about 2 more minutes, add the second tablespoon of water and replace cover to finish steaming the fish. Cook until fish is cooked through.

Serve immediately.

4 servings
Per serving: 134 Total calories; 4 Sat-fat calories

Q FISH IN WINE SAUCE

This delicate fish dish takes no time to make.

¾ pound of white fish fillets, such as flounder or sole	3 tablespoons minced shallot
¼–½ cup white wine or vermouth	Freshly ground black pepper to taste

Preheat oven to 400°F. Place the fillets in one layer so they fill a shallow baking pan and pour the wine over them. The wine should *not* cover them.

Sprinkle shallots over fish.

Depending on the thickness of the fish, bake for 5–20 minutes until it flakes easily.

Pepper liberally and serve.

3 servings
Per serving: 40 Total calories; 0 Sat-fat calories

SCALLOPS AND SHRIMP

Both scallops and shrimp are low sat-fat gems. They take only 3–5 minutes to cook, may be added to innumerable sauces with no fuss or bother, are extremely low in saturated fat (1 ounce of either contains only 1 sat-fat calorie), and are delicious.

You may have been told to avoid shrimp because it is higher in cholesterol than other shellfish. Don't worry. Shrimp contains only slightly more cholesterol than other meats, but is extremely low in saturated fat. It also contains risk-reducing omega-3 polyunsaturated fats. We recommend that you eat as much shrimp as you can afford unless you are wealthy or a shrimp fisherman.

Q SCALLOP OR SHRIMP CURRY

Delight your guests or family with this unusual curry. The apples and lime create a unique combination of sweet and sour tastes.

1 cup chopped onion
1 apple, peeled, cored, and
   diced
2 cloves garlic, minced
1–3 teaspoons curry powder
1 tablespoon olive oil
¼ cup unbleached white flour
½ teaspoon salt (optional)
¼ teaspoon cardamom
¼ teaspoon freshly ground
   black pepper

1 can chicken broth (10¾ oz),
   strained
1 tablespoon fresh lime juice
1¼ pounds bay scallops or
   shrimp, shelled and deveined
1 cup sliced mushrooms
10–15 snow peas (optional)
½–1 cup water

In a large skillet, sauté onion, apple, garlic, and curry powder in olive oil until tender.

Remove skillet from heat and blend in flour, salt, cardamom, and pepper.

Stir in chicken broth and lime juice until curry sauce is well blended.

Bring curry sauce to a boil, reduce heat, and simmer, uncovered, for about 5 minutes. Stir occasionally.

Meanwhile, place scallops or shrimp in a pot of boiling water and cook until just tender (5–10 minutes). Drain and set aside.

When curry sauce is finished cooking, add shellfish, mushrooms, and snow peas. If sauce is too thick, add water, ¼ cup at a time until desired consistency is achieved. Serve curry over rice.

6 servings
Per serving: 187 Total calories; 7 Sat-fat calories

Q **SCALLOPS PROVENÇAL**

It takes only about 15 minutes and very little effort to create this delightful combination of color, texture, and taste.

1 pound bay scallops	2 cups snow peas (about ½
¼ cup unbleached white flour	pound)
3 cloves garlic, minced	2 cups sliced red pepper
2 tablespoons olive oil	1 cup sliced mushrooms

Rinse scallops, dry with a paper towel, and roll scallops in flour.

In a wok or large skillet, sauté scallops and garlic in olive oil until tender (about 5–10 minutes).

Add snow peas, red peppers, and mushrooms and mix until heated through.

Serve over rice.

5 servings
Per serving: 190 Total calories; 8 Sat-fat calories

⬚ SCALLOP OR SHRIMP CARIBBEAN

¼ cup sugar
2 tablespoons cornstarch
⅛ teaspoon salt (optional)
½ cup orange juice
⅓ cup white vinegar
½ cup water
1 pound bay scallops or shrimp, shelled and deveined

2 teaspoons grated orange peel
½ pound mushrooms, sliced
1 medium orange, peeled and cut into bite-size pieces
¼ pound snow peas
¼ cup sliced green onions
3 cups cooked long-grain rice
3 tablespoons sliced almonds

In a large skillet, combine sugar, cornstarch, and salt. Slowly stir in orange juice, vinegar, and water.

Stir constantly over medium heat until mixture thickens.

Add scallops or shrimp and orange peel.

When shellfish is cooked through (5–10 minutes), add mushrooms, orange pieces, snow peas, and green onions.

Serve over rice, topped with almonds.

6 servings
Per serving: 170 Total calories; 3 Sat-fat calories

⬚ SCALLOP OR SHRIMP CREOLE

2 green peppers, chopped
1 cup chopped onion
2 cloves garlic, minced
1 tablespoon olive oil
1 teaspoon brown sugar
¼ teaspoon freshly ground black pepper
½ teaspoon thyme
¼ teaspoon cayenne pepper
1 bay leaf

½ teaspoon salt (optional)
2 large cans (28 oz each) tomatoes, drained, juiced, and chopped
½ cup sliced celery
1½ cups sliced mushrooms
3 tablespoons chopped parsley
1 pound bay scallops or shrimp, shelled and deveined

Sauté green peppers, onion, and garlic in olive oil until soft.

Add brown sugar, pepper, thyme, cayenne pepper, bay leaf, and salt and stir well.

Stir in tomatoes and cook over low heat for 30 minutes or until sauce is thick.

Add celery and mushrooms and cook for a few minutes more.

Mix in parsley and scallops or shrimp and cook for 5–10 minutes or until shellfish is cooked through.

Serve immediately so shellfish will not overcook.

Serve over rice.

6 servings
Per serving: 184 Total calories; 7 Sat-fat calories

SPICY SHRIMP LOUISIANA

1–1¼ pounds shrimp
¼ teaspoon ground white pepper
⅛ teaspoon freshly ground black pepper
¼ teaspoon cayenne pepper
½ teaspoon basil
¼ teaspoon thyme
¼ teaspoon salt (optional)
¼ cup water

¼ cup unbleached white flour
1 tablespoon olive oil
½ cup chopped onion
1 green pepper, chopped
2 stalks celery, chopped
2 cloves garlic, minced
1 can (10¾ oz) chicken broth, strained
1 tablespoon tomato paste
¼ cup chopped green onions

Shell, devein, and clean shrimp. Cook in boiling water for about 3 minutes. Discard water. Set shrimp aside.

Combine the white, black, and cayenne pepper, basil, thyme, and salt. Set aside.

Slowly add water to flour and mix into a paste. Set aside.

Heat oil in wok or large frying pan until hot.

Stir in onion, green pepper, celery, and garlic, and cook until soft.

Mix in spice mixture.

Stir in broth and tomato paste.

Stir in flour mixture and cook until sauce thickens.

Add shrimp and green onions and serve over rice.

6 servings
Per serving: 95 Total calories; 3 Sat-fat calories

Q SHRIMP WITH GREEN PEPPERS

1 pound shrimp, shelled and deveined	1 tablespoon cornstarch
2 tablespoons soy sauce	2 tablespoons + 1 cup water
2 tablespoons dry sherry	1–2 teaspoons chopped ginger root
1–2 teaspoons chili paste with garlic*	2 green onions, sliced
2 tablespoons tomato paste	2 teaspoons olive oil
½ teaspoon sugar	1 large green pepper, sliced
	¼ cup water

Put shrimp in a pot of boiling water and cook for 2–5 minutes until no longer raw. Drain and set aside. (Shrimp may be made a day in advance and refrigerated.)

Combine soy sauce, sherry, chili paste, tomato paste, and sugar. Set aside.

Combine cornstarch with 2 tablespoons water. Then stir in 1 cup water. Set aside.

In a large skillet or wok, sauté ginger and green onions in olive oil for a few seconds.

Remove skillet from heat and stir in soy sauce mixtures and cornstarch. Return skillet to high heat. When sauce begins to thicken, mix in cooked shrimp and green pepper until well coated. If sauce is too thick add more water, 1 tablespoon at a time.

4 servings
Per serving: 174 Total calories; 6 Sat-fat calories

*Available at Oriental food stores and some supermarkets

☑ HONEY-CURRY SCALLOPS

2 tablespoons honey
½–1 teaspoon curry powder
2 tablespoons Dijon mustard

1 teaspoon fresh lemon juice
1 pound sea scallops

Preheat broiler.

Mix honey, curry powder, Dijon mustard, and lemon juice in a medium bowl. Add scallops and mix until they are well coated with sauce.

Lay scallops on broiler pan and place about 5 inches from source of heat. Broil for 5–10 minutes or until scallops are no longer pink inside. Don't overcook or scallops will be rubbery.

4 servings (about 5 scallops each)
Per serving: 140 Total calories; 4 Sat-fat calories

VEGETABLES 18

Hooray for vegetables! Vegetables provide meals with texture, color, dietary fiber, vitamins, and minerals. They score high in a cancer prevention eating plan as well as a heart-healthy eating plan. And, in addition, they are delicious! They fill you up without filling you out.

One of the best ways to cook vegetables is also the easiest. Cook fresh vegetables in a steamer until they are just tender (a few minutes at most). Perhaps add some melted margarine or oil, vinegar, and herbs. Or, for a nonfat treat, sprinkle on vinegar or minced garlic. Steaming vegetables minimizes loss of vitamins. It also brings out the unique taste of each vegetable.

In addition to steaming, vegetables may be prepared in a variety of enticing ways, as you will find in the recipes below.

Q SWEET VEGETABLE MÉLANGE

2 large onions, sliced (about 2 cups)
1 tablespoon olive oil
2 cups sliced carrot
2 small sweet potatoes, cubed (about 2 cups)

1½ tablespoons brown sugar
1 teaspoon cinnamon
¼ cup raisins
½ cup water

In a medium casserole, sauté onions in olive oil until soft.

Cover with carrots, then sweet potatoes.

Mix brown sugar, cinnamon, and raisins and sprinkle over vegetables.

Pour water over vegetables.

Cover and bake at 400°F for 45 minutes or until vegetables are tender.

8 servings
Per serving: 90 Total calories; 2 Sat-fat calories

INDIAN VEGETABLES

Indian Vegetables is one of the Goors' all-time favorite recipes. This large pot of colorful, tasty vegetables may be eaten warm or cold. Try it as a main dish served over rice.

2 tablespoons olive oil
1 teaspoon black mustard seeds*
3 cloves garlic, chopped
1 medium onion, chopped
1 green pepper, chopped
2–3 potatoes, peeled and cubed
1 small eggplant, peeled and cubed
1½ teaspoons turmeric
1 teaspoon salt (optional)
¼ cup water
1 teaspoon cumin
1 teaspoon coriander

1 teaspoon garam masala*
Any vegetables, for example:
1 head broccoli, cut into flowerets (about 3 cups)
1 cup or more cauliflower flowerets
6 carrots, sliced
1 cup or more green beans, cut in half
1 cup sliced celery
1 zucchini, sliced
1 cup water

In a large pot, heat olive oil and add black mustard seeds.

When the mustard seeds begin to pop, add garlic, onion, and green pepper and cook until soft.

Stir in potatoes and eggplant.

Add turmeric and salt and mix until vegetables are covered with turmeric sauce.

Add ¼ cup water, reduce heat to low, cover the pot, and cook for 10 minutes.

Stir in cumin, coriander, garam marsala, and vegetables.

Add 1 cup water and increase heat to medium.

---

*Available at Indian or Mideast food stores

After 10 minutes, lower heat and cook until vegetables are tender.

12 servings
Per serving: 86 Total calories; 2 Sat-fat calories

VEGETABLE SOUFFLÉ
WITH TAHINI SAUCE

This recipe is a lot of work, but it's worth it. You may prepare the vegetable purée one or two days before serving and refrigerate it.

1 turnip, peeled and grated
6 carrots, peeled and grated
3 cups broccoli flowerets (about 1 head)
2 tablespoons margarine
2 tablespoons firmly packed brown sugar

1 tablespoon curry powder
½ teaspoon salt (optional)
¼ teaspoon freshly ground black pepper
⅛ teaspoon grated nutmeg

Tahini Sauce

1 clove garlic
1 tablespoon parsley
3 tablespoons tahini (sesame seed paste)*

1 cup nonfat yogurt
1 tablespoon fresh lemon juice
½ tablespoon fresh dill, or ½ teaspoon dried dillweed

4 egg whites

The Vegetable Purée

Steam turnip and carrot 2–3 minutes or until tender. Set aside.

Steam broccoli flowerets about 5 minutes or until tender.

Purée turnip, carrot, and broccoli in food processor or blender until smooth. Set aside.

Melt margarine in a large skillet over low heat.

Stir in brown sugar until well blended.

Stir in curry powder, salt, pepper, and nutmeg.

Add puréed vegetables and mix well, stirring frequently until most moisture has evaporated.

---

*Available at Mideast food stores and many supermarkets

Cool. (Cover and refrigerate if you wish to finish dish later.)
While vegetable purée is cooling, make tahini sauce.

The Tahini Sauce
Chop garlic and parsley in food processor or blender.
Add tahini, yogurt, lemon juice, and dill.
Blend until smooth. Chill.

The Soufflé
Preheat oven to 450°F. Grease a 1- or 2-quart casserole with margarine.
Beat egg whites until stiff but not dry.
Fold vegetable purée into egg whites, 1/3 at a time. Place in baking dish and bake at 450°F for 15 minutes.
Reduce heat to 350°F and bake for 30 minutes more or until puffed and golden brown.
Serve with tahini sauce.

8 servings

	Total calories	Sat-fat calories
Per serving:	75	5
Tahini sauce per tablespoon	20	1

Q MURIEL'S CHINESE VEGETABLES

2 ounces cellophane noodles*
3 cups broccoli flowerets (about 1 head)
2 cups cauliflower flowerets
2 cloves garlic, minced
1 red pepper, sliced

1 tablespoon olive oil
1 tablespoon sesame oil
2 tablespoons dry white wine or vermouth
1 teaspoon five-spice powder*
2 tablespoons soy sauce

Pour boiling water over cellophane noodles and let them soak for 15–30 minutes.
Steam broccoli and cauliflower in steamer until just tender. Set aside.
Sauté garlic and red pepper in oils for a few seconds.

---

*Available in Oriental food stores and some supermarkets

Mix in broccoli and cauliflower.
Stir in wine and five-spice powder.
Drain cellophane noodles and stir into vegetables.
Stir in soy sauce until vegetables are well coated with sauce.

9 servings
Per serving: 72 Total calories; 4 Sat-fat calories

ITALIC MIXED VEGETABLES

Q

ITALIAN MIXED VEGETABLES

1 clove garlic, minced
1 onion, sliced
1 tablespoon olive oil
3 cups combined red and/or
yellow and/or green sweet
peppers, sliced

2 zucchini, sliced (about 2 cups)
Salt to taste
1 teaspoon thyme, oregano, or
basil, or combination

In a large skillet, sauté garlic and onion in olive oil until tender.
Stir in peppers, zucchini, salt, and herbs.
Cover. Cook until tender.

8 servings
Per serving: 35 Total calories; 2 Sat-fat calories

RATATOUILLE

Add eggplant, bay leaf, and tomatoes to Italian mixed vegetables
and you have a French dish — ratatouille.

2 cloves garlic, minced
1 onion, sliced
1 tablespoon olive oil
3 cups combined red and/or
yellow and/or green sweet
peppers, sliced
2 zucchini, sliced (about 2 cups)
4 fresh tomatoes, cubed, or 1
large can (28 oz) Italian plum
tomatoes, drained

Salt to taste
1 bay leaf
1 teaspoon dried basil, or 2
tablespoons fresh basil,
chopped
1 small eggplant, cubed and
steamed (about 2 cups)*

---

*See page 296 for eggplant preparation.

Sauté garlic and onion in olive oil in a medium-large casserole.
Add peppers, zucchini, tomatoes, salt, bay leaf, and basil.

Cover and simmer until vegetables are tender (about 15–20 minutes).

Add steamed eggplant and cook for 5 minutes more.

10 servings
Per serving: 36 Total calories; 2 Sat-fat calories

Q   # ARTICHOKE

Artichokes make a great appetizer. Watch your family gobble them up and then fight for the delectable hearts.

1 artichoke for two people   Margarine

Trim the stem and pull off the small leaves at the base of the artichoke.

With scissors, cut off the tips of the bottom leaves.

Drop artichoke into a large pot of boiling water and boil slowly for 40–45 minutes or until a leaf will pull off easily.

To eat artichoke, pull off a leaf, dip the bottom in a small bowl of melted margarine, and scrape the leaf between your teeth to extract the "meat." Discard the leaf.

When no more edible leaves are left, you have reached the heart. Remove excess leaves and scrape off the hairy fibers above the heart. Dip the heart in margarine.

Per serving:	*Total calories*	*Sat-fat calories*
Artichoke	26	0
Margarine per tablespoon	90	18

BEANS

If you have been avoiding beans because eating them produces more gas than you care to discuss, here is a way to prepare dried beans (except lentil and split peas) that reduces their gas-producing potential.

1. Rinse beans and pick out foreign matter.
2. Pour boiling water over beans and let them soak for four hours.
3. Drain beans and cook them in fresh water.

CURRIED BEANS

2 cups dried beans (½ cup each chickpeas, black-eyed peas, pinto beans, small red chili beans, or any combination)
1 teaspoon minced ginger root
1 cup chopped onion
2 tablespoons olive oil

1 cup chopped tomato
1 teaspoon coriander
2 teaspoons cumin
1 teaspoon turmeric
¼ teaspoon cayenne pepper
1 teaspoon salt (optional)
2 tablespoons tomato paste

Place dried beans in a large bowl or casserole. Rinse and remove any foreign matter.

Cover beans with boiling water and let them soak for at least 4 hours.

Drain water. Cover beans with fresh water and simmer for 40–60 minutes or until tender.

In a skillet, sauté ginger and onion in olive oil until soft.

Stir in tomato, coriander, cumin, turmeric, cayenne pepper, salt, and tomato paste.

Stir periodically for about 5 minutes. If beans become too dry, add a few tablespoons of water.

11 half-cup servings
Per serving: 155 Total calories; 4 Sat-fat calories

CHICKPEAS WITH LEMON AND HERBS

This dish also tastes good when made with black-eyed peas instead of chickpeas, and parsley instead of oregano.

2 cups dried chickpeas	1 teaspoon salt (optional)
½ cup fresh lemon juice	2 teaspoons oregano
2 tablespoons olive oil	4 green onions, sliced

Place chickpeas in a large bowl or casserole. Rinse and remove any foreign matter.

Cover chickpeas with boiling water and let them soak for at least 4 hours.

Drain water. Cover chickpeas with fresh water and simmer for 40–60 minutes or until tender.

Combine lemon juice, olive oil, salt, oregano, and green onions and pour over chickpeas. Mix thoroughly.

10 half-cup servings
Per serving: 170 Total calories; 5 Sat-fat calories

Q GREEN BEANS BASILICO

3 cups green beans, trimmed, and cut in half	1 tablespoon olive oil
1 clove garlic, minced	1 teaspoon basil
½ cup chopped onion	½ teaspoon oregano
½ cup chopped green pepper	½ teaspoon salt (optional)

In a pot of boiling water, cook green beans 5–10 minutes until tender but still crisp and bright green. Drain and set aside.

In a large skillet, sauté garlic, onion, and green pepper in olive oil until soft.

Stir in basil, oregano, and salt.

Stir in green beans.

6 servings
Per serving: 49 Total calories; 4 Sat-fat calories

⊡ BROCCOLI AND MUSHROOMS

Because broccoli is a cruciferous vegetable, it is highly recommended in both heart-healthy and cancer-healthy eating. Even if it were not so healthy it would still be a pleasure to eat.

1 tablespoon olive oil   ½ pound mushrooms, sliced
2 cloves garlic, minced
2 heads broccoli, cut into
   flowerets

In a large skillet or wok, heat olive oil.
Add garlic, broccoli, and mushrooms and stir for about 1 minute.
Add 2 tablespoons of water, cover, and cook over low heat until broccoli is just tender (about 5–10 minutes).

6 servings
Per serving: 65 Total calories; 5 Sat-fat calories

⊡ SESAME BROCCOLI

1 tablespoon soy sauce   2 heads broccoli, cut in
1 tablespoon sesame oil   flowerets
¼ cup dry sake or vermouth   1 tablespoon sesame seeds,
2 teaspoons honey   toasted

Combine soy sauce, sesame oil, wine, and honey in bowl. Set aside.
Steam broccoli until tender.
Toss broccoli and dressing together.
Sprinkle sesame seeds over broccoli and serve.

8 servings
Per serving: 50 Total calories; 3 Sat-fat calories

Q

CARAWAY CARROTS

Carrots are an excellent source of vitamin A. They keep well in the refrigerator and make great snacks. They are perfect for last-minute chefs because they cook quickly and taste wonderful with very little embellishment.

6 carrots, sliced (about 3 cups)   2 teaspoons caraway seeds
2 teaspoons margarine

Place sliced carrots in a small saucepan with water to cover.
Gently simmer until carrots are soft. Drain.
Add margarine and mix until carrots are covered.
Stir in caraway seeds.

6 servings
Per serving: 40 Total calories; 2 Sat-fat calories

Q

CARROTS AND LEEKS

1 leek, cleaned thoroughly and   2 cups sliced carrots
   the white bulb sliced   ¼ teaspoon thyme
2 teaspoons olive oil

In a small saucepan, sauté leeks in olive oil until tender.
Add carrots and thyme.
Cover and cook over low heat until carrots are tender.

4 servings
Per serving: 61 Total calories; 3 Sat-fat calories

Q

CAULIFLOWER SAUTÉ

2 cups cauliflower flowerets   1 cup snow peas
2 cloves garlic, minced   1 red pepper, sliced
1 small onion, sliced (about ¼   1 cup sliced mushrooms
   cup)   1 teaspoon oregano
1½ tablespoons olive oil

Steam cauliflower until just tender. Set aside.
In large skillet or wok, sauté garlic and onion in olive oil until soft.

Add steamed cauliflower, snow peas, red pepper, mushrooms, and oregano and stir until heated through.

6 servings
Per serving: 57 Total calories; 4 Sat-fat calories

[Q] ## CELERY-MUSHROOMS

3 cups sliced celery	1 cup sliced onions
½ teaspoon salt (optional)	1 cup sliced mushrooms
2 tablespoons margarine	

Place celery and salt in a medium saucepan with water to cover.

Bring to a boil, reduce heat, and simmer for 8–10 minutes or until celery is tender.

Meanwhile, melt margarine in a medium skillet over low heat. Sauté onions in margarine until golden.

Add mushrooms and stir for several minutes to blend flavors.

Drain celery and stir it into onion-mushroom mixture.

6 servings
Per serving: 44 Total calories; 5 Sat-fat calories

Cooking with Eggplant

Choose the blackest eggplant you can find. Peel it, cut it into bite-size pieces, and salt them heavily. Place a heavy plate on top of the pieces to help squeeze out the bitter juices. In 30–60 minutes, wash off the salt and gently squeeze eggplant pieces to rid them of bitter juices.

Steam eggplant in a vegetable steamer until tender. There are two advantages to steaming eggplant: steamed eggplant needs no oil (eggplant absorbs an enormous amount of oil) and thus has fewer sat-fat and total calories; and you can test the pre-cooked eggplant for bitterness before using it in a recipe.

Q KEEMA EGGPLANT

1 medium eggplant, cubed (about 4 cups)
1 cup sliced onion
1 tablespoon olive oil
2 teaspoons curry powder

3 tablespoons fresh lemon juice
1 tablespoon brown sugar
1 tablespoon ketchup
¼ cup water
1 cup canned chickpeas

Prepare eggplant as explained above.
Meanwhile, sauté onion slices in olive oil until tender.
Stir in curry powder.
Combine lemon juice, brown sugar, ketchup, and water and stir into eggplant mixture. Cook for 5 minutes.
Add chickpeas and cook for 2 minutes more.

6 servings
Per serving: 100 Total calories; 4 Sat-fat calories

⬚ HOT AND GARLICKY EGGPLANT

1 medium eggplant (about 1
pound)
5 small, dried black Chinese
mushrooms*
1 tablespoon chili paste with
garlic*
1 tablespoon vinegar

½ tablespoon soy sauce
½ tablespoon double black soy
sauce*
2 tablespoons dry sherry
½ teaspoon sugar
1 large green pepper, chopped
1 tablespoon olive oil
½ cup water

Prepare eggplant as explained on page 296.

Place mushrooms in a small bowl and cover with boiling water.

After about 15 minutes remove mushrooms. Squeeze out the excess water and discard stems. Slice mushrooms. Set aside.

Combine chili paste with garlic, vinegar, soy sauces, sherry, and sugar and set aside.

In a large skillet, sauté green pepper and mushrooms in oil until tender.

Stir in eggplant.

Mix in soy sauce mixture until vegetables are covered and then stir in water.

Simmer for about 5 minutes.

8 half-cup servings
Per serving: 35 Total calories; 2 Sat-fat calories

⬚ EGGPLANT WITH A GREEK INFLUENCE

1 large or 2 small eggplants
1 tablespoon olive oil
¼ cup fresh lemon juice

12 pitted black olives
1 teaspoon capers
½ teaspoon oregano

Prepare eggplant as explained on page 296. Taste steamed eggplant. If not bitter, proceed.

In a saucepan, combine eggplant, olive oil, lemon juice, olives, capers, and oregano.

---

*Available at Oriental food stores

Cook over low heat for 10 minutes or until heated through.

6 servings
Per serving: 51 Total calories; 4 Sat-fat calories

Q   ## LENTILS AND POTATOES

Lentils, a type of legume, are both delicious and nutritious. They are rich in vitamin C, folic acid, and many minerals, including iron and calcium. They are a good source of soluble fiber, which has been shown to lower blood cholesterol.

Lentils and Potatoes may be served at room temperature on a bed of lettuce or warm as a side dish.

1 cup lentils
1 cup peeled and cubed potato
    (about 1 medium potato)
½ teaspoon salt (optional)

2 cloves garlic, minced
⅓ cup chopped onion
1 tablespoon olive oil

Wash lentils and place them in a medium saucepan with potatoes, salt, and water to cover.

Bring to a boil. Reduce heat, cover, and simmer for about 20–25 minutes or until vegetables are tender.

Drain and set aside.

In a large skillet, sauté garlic and onion in olive oil.

Stir in cooked lentils and potatoes and serve or refrigerate.

6 servings
Per serving: 55 Total calories; 3 Sat-fat calories

Q   ## BRAISED MUSHROOMS ORIENTAL

These mushrooms make a tasty hors d'oeuvre or side dish.

1 pound mushrooms, sliced
2 tablespoons olive oil
2 teaspoons sugar

4 teaspoons soy sauce
1 cup water
2 teaspoons sesame oil

Sauté mushrooms in olive oil until tender.

Stir in sugar, soy sauce, and water.

Cover and simmer for 25 minutes or until water is absorbed. Add sesame oil.

6 side-dish servings
Per serving: 83 Total calories; 6 Sat-fat calories

POTATOES

Of all vegetables, potatoes are probably the most maligned. Many people consider them highly caloric and devoid of nutritional value. What injustice! Potatoes are filled with vitamins (particularly vitamin C), minerals, and protein. Eaten plain they have no fat and are extremely filling and delicious.

Q

POTATO SKINS

Leslie Goodman-Malamuth of the Center for Science in the Public Interest devised this recipe as a substitute for the highly saturated potato skins you often find in restaurants. Not only is this recipe quick and easy, the resulting potatoes are scrumptious.

4 large potatoes   Paprika to taste
1 tablespoon olive oil

Preheat oven to 450°F.
Scrub potatoes well, cut them lengthwise into six wedges the size and shape of dill pickle spears, and dry them on a paper towel.
In a large bowl, toss potato spears with olive oil until they are well covered.
Spread potatoes on a baking sheet, dust them with paprika, and bake for 20–30 minutes or until fork-tender.

6 servings (So good, 2 people can easily finish them off!)
Per serving: 79 Total calories; 3 Sat-fat calories

POTATOES LYONNAISE

2 pounds boiling or all-purpose potatoes (about 4 large)
2 tablespoons margarine
½ teaspoon salt (optional)
¼ teaspoon freshly ground pepper

1½ cups sliced onion (about 2 onions)
1 tablespoon olive oil
¼ cup chopped parsley

Peel and halve potatoes, then steam or boil them until just tender (about 10 minutes).

Cut potatoes into ¼-inch-thick slices.

Melt margarine in a large skillet. Add potato slices and cook for 15 minutes, shaking pan periodically. After 10 minutes, add salt and pepper and turn potatoes.

In a small skillet, sauté onions in olive oil until browned.

Add onions and parsley to potatoes and cook for 5 minutes more.

8 servings
Per serving: 90 Total calories; 7 Sat-fat calories

Q # BOUILLON POTATOES

4 medium potatoes, peeled and cut into ⅜-inch-thick slices
½ cup canned beef broth or beef stock
1 teaspoon vinegar
1 tablespoon minced carrot
1 small onion, quartered

2 cloves garlic, peeled
2 sprigs parsley
1 bay leaf
½ teaspoon thyme
3 sprigs parsley chopped
1 teaspoon garlic minced

Line the bottom of a large skillet with the sliced potatoes.

Combine the broth, vinegar, carrot, onion, whole garlic, cloves, parsley sprigs, bay leaf, and thyme, and pour over potatoes. Add water just to cover potatoes.

Bring to a boil and continue to boil until the liquid is completely evaporated (about 20 minutes). Check frequently, as the liquid's final evaporation occurs suddenly.

Sprinkle with chopped parsley and minced garlic and serve.

4 servings
Per serving: 106 Total calories; 0 Sat-fat calories

Q CURRIED WHIPPED POTATOES

You need not add butter or margarine to make delectable whipped potatoes. In this recipe, sautéed onions, mustard seed, and cumin make them special and exotic. Leave the onions out of this recipe and you have plain but scrumptious whipped potatoes.

4 potatoes (about 2 pounds)	½ teaspoon cumin
¾ cup chopped onions	1–4 tablespoons skim milk
2 teaspoons olive oil	Salt and freshly ground black
½ teaspoon mustard seed	pepper to taste

Peel potatoes, slice thinly, and place in a medium saucepan with water to cover. Bring to a boil and boil until tender.

Meanwhile, sauté onions in olive oil. Lower heat to medium and stir in mustard seed and cumin. Cook a few moments until onions are soft.

Drain potatoes. Beat potatoes with an electric mixer. Add milk, one tablespoon at a time, until potatoes are whipped.

Mix in onions and salt and pepper to taste.

4 servings
Per serving: 178 Total calories; 3 Sat-fat calories

SWEET POTATOES

Sweet potatoes are often considered a fattening treat. They are a healthy treat, but not fattening. One sweet potato has only 115 calories and is chock-full of vitamins A and C and many minerals.

▣ SWEET POTATOES WITH ORANGES, APPLES, AND SWEET WINE

4 cups sweet potatoes cut into
½-inch slices
1 cup diced apple
1 orange, peeled and cut into
bite-size pieces

1 tablespoon fresh lemon juice
2 tablespoons brown sugar
¼ cup plum wine or other
sweet wine
3 whole cloves

Preheat oven to 375°F.

Place sweet potato slices in a saucepan with water to cover. Bring to a boil. Reduce heat, cover, and simmer until just tender when pierced with a fork.

Drain sweet potatoes and place in a casserole.

Mix apple, orange, lemon juice, brown sugar, wine, and cloves. Pour mixture over sweet potatoes.

Bake, covered, for 30 minutes or until apples are tender.

6 servings
Per serving: 180 Total calories; 0 Sat-fat calories

FLUFFY SWEET POTATOES

3 sweet potatoes (to make 2
cups mashed)
⅔ cup orange juice
½ teaspoon grated orange peel

2 tablespoons brown sugar
2 tablespoons margarine, melted
1 egg yolk
2 egg whites

Peel sweet potatoes, cut into chunks, place in a medium saucepan, and cover with water.

Bring to a boil, then reduce heat and simmer until tender (about 10–15 minutes).

Preheat oven to 375°F. Grease a casserole with margarine.

Drain potatoes and mash in a large bowl.

Mix in juice, peel, sugar, melted margarine, and egg yolk.

Whip egg whites until stiff but not dry. Fold into sweet potato.

Pour sweet potato mixture into casserole and bake for 30 minutes.

6 servings
Per serving: 133 Total calories; 9 Sat-fat calories

⧈ SPICED SWEET POTATOES

This sweet potato recipe needs no fat to make it delicious.

2 large sweet potatoes
1 tablespoon brown sugar
¼ teaspoon ground cloves

¼–½ teaspoon cinnamon
¼–½ teaspoon salt (optional)
2 tablespoons orange juice

Peel and thinly slice sweet potatoes. Place in saucepan, cover with water, and boil until tender (about 10–20 minutes).
Drain and place in the bowl of an electric mixer.
Add sugar, spices, salt, and 1 tablespoon of the orange juice. Beat until fluffy.
Add more orange juice if necessary for puréed consistency.

4 servings
Per serving: 75 Total calories; 0 Sat-fat calories

⧈ SPINACH AND TOMATOES

Spinach is an excellent source of vitamin A. It is also rich in vitamin C and iron. It may be eaten raw in a salad or cooked in many interesting ways.

10 ounces fresh spinach,
  washed and shredded
2 cloves garlic, minced

1 tablespoon olive oil
1 tomato, diced
1 tablespoon raisins

In a medium saucepan, cook spinach in boiling water to cover until tender (about 2 minutes). Drain well and chop coarsely.
Sauté garlic in olive oil.
Mix in spinach.
Add tomatoes and raisins and heat through.

4 servings
Per serving: 60 Total calories; 4 Sat-fat calories

Q

SPINACH ORIENTAL

10 ounces fresh spinach, washed and shredded

1 tablespoon olive oil

1 teaspoon chopped ginger root

1 teaspoon double black soy sauce*

In a large skillet, lightly sauté spinach in oil until soft.
Stir in ginger and soy sauce.

4 servings
Per serving: 50 Total calories; 4 Sat-fat calories

SQUASH

Squash, both winter and summer varieties, is rich in vitamin A, vitamin C, niacin, and iron. Squash is delicious when simply baked, boiled, or steamed and enhanced with a little margarine and freshly ground pepper. Or it may be prepared in a variety of other interesting ways.

Q

ACORN SQUASH

3 medium acorn squash**

1 cup boiling water

3 teaspoons margarine

Freshly ground black pepper to taste

Preheat oven to 400°F.
Cut each squash in half and scoop out seeds and fibers.
Slice a small piece off the bottom of each half so that they will not roll over.
Place squash halves, cut-side down, in a shallow casserole.
Pour boiling water into the casserole and cover it tightly with aluminum foil.
Bake for 45 minutes or until squash is soft when pierced with a fork.

---

*Available at Oriental food stores and some supermarkets
**Butternut squash may also be cooked this way and is delicious. Its dull cream exterior conceals a beautiful, deep orange interior.

Turn squash cut-side up and fill each half with ½ teaspoon margarine.

Bake for 5 minutes more.

Grind pepper over squash and serve.

6 servings
Per serving: 55 Total calories; 3 Sat-fat calories

Q # GLAZED ACORN SQUASH

2 acorn squash   ¾ cup orange juice
2 tablespoons brown sugar

Cut squash crosswise (not through the stem) into ½-inch slices. Clean out fibers and seeds and peel.

Place squash in a large skillet.

Combine brown sugar and orange juice and pour over squash.

Cover and cook over medium heat for 15 minutes. Turn squash.

Raise heat and cook, uncovered, for 10 minutes more or until squash is tender and sauce is reduced.

6 servings
Per serving: 58 Total calories; 0 Sat-fat calories

Q AFGHAN SQUASH

½ cup sliced onion
2 teaspoons olive oil
½ teaspoon salt
½ teaspoon cumin
½ teaspoon coriander

¼ teaspoon cardamom
¼ teaspoon ground cloves
1 butternut squash, peeled and
cubed (about 3 cups)

Sauté onion in olive oil in a small casserole.
Stir in salt, cumin, coriander, cardamom, and cloves.
Add squash and 1 cup water.
Cook until tender (about 25 minutes).

8 servings
Per serving: 30 Total calories; 2 Sat-fat calories

SPAGHETTI SQUASH WITH TOMATO SAUCE

Spaghetti squash looks like an ordinary yellow squash — until
you bake it. Inside, the pulp separates into long, thin strands like
spaghetti. Use spaghetti squash as a healthy, vitamin-rich, delicious
pasta. Top the squash with the tasty sauce below or Sweet Red Pepper Sauce (page 259).

1 spaghetti squash (about 3 pounds)

Tomato Sauce

¼ cup sliced onion
1–2 teaspoons minced garlic
2 teaspoons olive oil
¼ cup chopped parsley
2 cups chopped cherry tomatoes
(or regular tomatoes)
¼ teaspoon oregano

¼ teaspoon basil
¼ teaspoon cumin
¼–½ teaspoon red pepper
flakes
¼–½ freshly ground black
pepper
Salt to taste (optional)

The Squash

Preheat oven to 350°F.
Cut squash in half lengthwise and scoop out seeds.
Place halves face down in shallow baking pan.
Bake for 45 minutes or until tender when poked with a fork.

The Sauce

Meanwhile, in an 8-inch skillet, sauté onion and garlic in olive oil until soft. Lower heat to medium and stir in parsley.

Stir in tomatoes. Add oregano, basil, cumin, red pepper flakes, black pepper, and salt. Cook on medium heat, stirring occasionally, for about 10 minutes. Turn to low and let flavors blend for about 5–10 minutes. Set aside.

When squash is cooked, scrape inside with a fork to release spaghetti strands. Pile onto a plate (as you would spaghetti) and top with tomato sauce.

4 servings
Per serving: 127 Total calories; 3 Sat-fat calories

Q   STEAMED ZUCCHINI MATCHSTICKS

So light, so tasty — you don't even need to add salt, spices, or fat. But you may want to crush garlic into one teaspoon of melted margarine and combine it with the vegetables.

2 small zucchini (or ½ small zucchini per person)	1 thick carrot, peeled
	1 teaspoon margarine (optional)
	1 clove garlic (optional)

Cut zucchini and carrot into 2-inch lengths.

Place a zucchini section on a cutting surface, skin-side down.

Holding the sides of the section, slice lengthwise at ⅛-inch intervals. Hold the slices together.

Roll the section one-quarter turn, making sure the slices stay together.

Again, make parallel slices, ⅛-inch apart lengthwise.

Result: zucchini matchsticks.

Repeat for remaining sections of zucchini and carrot.

Place zucchini sticks on top of carrot sticks in a vegetable steamer and steam until just tender (about 1 or 2 minutes).

4 servings

	Total calories	Sat-fat calories
Per serving	17	0
With margarine	24	2

Q

CURRIED ZUCCHINI

You can use this basic recipe for any vegetable.

1 clove garlic, minced
½ cup chopped onion
1 ½ tablespoons olive oil
½ teaspoon salt
½–1 teaspoon turmeric

¼–½ teaspoon cumin
½ teaspoon red pepper flakes
  (optional)
3 zucchini, sliced (about 3 cups)
2 tomatoes, chopped

In a large skillet, sauté garlic and onion in olive oil until soft.
Add salt, turmeric, cumin, and red peppers. Blend well.
Stir in zucchini and cook until tender.
Stir in tomatoes and serve.

8 servings
Per serving: 43 Total calories; 3 Sat-fat calories

PIZZA, QUICHE, CHILI, AND TORTILLAS   19

"OH, WOE IS ME,'' says the sat-fat counter. "How can I go on without pizza and chili? Life will be bare." STOP! The following recipes for pizza, chili, quiche, and tortillas are delectable. The only thing they lack is saturated fat. So don't feel sorry for yourself. You *can* have your cake — or pizza — and eat it too!

PIZZA

You might think that a low-sat-fat diet would eliminate pizza, but the following recipes will prove to you how fabulous low-sat-fat pizzas can be. They make good snacks as well as main courses for lunch or dinner. Freeze leftovers (if there are any!). Then, in the future when you want a treat, heat the frozen slices in your toaster oven.

To make pizza with a crisper crust, buy four inexpensive unglazed quarry tiles (each about a 5-inch square) at a tile store or purchase a pizza tile at a store that sells kitchen supplies. Pizza baked directly on hot tiles has a crunchier crust.

To slide the pizza onto the tiles it helps to have a pizza peel. It looks like this:

You may devise other gizmos to slide the pizza onto the tiles if you wish, but a pizza peel really works well. Of course, you may forgo both the tiles and the pizza peel and use a metal pizza pan or cookie sheet instead.

PIZZA

Dough

1 tablespoon active dry yeast
¼ cup warm water
Pinch of sugar
4 cups unbleached white flour

1 teaspoon salt (optional)
1 cup warm water
2 tablespoons olive oil

Topping

2 cloves garlic
3 tablespoons olive oil
Salt to taste
1½ cups tomato sauce (page 312)
2 cups sliced mushrooms
1½ sliced green peppers (about 1½ cups)

1 cup sliced onion
1⅓ cups low-fat (1%) cottage cheese
3 teaspoons oregano
4 teaspoons olive oil

The Dough

Place yeast, the ¼ cup warm (but not hot) water, and sugar in a large bowl or the work bowl of your food processor. Let proof (become bubbly).

Mix in flour and salt.

Mix in the 1 cup warm (but not hot) water and olive oil.

Knead or process until dough is smooth and elastic, adding more flour if needed.

Place dough in a large greased bowl, cover with a towel, and let rise for about 45 minutes.

While the dough is rising, place tiles (see page 309) in oven and heat oven to 450°F.

After the dough has risen, divide it into four parts, form each into a smooth ball, and cover for 10 minutes.

Roll the dough into four small circles, 10 to 12 inches each. Wait 10 minutes more. Roll the dough thinner.

To Make Each Pizza

Cover pizza peel with a thin layer of cornmeal or grease pizza pan with oil.

Place one rolled circle of dough on the pizza peel or in the pizza pan.

Crush garlic into olive oil. Paint the surface of the dough with garlic oil and sprinkle with salt.

Spoon about ¼ cup tomato sauce over the dough.

Arrange mushrooms, green peppers, and onions over tomato sauce.

Put cottage cheese on top (as if it were mozzarella).

Sprinkle with ¾ teaspoon oregano and drizzle with olive oil.

Bake for 10–20 minutes or until crust is golden brown.

4 pizzas, 4 slices per pizza
Per slice: 148 Total calories; 4 Sat-fat calories

CALZONE

A recipe that you can enjoy with no pangs of remorse. This seems like a lot of work, but once you do it, it goes quickly and is quite delicious.

Dough

1 tablespoon active dry yeast
pinch of sugar
½ cup warm water
3–4½ cups unbleached white
    flour

1–1½ teaspoons salt (optional)
1 cup skim milk
1 tablespoon olive oil

Tomato Sauce*

1 tablespoon olive oil

1 cup chopped onion

4 large cans (28 oz each)
    tomatoes

1 can (6 oz) tomato paste

2 teaspoons basil

1 teaspoon salt

Filling

1 clove garlic

¼ cup olive oil

Salt to taste

1 cup low-fat (1%) cottage
    cheese

1 green pepper, sliced

1 cup sliced mushrooms

1 cup sliced onion

The Dough

Place yeast, sugar, and warm water in food processor or large bowl and let proof.

Add 3 cups flour and salt and mix.

Add skim milk and olive oil and process until dough masses into a ball or knead until smooth and elastic. Add more flour if dough is too sticky.

Place dough in a bowl greased with oil and cover with a towel. Let rise in a warm place for about 1 hour.

If you are using pizza tiles (see page 309), place them in preheated 450°F oven 30 minutes before baking pizza.

While dough is rising, make the tomato sauce.

The Tomato Sauce

Place olive oil in large saucepan.

Add onion and cook over low heat until tender.

Strain juice from canned tomatoes. (Freeze juice for soups.) Chop tomatoes (easily done in food processor).

Mix tomato paste into tomatoes. Add tomato mixture to saucepan.

Add basil and salt and cook until thick (about 45 minutes).

To Make the Calzone

When dough has risen, divide it into 8 parts and form each part into a smooth ball. Cover with a towel or plastic wrap for about 10

---

*This recipe makes 8 cups of tomato sauce. You will need only about one cup for calzone. Freeze the rest for future use in other recipes or as spaghetti sauce.

minutes. It is important that you let the dough "rest" or it will be difficult to roll flat.

Roll each ball into a flat circle. Wait 10 minutes more.

Make each circle thinner. Place dough on floured surface or pizza peel sprinkled with cornmeal (see page 309).

Crush garlic into olive oil. Brush dough with the garlic oil, then sprinkle it with salt.

Spread about 2 tablespoons of tomato sauce over half the dough, leaving a border of ½ inch.

Spread 2 tablespoons cottage cheese evenly over tomato sauce.

Top with a few slices of green pepper, mushroom, and onion.

Fold the top half of the dough over and pinch the top and bottom edges together. Paint the top with garlic oil and salt lightly.

Slide calzone onto hot tiles or onto cookie sheet.

Bake for about 10–20 minutes or until browned.

Makes 8 calzone
Per calzone: 366 Total calories; 11 Sat-fat calories

FOCACCIA

The whole-wheat flour in this pizza not only makes it healthier but also gives it a toasty taste and crunchy texture. Try it! It is easy and makes great snacks. Freeze it in snack-size slices.

Dough

1½ teaspoons dry active yeast	2½ cups whole-wheat flour
½ teaspoon honey	¾ teaspoon salt (optional)
1 cup warm water	1 tablespoon olive oil

Tomato Sauce

1 large can (28 oz) tomatoes, or	½ teaspoon oregano
3 large tomatoes	¼ teaspoon basil
2 cloves garlic, minced	Ground hot cherry peppers
1 small onion, chopped	(optional)
2 teaspoons olive oil	

The Dough

Place yeast, honey, and warm water in food processor or large bowl. Let proof.

Add flour, salt, and olive oil and process or knead until smooth and elastic, adding flour if needed.

Place dough in an oiled bowl, cover with a towel, and let rise in a warm place for about 1 hour.

Punch down dough and let it rest on floured counter for 10 minutes.

Grease a 10 × 15-inch cookie sheet with oil. Roll out dough (or press with your hands) onto the cookie sheet.

Pinch a rim around the edge. Cover with a towel and let rise for 30 minutes.

Meanwhile, make the tomato sauce.

The Tomato Sauce

If using canned tomatoes, drain liquid and chop tomatoes. If using whole tomatoes, chop fine.

In a medium skillet, sauté garlic and onion in olive oil until tender.

Stir in tomatoes, oregano, and basil and let simmer until thick (about 10–15 minutes).

Let cool.

Preheat oven to 400°F.
Spread the sauce over the dough.
Add hot cherry peppers, if desired.
Bake for 20–25 minutes.

Makes 12 pieces
Per piece: 117 Total calories; 3 Sat-fat calories

PISSALADIÈRE

An onion pizza of Provence. Pissaladière makes a perfect luncheon dish, snack, or light dinner. Although it looks as if it took a lot of work, it is quite simple to make. Cook the onions ahead to save time later.

Filling

3 cups chopped onion
2 cloves garlic, minced

2 tablespoons olive oil

Dough

1 teaspoon dry yeast
pinch of sugar
¼ cup water
2–3 cups unbleached white
    flour

¼ teaspoon salt (optional)
¾ cup warm water
2 tablespoons olive oil

12 pitted black olives, halved

6 anchovies

The Filling

Slowly cook onion and garlic in olive oil until soft (about 30 minutes). Set aside. (You can refrigerate cooked onions for a few days.)

The Dough

About 1 hour before serving, place yeast, sugar, and ¼ cup warm water in bowl or food processor. Let proof.

Mix in 2 cups of flour and salt.

Add ¾ cup warm water and olive oil and knead or process for 15 seconds.

Add more flour until dough is smooth and elastic.

Place dough in oiled bowl, cover with towel, and let rise for about 45 minutes.

After 35 minutes, preheat oven to 450°F.

On a greased round pizza pan or cookie sheet, roll out or push the dough into a 10-inch circle.

Spoon onions evenly over dough.

Starting from the center of the circle, place olives in lines like the spokes of a wheel.

Place anchovies between the lines of olives.
Bake for 20 minutes or until dough is slightly golden brown.

Makes 8 slices
Per slice: 241 Total calories; 10 Sat-fat calories

QUICHE

The word *quiche* conjures up images of dozens of eggs and tons of cream, ham, and cheese. The following wonderful quiches will expand your definition. They are made with only low-sat-fat ingredients and make perfect appetizers or light meals.

SPINACH QUICHE

Partially baked nonsweet quiche crust (page 396)
1 tablespoon chopped parsley
1 teaspoon basil
1 package (10 oz) fresh spinach (or frozen spinach, thawed)
1 cup low-fat (1%) cottage cheese
1 cup buttermilk

1 egg
1 egg white
1 tablespoon unbleached flour
½ teaspoon salt (optional)
¼ teaspoon freshly ground black pepper
¼ teaspoon grated nutmeg
2 tablespoons sliced green onion

Preheat oven to 375°F.

Combine parsley with basil (easily done in food processor) and set aside.

If using fresh spinach, wash leaves and tear off stems.

In a medium saucepan, cook fresh or thawed spinach for about 3 minutes in ½ cup boiling water. Drain. Squeeze all liquid out of spinach or quiche will be watery.

Combine cottage cheese, buttermilk, egg, egg white, flour, salt, pepper, and nutmeg in food processor or bowl.

If using processor, add spinach and process. If mixing in bowl, chop spinach finely and add to cottage cheese mixture.

Stir in green onion and parsley-basil mixture and pour into partially baked pie crust.

Bake for about 30 minutes.

Makes 9 slices
Per slice: 200 Total calories; 17 Sat-fat calories

TOMATO QUICHE

Here is another quiche you can eat with no qualms. It has an absolutely delicious Mediterranean flavor. If you are an anchovy-hater, do not avoid this recipe. The anchovies enhance the flavor but are not discernible.

Partially baked nonsweet quiche
  crust (page 396)
1/3 cup chopped onion
1 tablespoon olive oil
1 large can (28 oz) + 1 small
  can (16 oz) tomatoes
1 clove garlic, minced
1/4 teaspoon basil
1/2 teaspoon oregano

1/2 teaspoon salt (optional)
6 sprigs parsley, stems removed
1 tin (2 oz) anchovies
1 egg
1 egg white
3 tablespoons tomato paste
25 large pitted black olives, cut
  in half
1/2 tablespoon olive oil

In a medium skillet, sauté onion in olive oil until tender.

Meanwhile, drain the juice from the tomatoes. (Freeze the liquid for future use.) Chop tomatoes and add to onion.

Mix in garlic, basil, oregano, and salt.

Increase heat to high. When tomato mixture begins to bubble, reduce heat to medium.

Cook tomatoes for about 50 minutes or until thick, stirring occasionally. You may have to reduce heat if mixture begins to boil. Make sure there is no excess liquid.

When sauce is very thick, remove skillet from heat. Cool sauce slightly.

Preheat oven to 375°F.

In a food processor or blender, mix parsley, anchovies, egg, egg white, and tomato paste.

Fold anchovy mixture into tomato sauce and pour into partially baked pie crust.

Artistically arrange olive halves on top of tomato mixture.

Dribble oil over quiche and bake for 25–30 minutes or until puffy and browned on top.

Makes 9 slices
Per slice: 220 Total calories; 21 Sat-fat calories

Q ## TOMATO TART

Wonderful! So light and tasty.

Biscuit Crust

1 cup unbleached white flour
1½ teaspoons baking powder
½ teaspoon salt (optional)

3 tablespoons olive oil
¼ cup nonfat skim milk

Tomato Filling

1 pound fresh whole or cherry tomatoes or 1 large can tomatoes (28 oz)
¾ cup nonfat plain yogurt
1 small jar pimientos (2 oz), drained
2 teaspoons unbleached white flour

¾ teaspoon sugar
½ teaspoon salt
⅛–¼ teaspoon red pepper flakes
Freshly ground black pepper to taste
2 green onions, thinly sliced

The Crust

Preheat oven to 425°F and lightly oil a 9-inch tart pan.*

Combine flour, baking powder, and salt in a mixing bowl or food processor bowl.

Add oil and milk and mix until a ball of soft dough forms.

Place the dough on a floured piece of wax paper and roll into a ⅛-inch-thick circle, about 12 inches in diameter.

Flip the paper and dough onto the tart pan. Peel off the waxed paper and press the dough into the pan. If there is excess, roll it over the edge into a ridge.

Press a sheet of aluminum foil into the dough to keep it from forming large bubbles during baking.

Bake 5 minutes and remove foil.

Bake 5–10 more minutes until crust is evenly browned. Set aside.

The Filling

Meanwhile, slice the tomatoes in half and squeeze out their juices, or drain the canned tomatoes and squeeze out their juices.

Chop the tomatoes into small pieces (preferably by hand — you don't want a purée). Set aside.

Combine yogurt, pimientos, flour, sugar, salt, red pepper flakes, and black pepper. Mix in green onions and tomatoes.

Spread tomato filling evenly over crust.

Place metal rim of tart pan upside down so it covers the edges of the crust and prevents them from burning. Broil for about 4 minutes or until warmed.

Makes 6 slices
Per slice: 173 Total calories; 8 Sat-fat calories

---

*A 9-inch tart pan with a removable bottom makes a very pretty crust that is easy to pop out. If you don't have a tart pan, a 9-inch pie plate will also work.

CHILI

Chili is traditionally made with beef. You will not miss the beef in the following vegetarian recipes. They are delicious and filling — wonderful for a fall or winter day.

Q ## CHILI NON CARNE

This is one of the best chili recipes we have ever tasted. It is filled with nutritious vegetables that provide texture but do not interfere with the delicious chili taste. Eat it hot in a bowl mixed with chopped onions, tomatoes, and lettuce, or spoon it into pita bread with chopped onion, lettuce, and tomatoes. Dried beans such as kidney beans and navy beans have been shown to have a modest effect in lowering blood cholesterol.

¾ cup chopped onion
2 cloves garlic, minced
1 tablespoon olive oil
2 tablespoons chili powder
¼ teaspoon basil
¼ teaspoon oregano
¼ teaspoon cumin
2 cups finely chopped zucchini
1 cup finely chopped carrot
1 large can (28 oz) tomatoes +
    1 small can (14½ oz) toma-
    toes, drained and chopped

1 can (15 oz) kidney beans,
    undrained
2 cans (15 oz each) kidney
    beans, *drained* and thoroughly
    rinsed
Chopped onions, tomatoes,
    lettuce, or green peppers, for
    garnish

In a large pot, sauté onion and garlic in olive oil until soft.

Mix in chili powder, basil, oregano, and cumin.

Stir in zucchini and carrots until well blended. Cook for about 1 minute over low heat, stirring occasionally.

Stir in chopped tomatoes, undrained and drained kidney beans.

Bring to a boil. Reduce heat and simmer for 30–45 minutes or until thick.

Top with chopped onions, tomatoes, and lettuce or green peppers.

Makes 8 one-cup servings
Per serving: 127 Total calories; 3 Sat-fat calories

Q

PAWTUCKET CHILI

1 large can (40 oz) kidney beans, or 2 small cans (16 oz each)

1 can (15 oz) chickpeas

2 cloves garlic, minced

1 medium onion, chopped

2 teaspoons olive oil

1 can (8 oz) tomato sauce

1 large can (28 oz) whole tomatoes, drained and chopped

1–3 teaspoons oregano

½ teaspoon thyme

1 teaspoon cumin

½ teaspoon basil

1–2 tablespoons chili powder

Rinse kidney beans and chickpeas to remove salt. Set aside.

Sauté garlic and onion in olive oil.

Add beans, chickpeas, and remaining ingredients and bring to a boil.

Simmer for 20 minutes (or longer) until thick.

Makes 8 one-cup servings
Per serving: 110 Total calories; 3 Sat-fat calories

TORTILLAS

Who says you can't have tortillas on a low-sat-fat diet? Admittedly, these tortillas contain no meat or cheese, but they are spicy and great tasting, just like their Mexican counterparts. As a bonus, your arteries will be happier with these than with beef or cheese.

Corn Tortillas* Filling

1 cup dried lentils

2 cups water

2½ tablespoons raisins

3 cloves garlic, minced

¼ teaspoon red pepper flakes

2 teaspoons chili powder

½ teaspoon cumin

¼ teaspoon basil

7 tablespoons tomato paste

2 cups water

Toppings

Shredded zucchini

Nonfat yogurt

---

*Look for corn tortillas in the refrigerator section of your supermarket. Be sure they contain only corn, water, and lime — no lard or other saturated fat.

The Filling

In a large pot, combine lentils and 2 cups water and simmer for 10 minutes.

Add raisins, garlic, red pepper flakes, chili powder, cumin, basil, tomato paste, and 1 cup of the remaining 2 cups water and mix well.

Cook slowly for 15 minutes, adding additional 1 cup water when lentil mixture becomes too thick. Stir periodically.

Continue cooking, stirring occasionally (15–30 minutes more) until lentil mixture is thick.

Makes filling for 16 tortillas. Freeze half for future use.

Meanwhile, wrap tortillas completely in aluminum foil and bake at 350°F for 10–15 minutes.

Assembling the Tortillas

Place about 3 tablespoons lentil mixture in center of each tortilla.
Cover with about 1 tablespoon shredded zucchini.
Top with about 1 tablespoon yogurt. Serve.

Makes 8 tortillas
Per tortilla: 90 Total calories; trace Sat-fat calories

PASTA, RICE, AND OTHER GRAINS

20

P ASTA, BARLEY, rice, and bulgur are filling and low in saturated fat. As side dishes or complete meals, they add texture and variety to your eating.

☐ ASPARAGUS PASTA

Asparagus Pasta makes a delightful luncheon dish, first course for an elegant meal, or light dinner. No one consuming this dish will believe how incredibly simple it is to make.

1 pound asparagus, sliced on the diagonal into 1-inch pieces
2 tablespoons Dijon mustard
2 tablespoons olive oil
¼ cup thinly sliced shallots
1 clove garlic, minced

2 anchovy fillets
¼ teaspoon thyme
2 tablespoons chopped parsley
¾ pound very thin spaghetti or pasta of your choice
Salt and freshly ground black pepper to taste

In a large pot of boiling water, cook asparagus until tender and still bright green (about 3 minutes).

Combine mustard, olive oil, shallots, garlic, anchovies, thyme, and parsley. Set aside.

Cook pasta. Drain, but reserve 1 cup of the cooking water.

Combine pasta with dressing and asparagus. Mix well. Add some of the cooking water if pasta is too dry. Add salt and pepper to taste.

Variation: Follow the above recipe but add two boned and skinned chicken breast halves that have been steamed and cut into bite-size pieces.

4 servings

	Total calories	*Sat-fat calories*
Per serving	411	2
With chicken	476	4

Q # SALMON PASTA NIÇOISE

This delicious pasta may be eaten warm or cold. It is a meal in itself.

3 large fresh tomatoes
1 egg or 1 egg white
2 tablespoons olive oil
4 tablespoons wine vinegar
1 tin anchovy fillets
1 large clove garlic, minced
6 large black pitted olives, halved

Salt to taste (optional)
Freshly ground black pepper to taste
8 ounces thin spaghetti
1 can salmon (7½ oz)*
1–2 slices red onion, coarsely chopped

Cut tomatoes into slices about ¼–⅜-inch thick. Cut these in half or smaller.

Place egg in small pot, cover with water, and bring to boil. Let boil 1 minute or so. Cover pot, turn off heat, and let sit for 10 minutes until hard-boiled. Set aside or refrigerate. (You can do this step anytime during the day.)

Combine olive oil, vinegar, 4 smashed anchovy fillets, and garlic and pour over tomatoes. Mix in olives. Season with salt and pepper. Set aside to marinate for about 30 minutes or more.

Cook spaghetti, drain it, and place it in a large bowl. Stir tomato mixture into pasta. Break up salmon with a fork and add to pasta.

---

*You may also substitute canned tuna in water for many fewer total fat calories.
Per serving: 385 Total calories; 18 Sat-fat calories

Slice egg (or remove egg yolk and slice white) and add along with onion and remaining anchovies.

4 servings
Per serving: 408 Total calories; 22 Sat-fat calories

PEASANT PASTA

Any combination of vegetables will do. Try these:

2 cups broccoli flowerets
1 cup cauliflower flowerets
1 zucchini, sliced
5 spears asparagus
20 green beans
½ pound very thin sphaghetti
¼ cup chopped fresh parsley
2 cloves garlic

8 anchovy fillets
3 tablespoons olive oil
1 large tomato, coarsely chopped
1 sweet red pepper, coarsely chopped
10–15 snow peas
2 dried chili peppers or ½ teaspoon red pepper flakes

Steam broccoli, cauliflower, and zucchini until tender, and set aside.

Snap off the bottoms of the asparagus and boil for 1–2 minutes, until just tender. Set aside.

Submerge green beans in boiling water for 1–3 minutes, until just tender. Set aside.

While spaghetti is boiling (6 minutes), blend together parsley, garlic, anchovy fillets, and olive oil in a blender or food processor.

Drain spaghetti. Reserve 1 cup of water.

Stir anchovy sauce into spaghetti. If spaghetti is too dry, add a little water.

Stir in cooked vegetables, tomato, red pepper, and snow peas, until well covered with sauce.

Stir in red pepper flakes.

6 servings
Per serving: 260 Total calories; 11 Sat-fat calories

Q

PASTA MEXICALI

½ pound fancy pasta (fusilli,
   rigatoni, shells, etc.)
1 zucchini
½ cup chopped onion
2 teaspoons olive oil

1 teaspoon cumin
1 teaspoon chili powder
¼ teaspoon salt (optional)
1 red pepper, sliced
¼ cup tomato juice

Cook pasta according to package directions. Set aside.

Cut zucchini in quarters lengthwise. Slice into bite-size chunks.
Steam zucchini until just tender. Set aside.

In a small skillet, sauté onion in olive oil until soft.

Stir in cumin, chili powder, and salt.

Add onion mixture to pasta and mix well.

Add zucchini and red pepper. Add tomato juice and mix well.

Serve warm or at room temperature.

6 servings
Per serving: 168 Total calories; 3 Sat-fat calories

DAN-DAN NOODLES

½ pound fettuccine or linguine
1 teaspoon natural all-peanut
   peanut butter
2 teaspoons sesame oil
½ teaspoon minced garlic
½ teaspoon minced ginger root

½ teaspoon hot chili oil
2½ tablespoons white vinegar
1 teaspoon sugar
4 teaspoons soy sauce
2 green onions, chopped

Cook noodles according to package directions. Drain and re-frigerate.

Combine peanut butter and sesame oil until mixture is completely smooth.

Mix in garlic, ginger, chili oil, vinegar, sugar, and soy sauce. Pour sauce over noodles. Sprinkle green onions over the noodles and serve.

4 servings
Per serving: 252 Total calories; 5 Sat-fat calories

PASTA WITH PESTO

Pesto hails from Genova, Italy, where the salty soil makes the basil particularly wonderful. Even in the United States, pesto can be superb. It is easy to make and freezes well. This is the only recipe in this book that calls for hard cheese. If you don't have a food processor or blender, you can use a mortar and pestle.

2 cups fresh basil	2 tablespoons Parmesan cheese
3 cloves garlic	1 tablespoon Romano cheese
1 teaspoon salt	1 package (16 oz) very thin
3 tablespoons olive oil	spaghetti
2 tablespoons margarine	

Prepare basil by rinsing it and tearing off the leaves. Discard the stems.

Chop garlic in a food processor or blender.

Add basil and salt. Process.

Add olive oil. Process until smooth. At this point you can put pesto aside for later use or freeze.

When ready to serve, mix margarine into pesto with a fork and blend well.

Blend in cheeses. Set aside.

Make spaghetti according to package directions.

Drain, but reserve 1 cup of the cooking water.

Mix pesto into pasta. If pesto is too dry, carefully stir in a small amount of spaghetti water.

8 servings
Per serving: 313 Total calories; 17 Sat-fat calories

EASY SPAGHETTI SAUCE À LA SICILIA

Make a basic tomato sauce and add steamed eggplant and mushrooms for an appetizing spaghetti sauce that needs no ground meat.

1 small eggplant, peeled and cubed	2 cups sliced mushrooms
	12 ounces spaghetti
6 cups Basic Tomato Sauce (page 328) or Zesty Fresh Tomato Sauce (page 328)	

Prepare eggplant (see page 296) and steam until tender. Set aside.

In a medium saucepan, heat 6 cups of tomato sauce.

Stir in eggplant and mushrooms, cook 5 minutes more.

While spaghetti sauce is cooking, prepare spaghetti according to package directions.

Pour tomato sauce over spaghetti and serve.

6 servings
Per serving: 285 Total calories; 6 Sat-fat calories

BASIC TOMATO SAUCE

1 cup chopped onion	1 can (6 oz) tomato paste
1 tablespoon olive oil	2 teaspoons basil
4 large cans (28 oz each) tomatoes, drained	1 teaspoon salt

In a large saucepan, cook onion in olive oil until soft.

Chop tomatoes and add to onion.

Stir in tomato paste. (Tomatoes can easily be chopped and tomato paste blended in food processor.)

Stir in basil and salt.

Simmer until thick (at least 1 hour).

This tomato sauce freezes well.

Makes 8 cups
Per half-cup serving: 37 Total calories; 1 Sat-fat calorie

ZESTY FRESH TOMATO SAUCE

Fresh tomatoes make this sauce special. It's fragrant, tasty, and simple to make.

1 medium onion, sliced	$\frac{1}{2}$ teaspoon basil
2–3 cloves garlic, minced	$\frac{1}{2}$ teaspoon cumin
1 tablespoon olive oil	$\frac{1}{2}$–1 teaspoon red pepper flakes
$\frac{1}{2}$ cup chopped parsley	$\frac{1}{4}$–$\frac{1}{2}$ freshly ground black
4 cups chopped cherry tomatoes (or regular tomatoes)	pepper
$\frac{1}{2}$ teaspoon oregano	Salt to taste (optional)

In a large skillet, sauté onion and garlic in olive oil until soft. Lower heat to medium and stir in parsley.

Stir in tomatoes. Add oregano, basil, cumin, red pepper flakes, black pepper, and salt. Cook at medium heat, stirring occasionally, for about 10 minutes. Turn to low and let flavors blend for about 5–10 more minutes.

Makes 2½ cups (approximately)
Per half-cup serving: 64 Total calories; 3 Sat-fat calories

SPAGHETTI TOURAINE

1¼ pounds fresh tomatoes
4 cloves garlic, peeled
2 tablespoons olive oil
Salt to taste
1 tablespoon margarine
1 tablespoon minced carrot
1 tablespoon minced celery
1 tablespoon minced leek
1 tablespoon minced shallot
1 cup dry white wine or vermouth

Bouquet garni (2 parsley sprigs, ⅓ bay leaf, and ⅛ teaspoon thyme wrapped in cheese-cloth)
½ cup + 2 tablespoons evaporated skim milk
¼ teaspoon salt (optional)
1 tablespoon dried tarragon (or fresh, if available)
10 ounces spaghetti

Place tomatoes in a large saucepan of boiling water. Immediately pour out hot water and pour in cold water.

Peel tomatoes, cut them in half crosswise (not across the stem), squeeze out the seeds and juice, and coarsely chop.

In a medium skillet, cook tomatoes and garlic in olive oil until reduced to a thick sauce (about 20 minutes). Stir occasionally. Add salt.

Meanwhile, melt margarine in a small saucepan. Stir in carrot, celery, leek, and shallot.

Add wine and bouquet garni.

Reduce until thick and stir in evaporated skim milk.

Remove bouquet garni and pour mixture through a sieve to strain out the vegetables. Add tarragon.

Mix with tomato sauce and pour over pasta.

4 servings
Per serving: 208 Total calories; 13 Sat-fat calories

Ⓠ RICE PILAU WITH APRICOTS AND RAISINS

3 tablespoons slivered almonds
1 tablespoon margarine
1 teaspoon minced ginger root
1 clove garlic, minced
¼ cup chopped onion
1 teaspoon salt (optional)
2 whole cloves

½ cinnamon stick
1 teaspoon turmeric
1½ cups long-grain rice
3¾ cups water
¼ cup apricots, sliced
2 tablespoons raisins

In a medium casserole, sauté slivered almonds in margarine over medium heat until golden.

Add ginger, garlic, and onion and sauté until soft.

Mix in salt, cloves, cinnamon stick, and turmeric.

Add rice and stir until well coated.

Add water and bring to a boil. Cover, reduce heat to low (or off), and cook until water is absorbed (about 25 minutes).

Mix in apricots and raisins.

Makes 14 half-cup servings
Per serving: 100 Total calories; 3 Sat-fat calories

Q OLIVE-ARTICHOKE RICE

3¾ cups water
1½ cups long-grain rice
½ teaspoon salt (optional)
3 tablespoons olive oil
1 tin (2 oz) anchovies (omit if
   you hate anchovies)

1 red pepper, sliced
½ cup artichoke hearts, diced
12 pitted black olives, sliced

In a medium saucepan, bring water to a boil.

Add rice and salt, cover, reduce heat to low, and cook for 25 minutes or until all water is absorbed.

Mix in remaining ingredients and cool to lukewarm.

Makes 14 half-cup servings
Per serving: 105 Total calories; 5 Sat-fat calories

Q INDIAN RICE

1 tablespoon olive oil
2 cloves garlic, minced
1 tablespoon minced ginger root
¾ cup chopped onion
¼ teaspoon cardamom
¼ teaspoon caraway seeds

1 teaspoon coriander
¼ teaspoon cinnamon
¼ teaspoon ground cloves
¼ teaspoon salt (optional)
1½ cups long-grain rice
3¾ cups water

In a medium saucepan, heat olive oil.

Add garlic, ginger, and onion and cook until soft.

Mix in cardamom, caraway seeds, coriander, cinnamon, cloves, salt, and rice and blend well.

Add water, cover, and bring to a boil. Reduce heat and cook until all water is absorbed (about 25 minutes).

Makes 12 half-cup servings
Per serving: 97 Total calories; 2 Sat-fat calories

Q
LEMON RICE WITH SPINACH
AND RED PEPPER

⅓ cup chopped onion
2 teaspoons olive oil
1 cup long-grain rice
½ teaspoon salt (optional)
2½ cups water

1 cup chopped spinach
2 tablespoons fresh lemon juice
1 red pepper, chopped (about ½ cup)

In a medium saucepan, sauté onion in olive oil until soft.

Mix in the rice and salt. Add water and bring to a boil. Reduce heat to low or off and cover saucepan.

After 15 minutes, stir spinach and lemon juice into rice.

Cook for 10 minutes more or until liquid is completely absorbed.

Mix in red pepper and serve.

Makes 8 half-cup servings
Per serving: 95 Total calories; 1 Sat-fat calorie

Q
FRIED RICE

2 egg whites
½ egg yolk
1 tablespoon + 1 teaspoon olive oil
3 green onions, cut into ¼-inch pieces

3 cups boiled rice (cold)
1 tablespoon soy sauce
¼ teaspoon sugar
¼ cup cooked diced chicken, shrimp, turkey, or combination

Beat egg whites and yolk together.

In a small skillet, scramble eggs in 1 tablespoon of the olive oil. Set aside.

In a large skillet, sauté green onions in the remaining teaspoon oil.

Add rice and mix thoroughly.

Stir in soy sauce and sugar.

Stir in eggs and meat.

Makes 6 one-half cup servings
Per serving: 167 Total calories; 6 Sat-fat calories

Q BULGUR WITH TOMATOES AND OLIVES

1 cup bulgur (cracked wheat)
2 tablespoons margarine
1 cup tomato juice
1 cup water

1 tomato, chopped
¼ cup sliced green olives
2 stalks celery, chopped
3 green onions, sliced

In a large skillet, sauté bulgur in margarine until bulgur begins to color and crackle.

Add tomato juice, water, and tomato and simmer until most liquid is absorbed (about 35 minutes).

Add olives, celery, and green onions and mix until heated through.

Makes 9 half-cup servings
Per serving: 79 Total calories; 2 Sat-fat calories

Q BARLEY PLUS

An interesting alternative to rice.

¾ cup chopped onion
½ cup chopped mushrooms
1 tablespoon olive oil
1 cup pearl barley, rinsed

1 can (10¾ oz) chicken broth, strained
½ teaspoon salt (optional)

Sauté onion and mushrooms in olive oil until tender. Stir in barley.

Add 1 cup of the chicken broth plus salt and bring to a boil. Cover and simmer for 25 minutes.

Add remaining broth plus water to equal 1 cup. Cook 25 more minutes until liquid is absorbed.

Fluff barley with a fork before serving.

6 servings
Per serving: 157 Total calories; 4 Sat-fat calories

21 SALADS

S ALADS ARE refreshing. They can be quite nutritious and add texture and bulk to a meal. Salads by themselves generally contain very little fat. But beware of high-fat salad dressings! These culprits turn many a healthy salad into a fat-calorie extravaganza.

Gourmet food shops specialize in a variety of salads — pasta salad, rice salad, chicken, turkey, and fish salads. Here are a few you can make yourself and eat without hesitation.

Q TARRAGON-RAISIN CHICKEN SALAD

4 boned and skinned chicken breast halves
½ teaspoon salt
1 small onion
1 small carrot
4 whole peppercorns

2 tablespoons reduced-calorie mayonnaise
2 tablespoons nonfat yogurt
2 teaspoons tarragon
2 tablespoons golden raisins

In a medium saucepan, combine chicken, salt, onion, carrot, and peppercorns. Add water to cover and bring to a boil.
Reduce heat and simmer until chicken is cooked through.
Strain broth. (Freeze for future use.)
Cut chicken into large chunks and set aside.
Combine mayonnaise, yogurt, tarragon, and raisins.
Add to chicken and mix until chicken is well coated.

4 servings
Per serving: 180 Total calories; 12 Sat-fat calories

�926 CORIANDER CHICKEN SALAD

6 boned and skinned chicken breast halves	¼ teaspoon coriander
1 carrot	2 cups broccoli flowerets
2 cloves garlic	2 tablespoons reduced-calorie mayonnaise
1 bay leaf	2 tablespoons nonfat yogurt
½ teaspoon salt (optional)	2 teaspoons Dijon mustard

In a medium saucepan, combine chicken, carrot, garlic, bay leaf, and salt. Add water to cover and cook at slow boil until chicken breasts are completely cooked.

Strain broth and freeze for future use.

Cut chicken into large chunks, mix with coriander, and set aside to cool.

Steam broccoli until just tender.

Combine salad dressing, yogurt, and mustard.

Mix mustard-yogurt dressing with chicken.

Stir in broccoli until coated with dressing.

8 servings
Per serving: 90 Total calories; 12 Sat-fat calories

�926 CHICKEN SALAD WITH SHALLOTS AND MUSHROOMS

4 boned and skinned chicken breast halves	2 teaspoons minced shallot
2 tablespoons olive oil	1 cup sliced mushrooms
2 tablespoons white vinegar	1 teaspoon thyme
	¼ teaspoon salt (optional)

Cook chicken as in Tarragon-Raisin Chicken Salad (page 334).

Combine remaining ingredients and pour over chicken.

Mix until chicken is well coated.

6 servings
Per serving: 140 Total calories; 11 Sat-fat calories

Q DIJON CHICKEN-RICE SALAD

3¾ cups water
1½ cups long-grain rice
½ teaspoon salt (optional)
2 tablespoons Dijon mustard
2 tablespoons white vinegar
3 tablespoons olive oil

½–1 cup diced green and/or red
  pepper
¼ cup pitted black olives, sliced
¼ cup sliced green onion
2 cooked chicken breast halves,
  diced

In a medium saucepan, bring water to a boil.

Add rice and salt, reduce heat, cover, and simmer for 20–25 minutes or until water is absorbed.

Place rice in a bowl.

Combine mustard, vinegar, and olive oil and mix into rice.

Add green pepper, olives, green onion, and chicken and mix well. Tastes best when tepid.

6 servings
Per serving: 285 Total calories; 12 Sat-fat calories

Q ORIENTAL CHICKEN SALAD

4 boned and skinned chicken
  breast halves
1 carrot
¼ small onion
1 head broccoli, cut into
  flowerets (about 3 cups)
3 tablespoons walnut oil

3 tablespoons soy sauce
1 tablespoon dry vermouth
2 teaspoons minced ginger root
¼ cup chopped walnuts
½ pound mushrooms, sliced
1 head red-leaf or Boston
  lettuce

In a large pot, combine chicken, carrot, and onion. Cover with water and boil until chicken is cooked through.

Cut chicken into bite-size pieces. Set aside.

Steam broccoli flowerets until *just* tender.

Combine walnut oil, soy sauce, and ginger in a large bowl.

Add walnuts, mushrooms, and chicken and mix until all are coated with sauce. Stir in broccoli.

Place some lettuce on each salad plate. Top with chicken salad.

4 servings
Per serving: 325 Total calories; 20 Sat-fat calories

▣ CURRIED TUNA SALAD WITH PEARS

3 tablespoons reduced-calorie
  mayonnaise
1½ tablespoons nonfat yogurt
¾–1 teaspoon curry powder

2 cans (6½ oz each) water-
  packed tuna, drained
3 tablespoons diced pear
Lettuce

Combine mayonnaise, yogurt, and curry powder.
Mix into tuna fish.
Stir in pear.
Serve over lettuce.

3 servings
Per serving: 220 Total calories; 11 Sat-fat calories

SALADE NIÇOISE

A salad that is a meal in itself. Our Salade Niçoise is just like those
served on the Riviera, but the egg yolks have been removed. .

Dressing

1 clove garlic, minced
Juice of ½ lemon (about 2
  tablespoons)
2 tablespoons white vinegar

1 tablespoon Dijon mustard
1 teaspoon basil
½ teaspoon salt (optional)
½ cup olive oil

Salad

4 potatoes
3 cups green beans, tips
  removed and cut in half
1 medium head red-leaf or
  Boston lettuce, shredded
4 tomatoes, cut into eighths

Whites from 3 hard-boiled eggs
¼ cup pitted black olives
2 tablespoons capers
1 tin (2 oz) anchovy fillets
1 can (6½ oz) water-packed
  solid white tuna, drained

Combine all dressing ingredients in a jar and shake vigorously. Set
aside.
Steam potatoes until tender, peel, and cut into bite-size pieces.
Mix potatoes with ¼ cup dressing and set aside.
Cook green beans in boiling water for 5 minutes or until just ten-
der and bright green.

Mix green beans with 2 tablespoons dressing and set aside.

Put lettuce and tomatoes in a large salad bowl and toss them with the remaining dressing.

Add potatoes, green beans, egg whites, olives, capers, anchovies, and drained tuna and mix until well coated with dressing. Traditionally each vegetable is segregated on a plate. We prefer them mixed into the salad.

10 servings
Per serving: 195 Total calories; 11 Sat-fat calories

INDONESIAN VEGETABLE SALAD

2 cups shredded lettuce or
   Chinese celery cabbage
1 cup sliced carrot
1 cup green beans, cooked in
   boiling water until just tender

2 tomatoes, sliced
1 cucumber, peeled and sliced

Dressing

1 tablespoon sliced green onion
½ tablespoon olive oil
4 tablespoons natural all-peanut
   peanut butter
1 clove garlic, minced
½ teaspoon red pepper flakes

1 bay leaf
1 slice lemon
1 teaspoon sugar
½ teaspoon salt
¾ cup skim milk
2 tablespoons water

Place lettuce on a platter.

Artistically arrange carrots, green beans, tomatoes, and cucumber over lettuce. Cover with plastic wrap and chill in refrigerator.

In a small saucepan, sauté green onion in olive oil.

Mix in peanut butter, garlic, red pepper flakes, bay leaf, lemon, sugar, and salt until peanut butter starts to melt.

Gradually blend in skim milk. Cook over low heat, stirring constantly, until thick. Chill dressing.

Before serving, dilute dressing with water, if necessary.

Pass platter and dressing separately so everyone can take what they want.

Salad
6 servings
Per serving: 32 Total calories; 0 Sat-fat calories

Dressing
Makes ¾ cup
Per tablespoon: 43 Total calories; 5 Sat-fat calories

TABBOULI

1 cup bulgur (cracked wheat)
3 cups boiling water
1 can (15 oz) chickpeas, drained
¼ cup fresh mint, minced, or ½ teaspoon dried mint
1 teaspoon oregano
½ teaspoon salt (optional)
¼ teaspoon freshly ground pepper

2 cloves garlic, minced
1 small onion, chopped
½ cup chopped green pepper
2 medium tomatoes, chopped
2 tablespoons olive oil
2 tablespoons fresh lemon juice
¼ cup chopped parsley

Place bulgur in a large bowl and cover with boiling water.

Let stand for about 1 hour or until fluffy. Squeeze out excess water.

Combine bulgur with remaining ingredients.

Chill for at least 1 hour.

Makes 10 half-cup servings
Per serving: 135 Total calories; 5 Sat-fat calories

CUCUMBER SALAD

Q

2 cucumbers, peeled and sliced
thin
1 medium onion, sliced thin
½ teaspoon salt (optional)

1 teaspoon sugar
1 teaspoon dill weed
1 cup white vinegar

Mix cucumbers and onion together in a ceramic or glass bowl.
Add salt, sugar, and dill weed to vinegar and pour over cucumbers
and onion.
Chill 1 hour.

6 servings
Per serving: 20 Total calories; 0 Sat-fat calories

EASTERN SPINACH SALAD

Q

1 package (10 oz) fresh spinach,
washed and shredded
10 water chestnuts, sliced
3 green onions, sliced
1 cup sliced mushrooms
1 cucumber, peeled and sliced
thin

1 tablespoon olive oil
2 tablespoons soy sauce
3 tablespoons fresh lemon juice
1½ tablespoons honey
1 tablespoon sesame seeds,
toasted

In a salad bowl, combine spinach, water chestnuts, green onions,
mushrooms, and cucumber slices.
Mix together olive oil, soy sauce, lemon juice, and honey and pour
over salad.
Sprinkle with sesame seeds.

8 servings
Per serving: 55 Total calories; 3 Sat-fat calories

POTATO SALAD

Q

4–5 Russet (red) potatoes
½ cup nonfat yogurt
3 tablespoons reduced-calorie
mayonnaise

1 teaspoon tarragon
1 tablespoon white vinegar
1 teaspoon Dijon mustard
½ teaspoon salt (optional)

Scrub potatoes thoroughly. Steam until tender.
Meanwhile, combine remaining ingredients. Set aside.
Cut potatoes into chunks (do not remove skin).
Pour sauce over potatoes so they are thoroughly coated.
Serve warm or cold.

6 servings
Per serving: 105 Total calories; 5 Sat-fat calories

☒ FRUIT SALAD WITH COTTAGE CHEESE OR YOGURT

This high-protein, low-fat dish makes a filling lunch. Round it off
with a piece of Honey Whole-Wheat Bread (page 360) and, for dessert, air-popped popcorn.

Spring or Summer Fruits

¼ cantaloupe   1 peach
½ cup blueberries   ⅙ honeydew melon

Fall or Winter Fruits

½ Golden Delicious apple   ½ Bosc pear
1 kiwi fruit   ½ orange

½ cup low-fat (1%) cottage
   cheese or nonfat yogurt

Cut fruit into bite-size pieces and place in bowl.
Mix in cottage cheese or yogurt.

Serves 1

	Total calories	Sat-fat calories
Spring or summer salad:		
with cottage cheese	280	7
with nonfat yogurt	250	0
Fall or winter salad:		
with cottage cheese	270	7
with nonfat yogurt	245	0

22 SANDWICHES, DIPS, AND A DRINK

SOUR CREAM need not be the basis for your dips and sandwich spreads. Sour cream has 270 sat-fat calories per cup. In its place, use nonfat or low-fat yogurt, tofu, eggplant, chickpeas, or cottage cheese for delicious, low-fat dips and spreads.

▣ TOFU (MOCK EGG SALAD) SANDWICH

Fresh tofu is available at Oriental food stores, health food stores, and even some supermarkets. Tofu (bean curd) is an excellent source of protein. Although it has a negligible amount of saturated fat, it is surprisingly high in total fat and thus should be eaten with thought. Store tofu in water in a covered container in the refrigerator. Change the water daily to keep tofu fresh for up to a week.

1 cake fresh tofu (about 3 × 3 × 1¼ inches)
1 tablespoon reduced-calorie mayonnaise
½–1 teaspoon curry powder
1 green onion, sliced
½ tomato, chopped
2 six-inch whole-wheat pita bread pockets

In a small bowl, break up tofu with a fork.
Mix in mayonnaise, curry powder, green onions, and tomatoes.
Spoon tofu spread into pita bread pockets.

Makes 2 sandwiches

Double the amount of ingredients and use tofu spread as a dip with fresh raw vegetables.

Makes about 2 cups

	Total calories	Sat-fat calories
Per sandwich	150	9
Per tablespoon	9	1

Q BABA GHANOUSH

1 medium eggplant
¼ cup or more fresh lemon
  juice
3 tablespoons tahini (sesame
  seed paste)*

1–2 cloves garlic
¼ cup chopped parsley
Salt to taste

Peel eggplant, cut into bite-size pieces, and salt heavily. Set aside for 15 minutes. Rinse and squeeze eggplant and steam in vegetable steamer until soft.

Purée eggplant in food processor or blender.

Blend in lemon juice and tahini.

Just before you serve, crush garlic into purée and mix in parsley and salt.

Taste. Add more lemon juice if you wish.

Serve with whole-wheat or plain pita bread cut into pieces.

Makes about 2 cups
Per tablespoon: 12 Total calories; 1 Sat-fat calorie

Q CHICKPEA SANDWICH OR DIP

1 can chickpeas
2 cloves garlic
⅓ cup parsley
1 tablespoon tahini (sesame
  seed paste)*
Juice of 1 lemon (about ¼ cup)

4 six-inch whole-wheat pita
  bread pockets
Chopped tomatoes, green
  onions, and lettuce, for
  garnish

---

*Available at Mideast food shops and many supermarkets

Drain chickpeas. Reserve liquid. In blender or food processor, chop garlic and parsley.

Add chickpeas, tahini, and lemon juice.

Blend until smooth, adding more chickpea liquid if spread is too stiff.

Make sandwiches by spooning chickpea spread into pita bread pockets.

Garnish with chopped tomatoes, green onions, and lettuce.

Makes 4 sandwiches

Use as a dip for vegetables, crackers, squares of pita, etc.

Makes about 1½ cups

	Total calories	Sat-fat calories
Per sandwich	195	4
Per tablespoon	20	1

EGGPLANT APPETIZER

A tasty appetizer. Eat with quartered pita bread or crackers or heat and serve as a vegetable.

4 cups peeled, cubed eggplant	½ cup Spanish olives
½ cup chopped onion	½ cup black olives
4 cloves garlic, minced	2 teaspoons capers
2 stalks celery, sliced	2 teaspoons brown sugar
1 tablespoon olive oil	2 tablespoons white vinegar

Salt eggplant heavily and set aside for 15 minutes.

Rinse salt off eggplant under running water while squeezing out bitter juices.

Steam eggplant until tender.

Taste. If not bitter, set aside. If bitter, find a recipe without eggplant!

Sauté onion, garlic, and celery in olive oil until soft.

Mix in eggplant, olives, capers, brown sugar, and vinegar and heat until warm.

Eat hot, at room temperature, or chilled.

10 servings
Per serving: 46 Total calories; 6 Sat-fat calories

YOGURT CHEESE

Yogurt cheese made with nonfat yogurt may be substituted for sour cream and cream cheese in some recipes, greatly reducing the sat-fat and total fat calories. It is easy to make. Place nonfat yogurt (without gelatin) in a coffee filter (or cheesecloth) in a coffeepot or in a strainer over a bowl. Cover and refrigerate overnight. As the yogurt drains, it condenses. About half the yogurt will become cheese. Pour off whey and keep cheese in a covered container in the refrigerator. Add herbs, green onions, or Dijon mustard to make a flavored cheese.

Per tablespoon: 7 Total calories; 0 Sat-fat calories

FAUX GUACAMOLE

You guests will never imagine that the dip they are eagerly devouring was made with asparagus. What a buy. A great-tasting treat at a cost of 0 sat-fat and 0 total fat calories.

2 tablespoons yogurt cheese*	1 tablespoon fresh lemon juice
1 pound asparagus	2 ounces diced green chili
1 clove garlic, crushed	peppers**
¼ teaspoon cayenne pepper	1 cup chopped tomatoes
¼ teaspoon chili powder	1 tablespoon chopped onion
	Whole-wheat pita bread

Prepare yogurt cheese a day in advance (see box).

Snap off the bottom ends of the asparagus and discard. Find a frying pan that will hold the asparagus in one layer and fill it with an inch of water. Bring the water to a boil and add the asparagus. Cook until soft. Drain asparagus and purée with garlic in blender or food processor.

---

*See box above.
**Available in small cans in most supermarkets

Mix in cayenne pepper, chili powder, lemon juice, yogurt cheese, chili peppers, tomatoes, and onion. Chill for several hours.

Serve with toasted whole-wheat pita pockets divided into quarters or Bagel Chips (recipe follows).

Makes 1½ cups (approximately)

	Total calories	Sat-fat calories
Per tablespoon	7	0
With pita bread quarter	33	0

BAGEL CHIPS

A great crunchy snack — eat them alone or with dips.

Bagels (plain, onion, garlic, etc.)

Flavor Options

| 1 clove garlic | Cajun Spice Mix (page 247) |
| Chili powder | Cinnamon and sugar |

Preheat oven to 200°F.

Cut bagel into ¼–⅜-inch-thick slices. They will look like very thin bagels. (Halve or quarter slices if you want smaller bagel chips.) Place pieces on cookie sheet on one layer.

Either press garlic and spread over bagel slices, sprinkle chili powder or spice mix over them, leave them plain, or for a sweet treat, sprinkle on a mix of cinnamon and sugar.

Bake for 1–2 hours.

Per bagel chip: 38 Total calories; 0 Sat-fat calories

VEGEBURGERS

For those who crave hamburgers but do not want the saturated fat they contain, Vegeburgers are a meatless substitute. Worthington Foods sells a soy product called GranBurger. It may be used to make Vegeburgers, spaghetti sauce, soup — any food that calls for hamburger meat.

1 ⅓ cups hot water
1 ⅔ cups GranBurger
¼ cup chopped onion
2 tablespoons unbleached white flour
1 cup bread crumbs made from 2 slices bread

½ teaspoon salt
¼ teaspoon poultry seasoning
1 egg
2 egg whites
2 tablespoons skim milk
2 tablespoons olive oil

Add hot water to GranBurger and let sit for 3–5 minutes.

Stir in onion, flour, bread crumbs, salt, and poultry seasoning.

Beat together egg, egg whites, and skim milk and mix into GranBurger mixture.

Form patties. They will probably fall apart, so handle with care.

Heat olive oil in large frying pan.

Fry as with hamburgers.

Makes about 10 burgers
Per burger: 73 Total calories; 3 Sat-fat calories

FROTHY FRUIT SHAKE

Use your imagination and the fruit you have in the house to create refreshing fruit shakes of different flavors. Here's one example:

1 cup strawberries
1 ripe banana, peeled and quartered
1 orange, peeled and halved

Dash of salt (optional)
½ cup crushed ice or 4–5 ice cubes

Place fruit and salt in a blender and purée.

Combine purée with ½ cup of finely crushed ice. You can make crushed ice by placing ice cubes in a plastic bag and smashing them with a meat-tenderizing mallet or hammer until crushed evenly. You can also crush ice in an electric ice-crusher. You may add ice cubes to the purée in the blender and blend until cubes are crushed.

Makes 2 one-cup servings.
Per Serving: 105 Total calories; 0 Sat-fat calories

BREADS   23

STARCHES HAVE received bad press over the years. Bread, rice, pasta, and potatoes have been associated with weight gain. Weight problems begin not with starch but with the fat that is put on the starch: bread slathered with margarine, potatoes stuffed with sour cream. An ounce of carbohydrate has less than *half* as many calories as an ounce of fat. An average piece of bread has 9 fat calories. Cover it with margarine and the fat calorie value goes up to 109. And, of course, the saturated fat content also rises.

You can cut down on saturated fats and cholesterol by replacing fatty meats and high-fat dairy products with grains, potatoes, breads, and pasta. Many starchy foods (such as whole grains and potatoes with skin) provide fiber, bulk, vitamins, and minerals.

Many of the following recipes are for 1 loaf so that you can make them in your food processor. Double ingredients for 2 loaves.

You can make any loaf into baguettes by following the portion of the recipe for French Bread, page 352, beginning with "Divide dough in half."

We have chosen to use olive oil in baking most of our breads because olive oil lowers LDL-cholesterol without lowering HDL-cholesterol, as well as preventing the oxidation of LDL-cholesterol — the first step in the process of atherosclerosis. Choose a mild-tasting olive oil, and your taste buds won't notice the difference.

NOTE: The instruction "Let proof" means to wait for the yeast to ferment, swell, and get bubbly. This takes only a few minutes at most.

SHAKER DAILY LOAF

1 tablespoon active dry yeast
Pinch of sugar
¼ cup warm water
6 cups unbleached white flour
(approximately)

2¼ cups skim milk
2 tablespoons margarine
2 tablespoons maple syrup or
honey
2 teaspoons salt

Dissolve yeast and sugar in the warm water in a large bowl or a food processor. Let proof (become bubbly).

Mix in 3 cups of the flour.

In a small saucepan, scald skim milk. Remove from heat.

Add margarine, maple syrup, and salt to milk and mix until margarine melts.

When liquid has cooled to lukewarm, add to flour in bowl.

Stir in more flour, ½ cup at a time, until dough is fairly stiff.

Knead dough 10 minutes or process 15 seconds or until dough is smooth and elastic.

Place dough in a large oiled bowl, cover with a towel, and let rise in a warm place for 1 hour or until doubled in bulk.

Remove dough from bowl and divide it in half.

Let dough rest, covered, for 10 minutes.

Roll into two loaves and place in loaf pans greased with margarine.

Cover and let rise until doubled (1–2 hours).

Preheat oven to 350°F.

Bake loaves for 35–40 minutes or until they are golden brown and sound hollow when tapped.

Makes 2 loaves

	Total calories	*Sat-fat calories*
Per ½-inch slice	90	2
Per loaf	1512	28

CARDAMOM BREAD

1 tablespoon active dry yeast
2 tablespoons brown sugar
¼ cup warm water
2–4 cups unbleached white
  flour

1 teaspoon salt
¼–½ teaspoon cardamom*
2 tablespoons olive oil
1 cup skim milk

Combine yeast, brown sugar, and water in a large bowl or a food processor. Let proof.

Add 2 cups flour, salt, and cardamom and mix.

Mix in olive oil and skim milk. Add more flour until you produce a stiff dough.

Knead dough 10 minutes or process 15 seconds or until dough is smooth and elastic, adding more flour if necessary.

Place dough in a large oiled bowl, cover with a towel, and let rise in warm place for 1 hour or until doubled in bulk.

Roll into loaf and place in loaf pan greased with margarine.

Cover with a towel and let rise for 1 hour or until doubled in bulk.

Preheat oven to 425°F.

Bake loaves for 10 minutes.

Reduce heat to 350°F and bake for 30 minutes more or until loaves are golden brown and sound hollow when tapped.

Makes 1 loaf

	Total calories	Sat-fat calories
Per ½-inch slice	98	2
Per loaf	1663	41

*For a totally different taste, substitute 1 teaspoon cinnamon.

FRENCH BREAD I

A French bread of peasant stock. Give yourself a treat and eat it warm, straight from the oven. It also freezes well. Make smaller loaves for submarine sandwiches. Any bread is an impressive gift to bring to friends. And this bread is so easy you'll be embarrassed to answer yes when asked if you made it yourself.

1½ tablespoons active dry yeast	1 teaspoon salt
½ teaspoon sugar	2 tablespoons olive oil
¼ cup warm water	1 cup water
2–3 cups unbleached white flour	

Place yeast, sugar, and ¼ cup very warm, but *not hot*, water in a large bowl or a food processor. Let proof.

Mix in 2 cups flour and the salt.

Add olive oil and 1 cup water to flour and knead dough 10 minutes or process 15 seconds or until dough is smooth and elastic, adding more flour if necessary.

Place dough in large oiled bowl, cover with a towel, and let rise in a warm place for 1 hour or until doubled in bulk.

Divide dough in half.

Roll each half into a rectangle. Fold over in thirds like this:

1.   2.   3.

Press the edge into the dough after each fold.

Put into greased (with margarine) French bread pan that looks like this:

Cover and let rise for about 1 hour, or until doubled in bulk.
After 50 minutes, preheat oven to 450°F.
Uncover bread and slash with parallel or diagonal lines like this:

Place bread pan in oven on a diagonal to the right. Put 4 ice cubes in the bottom of the oven to create steam for crustier loaves.

In 5 minutes, add 4 more ice cubes.

In 10 minutes, shift pan so it is on a diagonal to the left, like this:

Reduce heat to 400°F and bake for 10 minutes more or until golden brown. Take loaves out of pan and cool or eat immediately.

Freezes nicely. If thawed, slice *before* reheating. Thawed French bread flakes like crazy when cut after reheating.

Makes 2 baguettes

	Total calories	Sat-fat calories
Per ½-inch slice	87	2
Per baguette	874	19

FRENCH BREAD II

There is almost nothing more satisfying and delicious than eating freshly baked bread hot from the oven — particularly French Bread II. This French bread is lighter than French Bread I. It takes a long time to rise, but it's worth the wait.

1 tablespoon active dry yeast	4+ cups unbleached white flour
1 tablespoon sugar	1–1½ teaspoons salt
⅓ cup warm water	1¼ cups water

Place yeast, sugar, and ⅓ cup warm water in large bowl or bowl of food processor and let proof.

Mix in 4 cups of flour and salt.

Add 1¼ cups water and knead dough 10 minutes or process about 15 seconds. Keep adding flour until dough is smooth and elastic.

Make dough into a ball and place in an oiled bowl approximately twice the size of the dough so you'll be able to see when the dough is doubled in size. Cover with a damp dish towel.

Place bowl in a warm place (on top of the refrigerator is often a nice, warm spot) and let rise until doubled in size. The dough will swell above the edge of the bowl. This will take at least 1½ hours.

When the dough has doubled in bulk, punch it down and knead it a few times. Let it rest a few minutes. If you have two French bread pans, which together hold 4 loaves, divide the bread into 4 equal pieces. If you have one French bread pan that holds 2 loaves, divide the dough in half, then divide one of the halves in half again. You will make 2 baguettes with the smaller pieces of dough and 1 round loaf with the larger piece.

For the baguettes: Grease the bread pan with margarine. Flatten the dough into an oval. Squeeze the dough into a long, thin rope with a diameter of about 1½ inches. Roll the dough with the palms of both of your hands (to resemble the clay coils you made as a kid) to lengthen and smooth it. Place in bread pan.

For the round bread: Grease the bottom of an 8-inch cake pan with margarine. Form a ball by folding the edges of the dough under itself. Place in cake pan.

Cover bread with towel and let rise until baguette dough fills out the bread pan.

When bread has completed its second rise (about 1½ hours), pre-heat oven to 450°F. Make 3 diagonal slashes in the baguettes, about

⅛–⅜ inches deep. In the round bread, make a 4-inch slash through the center of the top. Make another slash through the center perpendicular to the first slash.

Place bread pans in the oven. You will probably have to use 2 shelves or 2 ovens. Put 4 ice cubes on the oven floor to make the loaves crusty. Bake for 5 minutes. Add 4 more ice cubes. Bake for 5 more minutes. Shift the direction of the bread pans (see drawings on page 353) and bake for 10 more minutes or until golden brown.

Makes 4 baguettes or 2 baguettes and 1 round loaf

	Total calories	Sat-fat calories
Per baguette	471	2
Per 1½-inch slice	52	0
Per round loaf	942	4
Per ½-inch slice	94	0

BUTTERMILK HERB BREAD

1 tablespoon active dry yeast	¼ teaspoon marjoram
2 tablespoons sugar	¼ teaspoon oregano
¼ cup warm water	¼ teaspoon thyme
2–3 cups unbleached white flour	3 tablespoons margarine
	½ cup buttermilk
1 teaspoon salt	1 egg

Place yeast, sugar, and water in a large bowl or in your food processor. Let proof.

Mix in 2 cups flour, salt, marjoram, oregano, and thyme.

In a small saucepan, melt margarine. Add buttermilk. If liquid is cool, heat until warm but *not too hot.*

Add liquid to the flour. (If using a food processor, process at least 15 seconds.)

Mix in enough flour to make a stiff but soft dough.

Add egg. Knead dough 10 minutes or process 15 seconds or until dough is smooth and elastic.

Put dough in a large oiled bowl, cover with a towel, and let rise in a warm place for 1 hour or until doubled in bulk.

Form loaf and place in loaf pan greased with margarine. Cover and let rise 1 hour or until doubled in bulk.

Preheat oven to 375°F.

Bake loaf for about 35 minutes or until it is golden brown and sounds hollow when tapped.

Makes 1 loaf

	Total calories	Sat-fat calories
Per ½-inch slice	110	4
Per loaf	1874	75

GINGER-ORANGE BREAD

A very subtle taste of ginger pervades this whole-wheat bread.

1 tablespoon active dry yeast
2 tablespoons brown sugar
¼ cup warm water
1½ cups whole-wheat flour
1½ cups unbleached white flour
  (approximately)

1 teaspoon salt
2 teaspoons ground ginger
2 tablespoons olive oil
½ cup buttermilk
½ cup orange juice

Combine yeast, brown sugar, and warm water in a large bowl or a food processor. Let proof.

Mix in whole-wheat flour, white flour, salt, and ginger.

Add olive oil, buttermilk, and orange juice. Knead 10 minutes or process 15 seconds or until dough is smooth and elastic, adding more flour if necessary.

Place dough in a large oiled bowl, cover with a towel, and let rise in a warm place for 1 hour or until doubled in bulk.

Shape into a loaf and place in a loaf pan greased with margarine.

Cover with a towel and let rise in warm place for about 1 hour or until doubled in bulk.

Preheat oven to 400°F.

Bake loaf for 10 minutes.

Reduce heat to 350°F and bake for 30 minutes more or until golden brown.

Makes 1 loaf

	Total calories	Sat-fat calories
Per ½-inch slice	99	3
Per loaf	1678	46

CHALLAH

A delicious bread for the Jewish Sabbath or just for enjoyable eating.

1 tablespoon active dry yeast	½ teaspoon salt
2 tablespoons sugar	2 tablespoons olive oil
1 cup warm water	1 egg
2–4 cups unbleached white flour	

Place yeast, sugar, and ¼ cup warm water in a large bowl or a food processor. Let proof.

Mix in 2 cups flour and salt.

Add ¾ cup warm water, oil, and egg and mix or process for 15 seconds.

Knead dough 10 minutes or process 15 seconds or until dough is smooth and elastic, adding more flour if necessary.

Place dough in a large oiled bowl, cover with a towel, and let rise in warm place for 1 hour or until doubled in bulk.

Divide dough into two unequal portions, one-third and two-thirds.

Divide the smaller portion of the dough into three pieces. Roll each into a rope.

Divide the larger portion into three pieces. Roll each into a rope.

Braid the three larger ropes and place them on a greased cookie sheet.

Braid the three smaller ropes and place them on top of the larger braided pieces. Pinch the two together.

Cover with a towel and let rise for 1 hour or until doubled in bulk.

Preheat oven to 400°F.

Bake bread for 10 minutes.

Reduce heat to 375°F and bake for 30 minutes more or until golden brown.

Makes 1 large loaf or 2 small loaves

	Total calories	Sat-fat calories
Per ½-inch slice	70	2
Per loaf	1670	47

ANADAMA BREAD

This version of the New England bread has whole-wheat flour added to it to make it healthier while retaining its wonderful taste and texture.

1 tablespoon active dry yeast	1–1½ teaspoons salt
Pinch of sugar	2 tablespoons olive oil
¼ cup warm water	1 cup water
¾ cup corn meal	3 tablespoons molasses
1½ cups whole-wheat flour	
1½ cups unbleached white flour (approximately)	

Dissolve yeast with pinch of sugar in ¼ cup warm water in a large bowl or a food processor. Let proof.

Mix in corn meal, whole-wheat flour, 1 cup of the white flour, and salt.

Stir in olive oil, 1 cup water, and molasses.

Knead dough 10 minutes or process 15 seconds or until dough is smooth and elastic, adding more white flour if necessary.

Place dough in a large oiled bowl, cover with a towel, and let rise in a warm place for 1 hour or until doubled in bulk.

Form into a loaf and place in a loaf pan greased with margarine. Cover and let rise for 1 hour or until doubled in bulk.

Preheat oven to 400°F.

Bake loaf for 15 minutes.

Reduce heat to 350°F and bake about 30 minutes more or until loaf is golden brown and sounds hollow when tapped.

Makes 1 loaf

	Total calories	Sat-fat calories
Per ½-inch slice	113	2
Per loaf	1919	42

PEANUT BUTTER BREAD

A bread with a subtle peanut buttery taste and aroma.

1 tablespoon active dry yeast
2 tablespoons sugar
¼ cup warm water
2 cups whole-wheat flour
2½ cups unbleached white flour
  (approximately)

2 teaspoons salt
2 tablespoons olive oil
¼ cup natural all-peanut peanut
  butter
1 cup buttermilk

Place yeast, sugar, and warm water in a large bowl or a food processor. Let proof.

Mix in whole-wheat flour, white flour, and salt.

Stir in olive oil, peanut butter, and buttermilk. Knead 10 minutes or process 15 seconds or until dough is smooth and elastic, adding more white flour if necessary.

Place dough in a large oiled bowl, cover with a towel, and let rise in a warm place for about 1 hour or until doubled in bulk.

Divide dough in half and form loaves.

Place in loaf pans greased with margarine, cover, and let rise for about 1 hour or until doubled in bulk.

Preheat oven to 350°F.

Bake for 45–60 minutes or until loaves are golden brown and sound hollow when tapped.

Makes 2 small loaves

	Total calories	Sat-fat calories
Per ½-inch slice	78	3
Per loaf	1358	50

PUMPERNICKEL BREAD

1 tablespoon yeast
¼ cup warm water
Pinch of sugar
1 cup rye flour
2 cups whole-wheat flour
  (approximately)
2 cups unbleached white flour

1 teaspoon salt
2 tablespoons olive oil
2 tablespoons molasses
1¼ cups warm water
1 tablespoon caraway seeds
Corn flour

Place yeast in a large bowl or a food processor. Add ¼ cup warm water and sugar. Let proof.

Mix in rye flour, whole-wheat flour, 1½ cups white flour, and salt.

Add olive oil, molasses, and 1¼ cups warm water. Knead 10 minutes or process 15 seconds or until dough is smooth and elastic, adding more white flour if necessary.

Knead in caraway seeds.

Place dough in a large oiled bowl, cover with a towel, and let rise in a warm place for 1 hour or until doubled in bulk.

Sprinkle corn flour on a baking sheet.

Form dough into a round or loaf, place on baking sheet, cover, and let rise 1 hour or until doubled in bulk.

Preheat oven to 450°F.

Bake loaf for 10 minutes.

Reduce heat to 350°F and bake for 35 minutes more or until loaf sounds hollow when tapped.

Makes 1 large loaf

	Total calories	Sat-fat calories
Per ½-inch slice	92	2
Per loaf	2273	39

HONEY WHOLE-WHEAT BREAD

Whole-grain breads are much more nutritious than breads made with white flour. In whole-grain flours, the entire kernel is ground into flour so that vitamins, minerals, and fiber are not lost.

Honey Whole-Wheat Bread makes wonderful toast. Top it with bananas and cottage cheese and you have a filling, nutritious, and scrumptious breakfast. Honey Whole-Wheat Bread freezes well.

This recipe makes 4 loaves of bread. Freeze the ones you are not using.

2 tablespoons active dry yeast	½ cup honey
2 tablespoons salt	½ cup olive oil
1 quart-size package nonfat dry milk	2 teaspoons cinnamon
	½ teaspoon grated nutmeg
1 five-pound bag whole-wheat flour (about 16 cups)	1½ cups rolled oats
	½ cup raisins
6½ cups water	

In a mixing bowl, combine yeast, salt, nonfat dry milk, and 2 cups flour.

In a large saucepan, combine water, honey, and oil and heat until quite warm (about 115°F) but *not too hot* or you will kill the yeast.

Add liquid to dry ingredients in mixing bowl and beat for 4 minutes.

Mix in 4 cups flour.

Mix in the cinnamon, nutmeg, oats, and raisins.

Keep adding flour until you produce a stiff dough. Your mixer probably will not be large enough to handle all the dough. When the mixer reaches its limit, remove the dough to a pastry board or counter and add flour until the dough is stiff enough to knead.

Knead dough for 8–10 minutes or until smooth and elastic.

Place dough in large oiled bowl, cover with a towel, and let rise in warm place for about 1 hour or until doubled in bulk.

Form 4 loaves, place in loaf pans greased with margarine, cover with a towel, and let rise 1 hour or until doubled in bulk.

Preheat oven to 350°F.

Bake loaves for 45 minutes to 1 hour or until they are golden brown and sound hollow when tapped.

Makes 4 loaves

	Total calories	Sat-fat calories
Per ½-inch slice	130	2
Per loaf	2222	39

CUMIN WHEAT BREAD

Although this is a totally whole-wheat bread, it is not the least bit heavy. It is a favorite with young children as well as adults.

1 tablespoon dry yeast	1 teaspoon salt
¼ cup warm water	½ teaspoon whole cumin seeds
2 tablespoons honey	1½ tablespoons olive oil
3½ cups whole-wheat flour	1 cup skim milk

In a large mixing bowl or the bowl of a food processor, combine yeast, water, and honey. Let proof.

Mix in 2 cups of the flour, the salt, and cumin seeds.

Add oil and milk and mix or process well, adding more flour until dough is fairly stiff.

Knead dough 10 minutes or process for 15 seconds or until dough is smooth and elastic, adding more flour if necessary.

Form dough into a ball. Place in an oiled bowl. Cover and let rise for about 1 hour.

Roll dough into a loaf and place in loaf pan greased with margarine. Cover with towel and let rise for 1 hour.

Preheat oven to 375°F and bake for 50–60 minutes or until bread is golden and sounds hollow when tapped.

Makes 1 loaf

	Total calories	Sat-fat calories
Per ½-inch slice	107	2
Per loaf	1814	35

CINNAMON APPLESAUCE BREAD

1 tablespoon active dry yeast	1 teaspoon cinnamon
2 tablespoons brown sugar	⅔ cup applesauce
1 cup warm water	1 tablespoon olive oil
1½ cups whole-wheat flour	½ apple, peeled, cored, and
2 cups unbleached white flour	chopped (about ½ cup)
1 teaspoon salt	¼ cup raisins (optional)

Combine yeast, sugar, and water in a large bowl or a food processor. Let proof.

Mix in whole-wheat flour, 1 cup of white flour, salt, and cinnamon.

Mix in applesauce and olive oil.

Add remaining cup of white flour and more of either or both flours until dough is fairly stiff. Knead dough 10 minutes or process for 15 seconds or until dough is smooth and elastic, adding more flour if necessary.

Mix in apple and raisins.

Form dough into a ball. Place in an oiled bowl. Cover with towel and let rise for about 1 hour.

Roll dough into a loaf and place in loaf pan greased with margarine. Cover and let rise for an hour.

Preheat oven to 350°F. Bake for 50–60 minutes or until loaf sounds hollow when tapped.

Makes 1 large loaf

	Total calories	*Sat-fat calories*
Per ½-inch slice	143	1
Per loaf	2425	24

WHOLE-WHEAT BANANA RAISIN BREAD

This is a banana bread, not a banana cake. It is dense and delicious.

1 tablespoon yeast	2 ripe bananas, mashed
Pinch of sugar	2 tablespoons molasses
¼ cup warm water	1 tablespoon olive oil
1 cup unbleached white flour	1 cup nonfat buttermilk
2½ cups whole-wheat flour	¼ cup raisins (optional)
1 teaspoon salt	

Combine yeast, sugar, and water in a large bowl or the bowl of a food processor. Let proof.

Mix in white flour, 2 cups of whole-wheat flour, and salt.

Mix bananas, molasses, oil, and buttermilk together and add to the flours. Add more whole-wheat flour to make a dough you can knead.

Knead 10 minutes or process 15 seconds or until dough is smooth and elastic, adding more whole-wheat flour if necessary.

Add raisins.

Place dough in a large oiled bowl. Rotate dough to cover surface with a film of olive oil. Cover bowl with a towel and let rise in a warm place for about 1 hour or until doubled in bulk.

Form loaf and place in a loaf pan greased with margarine. Cover with a towel and let rise in a warm place for about 1 hour or until doubled in bulk.

Preheat oven to 350°F.

Bake for 45–55 minutes or until golden brown and hollow when tapped.

Makes 1 large loaf

	Total calories	Sat-fat calories
Per ½-inch slice	147	2
Per loaf	2494	30

OATMEAL BREAD

1 cup water	1 tablespoon active dry yeast
1 cup rolled oats	Pinch of sugar
2 tablespoons honey	⅓ cup warm water
1 tablespoon margarine	2½ cups unbleached white flour
1 teaspoon salt	(approximately)

In a small saucepan, boil 1 cup water and add oats, honey, margarine, and salt. Let cool.

Combine yeast, sugar, and ⅓ cup warm water in a large bowl or a food processor. Let proof.

Add 2 cups flour to the yeast mixture.

When oat mixture is warm, but *not hot,* add it to the flour mixture and knead dough 10 minutes or process 15 seconds or until dough is smooth and elastic, adding more flour if necessary.

Place dough in a large oiled bowl, cover with a towel, and let rise in a warm place for 1 hour or until doubled in bulk.

Form dough into a loaf and place in a loaf pan greased with margarine. Cover and let rise about 1 hour or until doubled in bulk.

Preheat oven to 350°F.

Bake for 45 minutes or until golden brown.

Makes 1 loaf

	Total calories	Sat-fat calories
Per ½-inch slice	94	2
Per loaf	1601	33

CRANBERRY BREAD

This tart but sweet loaf lies somewhere between bread and cake. To make sure you can bake it all year round, buy extra packages of cranberries at Thanksgiving and freeze them.

1½ cups cranberries
2 cups unbleached white flour
1½ teaspoons baking powder
½ teaspoon baking soda
1 teaspoon salt

¾ cup sugar
¾ cup orange juice
1 tablespoon grated orange peel
2 tablespoons margarine
1 egg

Preheat oven to 350°F and grease a loaf pan with margarine.

Chop cranberries in a food processor or hand chopper. Set aside.

In a large bowl, or the bowl of your electric mixer, combine flour, baking powder, baking soda, salt, and sugar.

Add orange juice, orange rind, margarine, and egg and mix until well blended.

Mix in cranberries.

Pour batter into loaf pan and bake for 45–55 minutes or until cake tester comes out clean.

Makes 1 loaf

	Total calories	Sat-fat calories
Per ½-inch slice	112	3
Per loaf	1899	55

ONION FLAT BREAD

1 tablespoon active dry yeast	1 teaspoon + a few shakes salt
1 pinch sugar	1 teaspoon margarine
1 cup warm water	1 cup chopped onions
2½–3 cups unbleached white flour*	1 teaspoon paprika

Place yeast, sugar, and water in large bowl or a food processor. Let proof.

Mix in 2 cups flour and salt. Knead for 10 minutes or process for 15 seconds, until smooth and elastic, adding flour if necessary.

Place dough in an oiled bowl, cover with a towel, and let rise in a warm place for an hour or until doubled in bulk.

Punch dough down and split in half. Let rest for 5 minutes.

Meanwhile, grease two 9-inch cake pans with margarine.

Melt 2 teaspoons of margarine.

Press dough into cake pans.

Spread margarine over the tops and press onion into the surface.

Let rise about 45 minutes or until doubled in bulk.

Preheat oven to 450°F.

Sprinkle tops with paprika and a few shakes of salt.

Bake 20–25 minutes, until lightly browned.

Makes 2 loaves, 8 slices per loaf

	Total calories	Sat-fat calories
Per slice	83	1
Per loaf	667	7

FOCACCIA GENOVESE

1 package active dry yeast	2¾ cups unbleached white flour
Pinch of sugar	1 teaspoon olive oil
1 cup warm water	1 teaspoon or more garlic slivers
2 teaspoons olive oil	1 teaspoon rosemary
1 teaspoon salt	¼ teaspoon salt

In a large bowl or food processor mix yeast, sugar, and water. Let proof.

---

*For a slightly different taste, use 1 cup of whole-wheat flour, along with 1½–2 cups unbleached white flour.

Stir in 2 teaspoons olive oil, 1 teaspoon salt, and 2 cups flour. Process 15 seconds or mix until smooth, adding more flour until dough is smooth and firm. Place in bowl lightly oiled with olive oil and cover with towel for about 1 hour or until doubled in size.

Grease 12-inch-round pizza pan with olive oil. Punch down dough and spread evenly over pan. Cover with towel and let rise 30 minutes.

Preheat oven to 375°F.

Brush dough with 1 teaspoon olive oil. Distribute garlic slivers evenly over surface and push them into the dough. Sprinkle dough evenly with rosemary and ¼ teaspoon salt.

Bake dough 30 minutes or until golden.

Makes 1 large flat loaf, 12 slices per loaf

	Total calories	Sat-fat calories
Per slice	116	2
Per loaf	1390	22

WHOLE-WHEAT BAGELS

1 tablespoon active dry yeast	1½ cups unbleached white flour
3 tablespoons sugar	1 teaspoon salt
1 cup warm water	2 tablespoons olive oil
1½ cups whole-wheat flour	

Mix yeast, sugar, and warm water in a large bowl or a food processor. Let proof.

Mix in whole-wheat flour, white flour, and salt.

Knead 8–10 minutes or process 15 seconds or until dough is smooth and elastic, adding more flour if necessary.

Place dough in a large oiled bowl, cover with a towel, and let rise in a warm place for 40 minutes. Punch down.

Roll into lengths about 5 inches long and ¾ inch wide. Pinch each into a circle to make a bagel.

Preheat oven to 350°F and grease cookie sheet with oil.

Fill a medium saucepan with water. Add oil and bring to a boil.

Drop a bagel into the boiling water.

When it rises to the top, remove it with a slotted spoon or spatula so the excess water can drip off.

Repeat this process with all the bagels.

Place bagels on cookie sheet and bake for 10 minutes.
Raise heat to 400°F and bake for 10 minutes more.

Makes 12 bagels
Per bagel: 115 Total calories; 1 Sat-fat calorie

PEPPERY BREADSTICKS

1 teaspoon peppercorns or freshly ground black pepper	1 teaspoon salt
	1 cup warm water
1 tablespoon yeast	1 teaspoon olive oil
Pinch of sugar	1 egg white
¼ cup warm water	1 tablespoon water
3 + cups unbleached white flour	

Place 1 teaspoon of peppercorns in food processor and process until coarsely ground or grind 1 teaspoon of freshly ground black pepper in large bowl.

Add yeast, sugar, and ¼ cup warm water. Let proof.

Mix in 3 cups of flour and salt.

Add oil and 1 cup warm water and knead about 10 minutes or process 15 seconds until dough is smooth and elastic, adding more flour if necessary.

Place dough in large oiled bowl, cover with a towel, and let rise for 1 hour or until doubled in bulk.

Push down dough. Let rest 5 minutes.

Preheat oven to 400°F.

Divide dough into 16 equal pieces.

Roll each piece into a long stick thickness and then divide into three breadsticks. Lay them on baking sheet. Let rest 15 minutes.

Beat egg white with a fork and mix with 1 tablespoon water. Paint breadsticks with egg white mixture.

Bake for 20–30 minutes or until browned.

Makes about 35 six-inch sticks
Per breadstick: 41 Total calories; 0 Sat-fat calories

SESAME BREADSTICKS

Beware! These breadsticks are habit-forming.

1 teaspoon active dry yeast
¼ cup warm water
⅔ cup whole-wheat flour
2 or more cups unbleached
   white flour
1 teaspoon salt, optional

⅔ cup nonfat skim milk
1 tablespoon olive oil
1 egg white
2 teaspoons water
1 tablespoon sesame seeds

Place yeast and warm water in large bowl or a food processor. Let proof.

Mix in flours and salt.

Add milk and olive oil, and knead for 10 minutes or process until dough is smooth and elastic, adding more flour if necessary.

Place dough in ungreased bowl, cover with a towel, and let rise 1 hour.

Preheat oven to 400°F.

On a lightly floured surface, roll the dough into a ¼-inch-thick rectangle. One dimension of the rectangle should be the length of your breadsticks.

Cut the dough into ½-inch strips. (If you prefer thicker breadsticks, cut the dough into one-inch strips.)

Roll each strip in your palms to make a breadstick and lay it on an ungreased baking sheet. Place the sticks in a line, about a ½-inch apart.

Beat the egg white and water together and brush onto breadsticks.

Sprinkle sesame seeds evenly over breadsticks.

Count the breadsticks so you can calculate their sat-fat calories.

Bake for 20–30 minutes or until golden brown. Cool on a rack.

Makes about 35 six-inch sticks
To determine the total calories and sat-fat calories for each breadstick, divide the number of breadsticks you made into the following numbers:
Total calories: 1423   Total sat-fat calories: 30
For example, 30 sat-fat calories divided by 35 breadsticks = 0.86 sat-fat calories each.

OAT BRAN MUFFINS

Oat bran, a food rich in soluble fiber, has a modest effect on lowering blood cholesterol levels.

[Q] APPLE OAT MUFFINS

1 ½ cups oat bran
½ cup whole-wheat flour
3 tablespoons brown sugar
2 teaspoons baking powder
½ teaspoon salt
1 teaspoon cinnamon
½ cup apple juice

¼ cup skim milk
1 egg
2 tablespoons olive oil
2 tablespoons honey
1 cup apples, peeled, cored, and diced
2 tablespoons raisins

Preheat oven to 400°F. Grease a 12-cup muffin tin with margarine.

Combine oat bran, flour, brown sugar, baking powder, salt, and cinnamon and set aside.

In a large mixing bowl, combine apple juice, skim milk, egg, oil, and honey.

Add flour mixture, apples, and raisins and combine until just moistened.

Fill muffin tin and bake at 400°F for about 20 minutes or until golden brown and a cake tester comes out clean.

Makes 12 muffins
Per muffin: 125 Total calories; 4 Sat-fat calories

Q MOTHER'S OAT BRAN MUFFINS

2¼ cups oat bran
¼ cup brown sugar
¼ cup chopped walnuts
¼ cup raisins
1 tablespoon baking powder

½ teaspoon salt
¾ cup skim milk
1 egg + 1 egg white, beaten
¼ cup honey
2 tablespoons olive oil

Preheat oven to 425°F. Grease a 12-cup muffin tin with margarine.

Combine oat bran, brown sugar, walnuts, raisins, baking powder, and salt.

Add skim milk, eggs, honey, and oil. Mix until ingredients are just moistened.

Fill muffin tin and bake for 15 minutes or until golden brown and a cake tester comes out clean.

Makes 12 muffins

	Total calories	Sat-fat calories
Per muffin	160	6
Without walnuts	144	5

Q ORANGE OAT MUFFINS

Can you believe it? Another oat bran muffin.

1 cup oat bran
½ cup wheat germ
½ cup whole-wheat flour
3 tablespoons brown sugar
2 tablespoons grated orange
  peel

2 teaspoons baking powder
1 egg
2 tablespoons olive oil
½ cup orange juice
¼ cup skim milk
2 tablespoons raisins

Preheat oven to 400°F. Grease a 12-cup muffin tin with margarine.

Combine oat bran, wheat germ, whole-wheat flour, brown sugar, orange peel, and baking powder. Set aside.

In a mixing bowl, mix egg, oil, orange juice, and skim milk.

Mix in dry ingredients until just moistened.

Carefully mix in raisins.

Fill muffin tin and bake for 15 minutes or until golden brown and a cake tester comes out clean.

Makes 12 muffins
Per muffin: 110 Total calories; 4 Sat-fat calories

Q   ## APRICOT OAT MUFFINS

Yet another oat muffin. Healthy and delicious — a good snack or breakfast on the run.

½ cup orange juice
1 cup dried apricots, chopped
  (easily done in food
  processor)
¼ cup brown sugar
1 cup oat bran

¼ cup wheat germ
¾ cup whole-wheat flour
2 teaspoons baking powder
2 tablespoons olive oil
½ cup skim milk
1 egg

Preheat oven to 400°F. Grease a 12-cup muffin tin with margarine.

In a small saucepan, heat orange juice until boiling. Mix in apricots and brown sugar.

Remove saucepan from heat and cool apricot mixture slightly.

In a medium bowl, combine oat bran, wheat germ, whole-wheat flour, and baking powder. Set aside.

In a mixing bowl, beat together oil, skim milk, and egg.

Add dry ingredients and apricot-orange juice mixture to milk mixture and mix until just moistened.

Fill muffin tin and bake for 15 minutes or until golden brown and a cake tester comes out clean.

Makes 12 muffins
Per muffin: 135 Total calories; 4 Sat-fat calories

BRAN MUFFINS

Wheat bran, made from the outer coverings of wheat kernels, is rich in vitamins, minerals, and insoluble dietary fiber. Insoluble dietary fiber promotes regularity and is believed to protect against colon cancer.

1 cup whole-wheat flour	1 cup buttermilk
1 cup wheat bran	1 egg, beaten
3 tablespoons brown sugar	3 tablespoons molasses
¼ teaspoon salt	2 tablespoons olive oil
1 teaspoon baking soda	⅓ cup raisins
½ teaspoon baking powder	

Preheat oven to 400°F. Grease a 12-cup muffin tin with margarine.
Combine whole-wheat flour, wheat bran, brown sugar, salt, baking soda, and baking powder. Set aside.
In a mixing bowl, mix buttermilk, egg, molasses, and oil.
Add dry ingredients and mix until just moistened.
Fold in raisins.
Fill muffin tin and bake for about 15 minutes or until golden brown and a cake tester comes out clean.

Makes 12 muffins
Per muffin: 116 Total calories; 4 Sat-fat calories

BANANA-CARROT MUFFINS

Not an oat bran muffin but tasty and healthy anyway. Eat as a snack or for a light breakfast.

3 medium carrots	2 teaspoons double-acting baking powder
2 medium bananas	
¼ cup margarine	¼ teaspoon salt
½ cup brown sugar	¼ teaspoon baking soda
1 large egg	1 teaspoon vanilla
2 cups whole-wheat flour	½ cup chopped walnuts

Preheat oven to 350°F. Grease a 12-cup muffin tin with margarine.
Grate carrots (a food processor does this well) and set aside.
Mash bananas with a fork and set aside.

In a mixing bowl, cream the margarine and brown sugar until fluffy. Add egg and beat well.

Stir in the mashed bananas.

In a small bowl, mix together flour, baking powder, salt, and baking soda.

Add flour mixture to banana mixture. Do not overmix.

Add grated carrots, vanilla, and nuts and combine carefully.

Fill muffin tin and bake for 20–25 minutes or until a cake tester comes out clean.

Makes 12 muffins
Per muffin: 195 Total calories; 11 Sat-fat calories

As an alternative, try substituting 1 cup oat bran + ½ cup wheat germ + ½ cup whole-wheat flour for the 2 cups of whole-wheat flour. Use only 2 tablespoons margarine and ¼ cup brown sugar.

Total calories: 155; Sat-fat calories: 8

GINGERBREAD MUFFINS

These muffins taste like cake. Use self-control! One muffin has only 9 sat-fat calories, but 12 have 108!!

1 cup unbleached white flour	¼ teaspoon allspice
¾ cup whole-wheat flour	¼ teaspoon grated nutmeg
¼ cup sugar	¾ cup buttermilk
¼ cup brown sugar	⅓ cup olive oil
1 teaspoon baking soda	1 egg
¼ teaspoon salt	1 egg white
1 teaspoon ginger	¼ cup light unsulphured
1 teaspoon cinnamon	molasses
¼ teaspoon cloves	

Preheat oven to 400°F and grease a 12-cup muffin tin with margarine.

Combine flours, sugars, baking soda, salt, and spices in a large bowl. Set aside.

In a large mixing bowl, combine buttermilk, oil, egg, egg white, and molasses.

Add flour mixture to buttermilk mixture. Do not overmix.

Pour into cups of muffin pan and bake for 15 minutes, or until cake tester comes out clean.

Makes 12 muffins
Per muffin: 177 Total calories; 9 Sat-fat calories

BUTTERMILK PANCAKES

Breakfast need not be a problem for those watching their sat-fat intake. In addition to the preceding bread and muffin recipes, try these pancakes, waffles, and the French toast that follows.

Instead of using sour cream (270 sat-fat calories per cup) or whole milk (45 sat-fat calories per cup), make your pancakes with buttermilk (0–12 sat-fat calories per cup). Buttermilk enhances the taste of waffles and pancakes. These delicious buttermilk pancakes will hardly make a dent in your sat-fat budget.

Use maple syrup or powdered sugar to sweeten pancakes and waffles. Butter adds only unneeded sat-fat calories.

HINT: Use a cast-iron griddle, and you will need little or no margarine to keep your pancakes from sticking to the surface.

½ cup unbleached white flour
¼ cup whole-wheat flour
½ teaspoon baking powder
½ teaspoon baking soda
½ cup buttermilk*

¼–½ cup skim milk*
1 egg white, lightly beaten
2 teaspoons olive oil (optional)
Margarine to grease grill

In a large bowl, combine the flours, baking powder, and baking soda.

Mix in buttermilk and skim milk, egg white, and oil. Do not overmix.

Lightly grease a hot griddle or skillet with margarine, making sure you keep track of the amount you use.

For each pancake, spread a tablespoon of batter on the griddle. When the pancake solidifies and the edges come away from the grid-

*For equally delicious pancakes, substitute ½ cup nonfat yogurt + ½ cup skim milk for the ½ cup buttermilk + ¼ cup skim milk at 33 total calories and 1 sat-fat calorie per pancake. The fat calorie count of this recipe is based on buttermilk containing no fat calories.

dle, turn the pancake. The bottom should be golden brown. Cook until other side is also golden.

Makes about 16 pancakes

	Total calories	Sat-fat calories
Total batter	495	13
Per pancake	31	1

(If you used more than 1 teaspoon of margarine to grease your griddle, add 1 sat-fat calorie for every 2 teaspoons you used. If you did not use olive oil, total batter: 415 Total calories, 2 sat-fat calories.)

BUTTERMILK WAFFLES

1 egg white at room
   temperature
1 cup whole-wheat flour
1 cup unbleached white flour
2 teaspoons baking powder
½ teaspoon salt
1 cup buttermilk
1 cup skim milk
2 tablespoons olive oil

Preheat waffle iron.

Beat egg white until stiff but not dry. Set aside.

In a medium bowl, combine whole-wheat flour, white flour, baking powder, and salt.

Add buttermilk and skim milk. *Do not overmix.*

Fold in egg white. Fold in oil.

Place batter on waffle iron in amounts specified by your waffle-iron instructions. Cook accordingly.

Makes 8 Belgian waffles

	Total calories	Sat-fat calories
Total batter	1261	40
Per square*	158	5

*Because waffle irons come in many sizes, this recipe may make more or less than 8 waffle squares. Divide 1261 by the number of waffle squares you make to figure out the total calories per square (for example, 1261 ÷ 8 = 158). Divide 40 by the number of waffle squares to figure out the sat-fat calories per square (for example, 40 ÷ 8 = 5).

CINNAMON FRENCH TOAST

2 egg whites
3 tablespoons skim milk
½ teaspoon vanilla
½ teaspoon ground cinnamon

Pinch of grated nutmeg
3 slices whole-wheat bread or
French bread
2 teaspoons margarine*

In a shallow dish, mix egg whites, skim milk, vanilla, cinnamon, and nutmeg.

Soak both sides of bread in mixture.

In a large frying pan, melt margarine over high heat.

Add bread. Reduce heat to medium.

Turn bread after 2 minutes. Cook until golden brown and crispy.

3 servings
Per serving: 106 Total calories; 8 Sat-fat calories

---

*Use a cast-iron pancake griddle, which requires little or no margarine to keep the waffles from sticking, to reduce the sat-fat and total fat even more.

24 DESSERTS

Y̶OU MIGHT think dessert would be the most difficult part of the meal to make low in saturated fat. This is not true. There are many desserts that not only are scrumptious and beautiful but fit perfectly into a low-sat-fat diet. (That is not to say they are necessarily low in total fat — so go easy.)

The trick to keeping desserts low in saturated fat is to substitute nonfat yogurt, buttermilk, or skim milk for sour cream, sweet cream, or whole milk and margarine or oil for butter; never to use lard, shortening, palm, or coconut oil; and to reduce eggs to no more than one and substitute egg whites for additional eggs.

You may be surprised that we use olive oil in making these desserts. Olive oil is the oil of choice because it lowers LDL-cholesterol without lowering HDL-cholesterol. Try using a mild-tasting olive oil in your baked goods. Only your arteries will be able to detect a difference.

You will notice that we recommend grated nutmeg in many recipes. Buy whole nutmegs at your grocery store and simply grate one when you need nutmeg in a recipe. The advantage is that each time you grate one it is fresh and thus has the taste it is supposed to have.

We recommend unbleached white flour because when a flour is bleached, it loses many of its important nutritional qualities.

APPLESAUCE CAKE

1 cup raisins	1 teaspoon vanilla
½ cup water	1½ cups unbleached white flour
1 cup chunky applesauce	1 teaspoon baking soda
⅓ cup margarine	½ teaspoon cinnamon
½ cup sugar	⅛ teaspoon ground cloves
1 egg	½ cup chopped walnuts

Preheat oven to 350°F. Grease a loaf pan with margarine.

In a small saucepan, combine raisins and water. Bring to a boil. Reduce heat, cover, and simmer for 1 minute.

Remove from heat. Stir in applesauce. Cool to lukewarm.

Cream margarine and sugar. Beat in egg and vanilla.

Combine flour, baking soda, cinnamon, and cloves and mix into batter.

Add applesauce mixture and nuts.

Pour into greased loaf pan and bake for 1 hour or until a cake tester comes out clean.

Cool for 10 minutes before removing from pan.

Makes 10 slices
Per slice: 250 Total calories; 14 Sat-fat calories

APPLE CAKE

A moist, hearty cake that is easy to make.

¾ cup brown sugar	½ teaspoon salt
½ cup olive oil	1 teaspoon baking soda
1 teaspoon vanilla	1½ teaspoons cinnamon
1 egg	¼ teaspoon grated nutmeg
1 egg white	4 cups Delicious apples, peeled
¾ cup unbleached white flour	and cut into chunks
1 cup whole-wheat flour	½ cup chopped walnuts

Preheat oven to 350°F. Grease an 8-inch springform pan with margarine and dust with flour.

In an electric mixer, beat together brown sugar and oil.

Add vanilla, egg, and egg white and beat until smooth.

Add flours, salt, baking soda, cinnamon, and nutmeg and beat until smooth.

With a large (wooden) spoon or rubber spatula, mix in apples and walnuts. The batter will be *very* sticky and stiff.

Spoon batter into pan and bake for 50–60 minutes or until a cake tester comes out clean.

Makes 12 slices
Per slice: 220 Total calories; 13 Sat-fat calories

BANANA CAKE

This banana cake is out of the ordinary. Rich and full-bodied.

1 cup whole-wheat flour	⅓ cup olive oil
½ cup unbleached white flour	½ cup brown sugar
¼ cup wheat germ	¾ teaspoon vanilla
1 teaspoon cinnamon	1 egg
½ teaspoon grated nutmeg	3 bananas, mashed
2 teaspoons baking powder	½ cup chopped walnuts
¼ teaspoon baking soda	5 prunes, chopped
¼ teaspoon salt	

Preheat oven to 350°F. Grease a loaf pan with margarine.

Mix flours, wheat germ, cinnamon, nutmeg, baking powder, baking soda, and salt and set aside.

In an electric mixer, mix oil and brown sugar. Add vanilla and egg and mix well.

Add bananas and blend until smooth. Mix in flour mixture.

Fold in nuts and prunes.

Pour batter into loaf pan and bake for 45–60 minutes or until a cake tester comes out clean.

Makes 10 slices
Per slice: 263 Total calories; 12 Sat-fat calories

LEMON LOAF

Crunchy, lemony goodness.

1 cup walnuts*
½ cup sugar
½ cup margarine
Grated peel of 1 lemon
2 cups unbleached white flour
¼ teaspoon salt

2 teaspoons baking powder
1 teaspoon baking soda
¾ cup buttermilk
¼ cup lemon juice
2 tablespoons fresh lemon juice
3 tablespoons sugar

Preheat oven to 375°F. Grease a loaf pan with margarine.

Chop walnuts with food processor or nut chopper. Set aside.

Cream ½ cup sugar and margarine with mixer.

Add grated lemon peel and mix until smooth.

Mix together flour, salt, baking powder, and baking soda and set aside.

Mix buttermilk and lemon juice and set aside.

Add flour mixture to creamed mixture alternately with buttermilk mixture. *Do not overmix.*

Stir in walnuts.

Pour into loaf pan and bake for 30–45 minutes or until a cake tester comes out clean.

Let cool in pan 10 minutes.

In a small saucepan, combine lemon juice and 3 tablespoons sugar and stir over low heat until sugar dissolves.

Pierce top of cake with a fork or skewer. Spoon lemon-sugar mixture into holes.

Let cool for easy slicing. (A whiff of lemon loaf may cause your impatient family to force you to slice the cake warm!)

Makes 10 slices
Per slice: 290 Total calories; 21 Sat-fat calories

---

*Lemon Loaf is delicious even without the walnuts. Eliminate walnuts and reduce total calories to 215, sat-fat calories to 15, per slice.

PHILIP WAGENAAR'S
RAISIN-GINGER-ORANGE CAKE

This is cake disguised as a quick bread. It is a sweet blending of textures and flavors. We are fortunate that Dr. Wagenaar occasionally takes time off from his biking expeditions around the world to bake.

1 ¾ cups unbleached white flour
2 teaspoons baking powder
½ teaspoon baking soda
½ teaspoon salt
⅓ cup margarine
¾ cup sugar
1 tablespoon grated orange
  peel*

1 tablespoon grated lemon peel*
4 egg whites
½ cup nonfat milk
½ teaspoon orange extract
2 tablespoons crystallized
  ginger**
2 cups raisins

Preheat oven to 350°F and lightly grease a loaf pan.

Combine flour, baking powder, baking soda, and salt. Set aside.

Cream together margarine, sugar, and orange and lemon peels.

Add egg whites, two at a time, beating well after each addition.

Combine milk and orange extract.

Add milk and flour mixtures alternately to batter and beat just to mix.

Stir in ginger and raisins.

Pour batter into loaf pan and bake for 45–60 minutes or until cake tester comes out clean.

Makes 12 slices
Per slice: 236 Total calories; 9 Sat-fat calories

---

*A dandy way to grate orange or lemon peel is to chop a few slices of the peel in a mini-chopper. Be sure to wash the fruit thoroughly before you cut the slices.
**Available in the spice section of most supermarkets

PUMPKIN CAKE

1 ¼ cups unbleached white flour   ½ cup raisins
½ cup rye flour   1 cup pumpkin purée
1 teaspoon baking soda   ¾ cup brown sugar
1 teaspoon baking powder   6 tablespoons margarine
½ teaspoon salt   ¼ cup skim milk
1 ½ teaspoons cinnamon   1 egg
1 teaspoon cardamom   1 egg white

Preheat oven to 350°F. Grease a loaf pan with margarine and lightly flour.

Combine flours, baking soda, baking powder, salt, cinnamon, cardamom, and raisins. Set aside.

In a large mixing bowl, mix together pumpkin purée, brown sugar, and margarine. Add skim milk, whole egg, and egg white and mix until smooth.

Stir in flour mixture.

Pour batter into loaf pan and bake for 45–60 minutes or until a cake tester comes out clean.

Makes 18 ½-inch slices
Per slice: 128 Total calories; 7 Sat-fat calories

THE YORK BLUEBERRY CAKE

½ cup brown sugar   ½ cup margarine
½ cup chopped walnuts   ¾ cup sugar
1 teaspoon cinnamon   1 egg
2 cups unbleached white flour 2 egg whites
1 teaspoon baking soda   1 cup nonfat yogurt
½ teaspoon salt   1 teaspoon vanilla
2 cups blueberries

Preheat oven to 350°F and grease a 13 × 9-inch baking pan with margarine.

Combine brown sugar, nuts, and cinnamon and set aside.

In a large bowl, combine flour, baking soda, and salt.

Mix ¼ cup of the flour mixture with the blueberries and set aside.

In a large mixing bowl, cream margarine and sugar until fluffy.

Beat in egg and egg whites.

Stir in yogurt and vanilla.

Add remaining flour to batter and beat until smooth.

Stir in floured blueberries.

Spread half of the batter into the baking pan and sprinkle half of the brown sugar mixture over it.

Cover with remaining batter (it will barely cover the entire surface) and top with remaining brown sugar mixture.

Bake for 40–45 minutes until cake tester comes out clean.

Makes 24 squares
Per square: 141 Total calories; 8 Sat-fat calories

CARROT CAKE SANS OEUFS

It is difficult to believe that this delicious, rich carrot cake has no eggs, but believe it! Carrot Cake sans Oeufs does not even contain an egg white.

¾ cup sugar
1 cup grated carrot (food processor grates quickly)
1 cup raisins
1 teaspoon cinnamon
1 teaspoon grated nutmeg
1 teaspoon ground cloves

1½ cups water
3 tablespoons margarine
2 cups flour
2 teaspoons baking soda
¼ teaspoon salt
1 cup chopped walnuts

Preheat oven to 325°F. Grease a 13 × 9-inch baking pan with margarine.

In a small saucepan, combine sugar, carrot, raisins, cinnamon, nutmeg, cloves, water, and margarine. Bring to a boil. Reduce heat, and simmer for 5 minutes.

Pour into a mixing bowl and cool to lukewarm.

Add flour, baking soda, and salt. Mix well.

Stir in walnuts.

Pour into pan and bake for 45–60 minutes or until a cake tester comes out clean.

Makes 24 squares
Per square: 122 Total calories; 5 Sat-fat calories

GINGER CAKE WITH PEAR SAUCE

Ginger Cake tastes good with or without pear sauce.

⅓ cup margarine	½ teaspoon salt
2 tablespoons maple syrup	1 teaspoon cinnamon
⅓ cup sugar	1½ teaspoons ginger
1 egg	½ teaspoon allspice
1½ cups unbleached white flour	¼ teaspoon grated nutmeg
½ teaspoon baking powder	1 cup buttermilk
½ teaspoon baking soda	

Pear Sauce

2 cups water	3 ripe Anjou or other pears
¼ cup sugar	1 tablespoon sugar

The Ginger Cake

Preheat oven to 350°F. Grease an 8 × 8-inch baking pan with margarine.

Cream margarine, maple syrup, and sugar until smooth.

Mix in egg.

Combine flour, baking powder, baking soda, salt, cinnamon, ginger, allspice, and nutmeg. Add to batter, alternating with buttermilk. Mix until smooth. Pour batter into baking pan and bake for 30 minutes or until a cake tester comes out clean.

Meanwhile, make the pear sauce.

The Pear Sauce

In a large saucepan, combine water and ¼ cup sugar and bring to a simmer.

Poach pears in simmering sugar water for about 10 minutes or until soft.

Drain pears and purée them with 1 tablespoon sugar in a blender until smooth.

Serve over cooled cake.

Makes 9 squares

	Total calories	Sat-fat calories
Per square	183	14
with Pear Sauce	194	14

PINEAPPLE POUND CAKE

This pound cake and the next one will remind you of cakes that are made with a pound of butter and 6 eggs. Nonfat yogurt and margarine make the difference in the saturated fat content of our pound cakes, but not in their taste and appearance.

2½ cups flour
1½ teaspoons baking soda
½ teaspoon salt
1 can (20 oz) pineapple chunks
   in heavy syrup
½ cup margarine

¾ cup sugar
3 egg whites
1 tablespoon grated orange peel
1 teaspoon vanilla
1 cup nonfat yogurt
¼ cup sugar

Preheat oven to 375°F. Grease a 10-inch tube pan with margarine.

Mix flour, baking soda, and salt and set aside.

Drain syrup from can of pineapples, reserving ¼ cup.

Cream margarine and ¾ cup of the sugar.

Add egg whites, orange peel, and vanilla and beat well.

Add flour mixture and yogurt alternately to sugar mixture and mix well.

Pour half the batter into pan. Spread 1 cup (or more) of pineapples evenly over batter. Cover with remaining batter.

Bake for 40 minutes or until a cake tester comes out clean.

Let the cake cool for 5 minutes.

Meanwhile, in a small saucepan, combine ¼ cup sugar with reserved pineapple syrup.

Bring to a boil, reduce heat, and simmer for 3–5 minutes or until syrup thickens slightly.

Remove cake from pan. Pierce it with a fork and spoon pineapple juice mixture into holes and over the top of the cake.

Makes 16 slices
Per slice: 177 Total calories; 9 Sat-fat calories

PEACH POUND CAKE

1 tablespoon unbleached white
  flour
2 tablespoons brown sugar
2 peaches,* sliced
¾ cup margarine
1 cup sugar
2½ cups unbleached white flour
¼ teaspoon salt

½ teaspoon baking soda
1 teaspoon baking powder
1 teaspoon vanilla
1 carton (8 oz) low-fat lemon
  yogurt
1 egg
1 egg white

Preheat oven to 325°F. Grease a 12-cup bundt pan with margarine and dust with flour.

In a medium bowl, mix 1 tablespoon flour and the brown sugar.

Add peaches and mix until covered with sugar.

Spread peaches around bottom of bundt pan.

In a large mixing bowl, cream margarine and sugar.

Stir in 2½ cups flour, salt, baking soda, and baking powder.

Add vanilla, yogurt, egg, and egg white and beat for 3 minutes at medium speed.

Pour batter over peaches and bake for about 45–60 minutes or until a cake tester comes out clean.

Cool for 10 minutes before removing from pan.

Makes 16 slices
Per slice: 210 Total calories; 16 Sat-fat calories

*If it is winter and no fresh peaches are available, use canned peaches or peel, core, and dice two pears instead. Add ¼ teaspoon grated nutmeg to the brown sugar and flour mixture.

ORANGE CAKE

1 ½ cups unbleached white flour | ½ cup sugar
2 teaspoons baking powder | ½ cup orange juice
¼ teaspoon salt | 3 egg whites
½ cup margarine | 2 tablespoons orange juice

Preheat oven to 350°F. Grease a loaf pan with margarine.

Combine flour, baking powder, and salt. Set aside.

In a large mixing bowl, beat margarine until soft. Gradually add sugar until creamy.

Add flour mixture, alternating with ½ cup orange juice, until batter is smooth.

In another bowl, whip egg whites until stiff but not dry.

Fold egg whites into batter.

Pour batter into loaf pan and bake for 40–50 minutes or until a cake tester comes out clean.

Cool in pan for 10 minutes.

Poke holes in top of cake. Pour 2 tablespoons orange juice into holes.

Makes 10 slices
Per slice: 180 Total calories; 15 Sat-fat calories

COCOA ANGEL FOOD CAKE

¾ cup cake flour | 1 teaspoon cream of tartar
¼ cup unsweetened cocoa | 1 teaspoon vanilla
1 ¼ cups sugar | ½ teaspoon almond extract
1 ¼–1 ½ cups egg whites (about 10–12)

Preheat oven to 350°F.

Sift together three times: cake flour, cocoa, and ¼ cup of the sugar. Set aside.

Sift remaining 1 cup sugar and set aside.

Whip egg whites until foamy. Add cream of tartar. Continue beating until whites are stiff but not dry.

Fold in sugar a little at a time.

Fold in vanilla and almond extract.

Sift flour-cocoa mixture over batter (¼ at a time) and fold into batter.

Pour batter into an ungreased 10-inch tube pan and bake for 45 minutes or until a cake tester comes out clean.

Invert the tube pan and let cake cool.

Makes 12 slices
Per slice: 119 Total calories; trace Sat-fat calories

MARBLE CAKE

To make a special occasion even more special, bake a marble cake and ice it with Cocoa Frosting (page 392).

3½ cups cake flour	1 tablespoon unsweetened
½ teaspoon baking soda	cocoa
2½ teaspoons baking powder	1 tablespoon sugar
½ cup buttermilk	1 teaspoon cinnamon
½ cup skim milk	⅛ teaspoon ground cloves
1 teaspoon vanilla	⅛ teaspoon baking soda
½ cup margarine	1 tablespoon margarine
¾ cup sugar	4 egg whites, at room
1 egg yolk	temperature

Preheat oven to 375°F. Grease a 10-inch tube pan with margarine.

Combine cake flour, baking soda, and baking powder and set aside.

Combine buttermilk, skim milk, and vanilla and set aside.

In a large mixing bowl, cream ½ cup margarine and ¾ cup sugar. Mix in egg yolk.

Add half the flour mixture and half the milk mixture and stir until smooth.

Add remaining flour mixture and milk mixture and stir until smooth.

Combine cocoa, cinnamon, cloves, baking soda, and 1 tablespoon sugar.

In a small saucepan, melt 1 tablespoon margarine and blend into cocoa-sugar mixture. Blend 1 cup of batter into cocoa mixture.

Whip egg whites until stiff but not dry.

Fold ⅔ of the egg whites into plain batter and remaining ⅓ egg whites into cocoa batter.

Pour plain batter into tube pan.

Drop spoonfuls of cocoa batter onto plain batter.

With a knife, swirl the cocoa batter through the plain batter.

Bake for 30 minutes or until a cake tester comes out clean.

Makes 12 slices
Per slice: 238 Total calories; 15 Sat-fat calories

DIVINE BUTTERMILK POUND CAKE

You will not believe how light and fine-grained this cake is.

1¾ cup cake flour
½ teaspoon baking soda
1 teaspoon baking powder
¼ teaspoon salt
½ cup margarine

¾ cup sugar
1 egg + 2 egg whites
½ teaspoon vanilla
¼ teaspoon almond extract
¾ cup buttermilk

Preheat oven to 375°F and grease an 8-inch springform pan with margarine.

Combine flour, baking soda, baking powder, and salt, and set aside.

In an electric mixer, cream margarine and sugar.

Add egg and egg whites, vanilla, and almond extract, and mix until smooth.

Add flour mixture and buttermilk, and mix until smooth.

Pour into springform pan and bake for 30–40 minutes, or until cake tester comes out clean.

When cool, frost it with our number-one favorite choice, Mocha Frosting (page 393). The following Walnut Glaze also tastes good.

Walnut Glaze

¼ cup brown sugar
½ tablespoon cornstarch
¼ cup cold water

½ teaspoon margarine
1 tablespoon chopped walnuts

In a small saucepan, mix together brown sugar and cornstarch. Slowly add water, making sure mixture is smooth.

At medium-high temperature, stir for 3–4 minutes, until mixture is thick and begins to boil.

Stir in margarine and walnuts. Spoon over cool cake.

Makes 12 slices

	Total calories	Sat-fat calories
Per slice	175	13
With Mocha Frosting	225	18
With Walnut Glaze	199	14

SPICE CAKE

2⅓ cups cake flour	½ teaspoon salt
1½ teaspoons baking powder	¾ cup margarine
½ teaspoon soda	1 cup sugar
1 teaspoon grated nutmeg	1 egg yolk
1 teaspoon cinnamon	1 cup less 2 tablespoons
½ teaspoon cloves	buttermilk
	3 egg whites

Preheat oven to 350°F and grease 10-inch tube pan with margarine.

Mix together flour, baking powder, baking soda, nutmeg, cinnamon cloves, and salt, and set aside.

In a large mixing bowl, cream margarine and sugar until fluffy.

Mix in 1 egg yolk.

Add dry mixture alternately with buttermilk.

Whip 3 egg whites until stiff but not dry and fold them into batter.

Pour into prepared pan and bake for 45–60 minutes, or until cake tester comes out clean.

Cool and ice with Cocoa Frosting (page 392) or Mocha Frosting (page 393).

Makes 12 slices

	Total calories	Sat-fat calories
Per slice	238	19
With frosting	288	24

CHOCOLATEY-CHOCOLATE COCOA CAKE

3 tablespoons unsweetened
  cocoa
4 tablespoons margarine
1 cup boiling water
1 cup sugar
1 teaspoon vanilla
1 egg yolk

1 teaspoon baking soda
½ cup buttermilk
2 cups unbleached white flour
1 teaspoon baking powder
2 egg whites

Cocoa Frosting

3 tablespoons margarine
3 tablespoons unsweetened
  cocoa
1 teaspoon vanilla

1½ cups confectioners' sugar
1 tablespoon skim milk

Preheat oven to 350°F. Grease a 10-inch tube pan with margarine and dust with flour.

Place cocoa and margarine in a large mixing bowl and add boiling water.

When margarine is melted, stir in sugar and vanilla and beat until smooth.

Stir in egg yolk and beat until smooth.

Stir baking soda into buttermilk. Add to batter and mix well.

Add flour and baking powder and mix well.

Whip egg whites until stiff but not dry and fold into batter.

Pour batter into pan and bake on middle rack of oven for 40–50 minutes or until a cake tester comes out clean.

Cool. Then make cocoa frosting.

The Cocoa Frosting

In a mixing bowl, blend margarine and cocoa.
Add vanilla.
Beat in confectioners' sugar.
Add milk.
If too stiff, add more milk. If too runny, add more sugar.
Frost top and sides of cake.

Makes 10 slices
Per slice: 273 Total calories; 13 Sat-fat calories

MOCHA CAKE

A rich, dark chocolate cake with a taste of mocha.

1¾ cups unbleached white flour ¾ cup sugar
⅓ cup unsweetened cocoa   1 egg
1 teaspoon baking soda   1 egg white
½ teaspoon baking powder   ⅔ cup buttermilk
¼ teaspoon salt   ⅔ cup brewed coffee
1 teaspoon cinnamon   1 teaspoon vanilla
½ cup margarine

Mocha Frosting

2 tablespoons margarine   Dash of salt
1 cup confectioners' sugar   1 tablespoon brewed coffee
2 tablespoons unsweetened   ¼ teaspoon vanilla
  cocoa

Preheat oven to 350°F. Grease an 8 × 8-inch baking pan or an 8-inch springform pan with margarine.

Combine flour, cocoa, baking soda, baking powder, salt, and cinnamon. Set aside.

In a large mixing bowl, cream margarine and sugar.

Add egg and egg white and beat well.

Combine buttermilk, coffee, and vanilla.

Alternately add flour mixture and buttermilk mixture to sugar mixture, beating until smooth. Pour into baking pan and bake for 40 minutes or until a cake tester comes out clean.

Cool. Then make the frosting.

The Mocha Frosting

Cream margarine. Add confectioners' sugar. Beat until smooth.

Add cocoa, salt, coffee, and vanilla. Beat until smooth.

Add more sugar if frosting is too thin.

Add more coffee if frosting is too thick.

Frost top and sides of cake.

Makes 16 squares

	Total calories	Sat-fat calories
Per square	140	10
With icing	174	13

CINNAMON SUGAR COFFEE CAKE

This coffee cake is moist and delicious.

1 ½ cups unbleached white flour
1 ½ teaspoons baking powder
1 teaspoon baking soda
½ teaspoon salt
¼ cup brown sugar
¾ cup sugar

1 teaspoon cinnamon
½ cup margarine
1 egg
1 egg white
1 teaspoon vanilla
1 cup nonfat yogurt

Preheat oven to 350°F. Grease an 8-inch springform pan with margarine.

Combine flour, baking powder, baking soda, and salt together in a bowl. Set aside.

In small bowl combine ¼ cup brown sugar, ¼ cup of the granulated sugar, and cinnamon and set aside.

Cream the remaining ½ cup sugar with margarine until light and fluffy.

Add egg and egg white and vanilla and mix until batter is smooth.

Add flour and yogurt alternately and mix until batter is smooth.

Pour batter into baking pan.

Pour sugar mixture on top of the batter and, with a knife, swirl the sugar into the batter.

Bake for 45–50 minutes or until cake tester comes out clean.

Makes 8 slices
Per slice: 299 Total calories; 20 Sat-fat calories

NUTMEG TORTE

This is a very rich cake. It is rather silly-looking because it is so flat, but it tastes delicious.

¾ cup brown sugar
1 cup unbleached white flour
¼ cup margarine
1 cup nonfat yogurt

1 egg
½ teaspoon freshly grated nutmeg
1 teaspoon baking soda
1 walnut half

Grease an 8-inch springform pan with margarine and preheat oven to 350°F.

With pastry blender or your fingers combine sugar, flour, and margarine to make a crumbly mixture.

Press 1¼ cups of the crumbs into the bottom of the pan. Reserve the rest.

Combine yogurt, egg, nutmeg, and baking soda.

Stir yogurt mixture into reserved crumb mixture to make a batter.

Pour batter over crumb crust.

Bake for about 40–50 minutes or until cake tester comes out clean.

Place walnut half in the center of the torte.

Makes 8 slices
Per slice: 204 Total calories; 11 Sat-fat calories

TANTE NANCY'S APPLE CRUMB CAKE

Apple Crumb Cake is luscious. The crust is thick, crunchy, and sweet. The slightly tart apples melt in your mouth.

2–2½ pounds tart apples*
(about 6–7 large), peeled,
cored, and sliced
⅓ cup water
¼ cup sugar
2 cups unbleached white flour

¾ cups sugar
1½ teaspoons baking powder
½ cup margarine
1 egg yolk
2 teaspoons margarine

Preheat oven to 350°F. Grease an 8-inch springform pan with margarine.

In a large pot, cook apple slices with water and ¼ cup sugar until apples are tender but not mushy. Drain and reserve.

In a small bowl, mix flour, ¾ cup sugar, and baking powder.

With a pastry blender, cut in ½ cup margarine.

Cut in egg yolk.

Reserve 1 cup of flour mixture for the topping. Press remainder into bottom and sides of pan.

Spoon drained apples into pan.

Cover with reserved topping and dot with 2 teaspoons margarine.

Bake for about 1 hour or until crust is golden brown.

Makes 12 slices
Per slice: 225 Total calories; 15 Sat-fat calories

PIE, TART, OR QUICHE CRUST

1 ice cube
⅓–½ cup cold water
1½ cups unbleached white flour
2 tablespoons sugar
Pinch of salt

¼ cup tub margarine, frozen
1½ tablespoons olive oil
(For nonsweet pie dough,
eliminate sugar and add ¾
teaspoon salt)

Place ice cube in the cold water. Set aside.

---

*You can use as few as 5 large apples, but more is better. Or substitute 2–2½ pounds peaches or 4 cups blueberries.

Place 1½ cups flour in food processor fitted with steel blade or in a mixing bowl.

Add sugar and salt and mix until well blended.

Cut margarine into ½-inch pieces and add to flour mixture.

Process briefly or use pastry blender until flour mixture resembles coarse meal or oatmeal flakes.

Add oil and ⅓ cup of ice water (without ice cube).

Process 2–3 seconds or blend until dough begins to collect into a ball. *Do not overprocess.*

If dough is too dry, carefully add a few drops more cold water and blend briefly.

Remove ball of dough, lightly flour, and wrap in wax paper. Place in a plastic bag and chill in refrigerator for at least 2 hours. (Dough will keep 2–3 days in refrigerator or for several months in freezer.)

To Bake

Preheat oven to 450°F. Grease an 8- or 9-inch pie or quiche pan with margarine.

On a piece of wax paper, roll dough into an ⅛-inch-thick circle slightly larger than the pie pan.

Turn over the wax paper so the dough is facing downward and lay it over the pan. Peel wax paper off the dough.

Gently push the dough to conform to the shape of the pan.

Trim excess dough, except for about ¼ inch above the rim of the pan. Form a ridge.

Spread margarine on a piece of aluminum foil larger than the pan.

Set foil, greased-side down, onto pie dough.

Fill with dried beans or aluminum pie weights to keep the crust from bubbling up.

Bake for 7–8 minutes.

Remove foil and beans. Prick crust with a fork to release air bubbles.

For partially baked pie crust, bake 3–4 minutes more or until crust is just beginning to brown and shrink from the edges.

For fully baked pie crust, bake 7–10 minutes more or until lightly browned.

	Total calories	*Sat-fat calories*
Sweet pie crust	1260	95
Nonsweet pie crust	1170	95

GRAHAM CRACKER CRUST

Not only do Honey Graham Crackers make a delicious cookie, Honey Graham Cracker crumbs make a delicious pie crust, particularly for lemon meringue or Key lime pie. Commercial graham crackers, graham cracker crumbs, and ready-to-bake graham cracker crusts are often made with lard or hydrogenated vegetable oil. Make your own using the Honey Graham Crackers recipe on page 406.

8 homemade graham cracker crumbs (1¼ cups)	1 teaspoon sugar 2 tablespoons margarine

Preheat oven to 375°F.
In food processor or blender, finely crush 8 graham crackers.
Combine crumbs and sugar and pour into pie plate.
Melt margarine and mix into crumbs.
Press crumbs into pie plate to make a crust.
Bake 8 minutes, or until lightly browned.

Makes one pie crust
Per crust: 690 Total calories; 52 Sat-fat calories

KEY LIME PIE

This pie is as pretty to look at as it is delightful to eat. It never fails to wow guests and please the most discriminating palate. Many Key lime pies call for 3 egg yolks and butter. You will use only 1 egg yolk and margarine to create this divine dessert. You can use lemon juice instead of lime juice and call this Lemon Meringue Pie.

Partially baked sweet pie crust (page 396) or
  Graham Cracker Crust (above)

Filling

¾ cup sugar
¼ cup unbleached white flour
3 tablespoons cornstarch
¼ teaspoon salt

½–⅔ cup fresh lime juice +
   water to equal 2¼ cups
1 egg yolk
1 teaspoon margarine

Meringue

5 egg whites, at room
   temperature

¼ teaspoon cream of tartar
½ cup + 2 tablespoons sugar

The Filling

In a medium saucepan, thoroughly mix sugar, flour, cornstarch, and salt.

Add ¼ cup lime water and blend into a smooth paste.

Add remaining lime water and mix until smooth.

Stir filling over medium heat until it begins to boil and thicken. Remove saucepan from heat.

In a small bowl, combine egg yolk with a small amount of filling and blend until smooth. Mix back into filling in saucepan. (This step is important. If you were to add the egg yolk directly into the hot filling, the egg yolk would curdle.) Stir margarine into the filling and pour into crust. Cool until filling gels.

The Meringue

Preheat oven to 375°F.

Whip egg whites with cream of tartar until stiff but not dry.

Add sugar and continue beating until whites form stiff peaks.

Gently cover lime filling with egg whites, making sure whites cover pie completely.

Bake for 8–10 minutes or until meringue is golden brown.

Cool at room temperature.

Makes 10 slices

	Total calories	Sat-fat calories
Per slice		
With pastry crust	270	12
With Graham Cracker Crust	210	8

STRAWBERRY TART

Another pièce de résistance to end any meal on a high note. Make this tart with strawberries, kiwi fruit, peaches, or most any other fruit, even lemons. Try a combination of many fruits on one tart. Tarts are typically filled with crème patissière. Instead of the 6 egg yolks normally used in this French custard, this strawberry tart uses packaged vanilla pudding and pie filling.

Fully baked sweet pie crust
(page 396)
2 quarts strawberries
·1 package vanilla pudding and
pie filling

1¾ cups skim milk
1 scant tablespoon vanilla
½ cup apricot preserves
1 tablespoon sugar

Wash and hull strawberries.

On a plate the size of your tart pan, make a pleasing arrangement of strawberries.

Make vanilla pudding according to package instructions but use 1¾ cups skim milk and 1 scant tablespoon of vanilla instead of the ingredients listed on the box.

Spread pudding evenly over the bottom of the pie crust.

Immediately arrange fruit on crust.

Combine apricot jam and sugar and heat until syrup is thick and forms a ball at the end of your spoon.

Paint fruit with glaze. Refrigerate tart.

Makes 10 slices
Per slice: 215 Total calories; 10 Sat-fat calories

STRAWBERRY-RHUBARB PIE

Rhubarb gives this pie a wonderful blending of sweet and sour.

Partially baked sweet pie crust
(page 396)
3 stalks rhubarb
2 pints strawberries, washed
and hulled

2½ teaspoons margarine
¾–1 cup sugar
2⅔ tablespoons quick-cooking
tapioca

Prepare partially baked sweet pastry for pie bottom crust, but use 1¾ cups flour.

Refrigerate extra pastry.

Preheat oven to 400°F.

Slice rhubarb into ¼-inch pieces. Cut strawberries into quarters.

Gently sauté rhubarb in 2 teaspoons of the margarine until slightly softened (about 5 minutes).

Combine rhubarb, strawberries, sugar, and tapioca, and set aside for 15 minutes.

Fill crust with fruit mixture.

Dot with the remaining ½ teaspoon margarine.

Roll out remaining pastry and cut into strips. Cover pie with lattice top. Bake for 25–40 minutes or until crust is browned.

Makes 10 slices
Per slice: 240 Total calories; 11 Sat-fat calories

APPLE PANDOWDY

1¼ cups unbleached white flour	½ cup brown sugar
1 tablespoon sugar	1 tablespoon flour
¼ teaspoon salt	1 teaspoon cinnamon
3 tablespoons margarine	3 tablespoons molasses
1 tablespoon olive oil	7 cups tart apples (about 7),
3 tablespoons + 1 teaspoon	peeled and sliced
skim milk	½ cup chopped walnuts

Preheat oven to 400°F. Grease a 2-quart shallow baking pan with margarine.

In a small bowl, combine flour, sugar, and salt.

Cut in margarine with a pastry blender until margarine is the size of small peas.

Add oil and 3 tablespoons of skim milk. Mix until dough forms a ball. If too dry, add 1 teaspoon of milk.

Wrap dough in wax paper, place in a plastic bag, and refrigerate for 30 minutes.

In a large bowl, combine brown sugar, flour, and cinnamon.

Mix in molasses. Mixture will be sticky.

Mix in apples and walnuts. Molasses mixture will clump. Don't worry.

Pour into pan. Spread molasses mixture over apples as evenly as possible.

Roll out pastry into a rectangle and place over apples.

Bake for 30–40 minutes or until crust is golden brown.

Makes 10 pieces
Per piece: 243 Total calories; 11 Sat-fat calories

DEEP-DISH PEAR PIE

This pie is absolutely scrumptious! Your fortunate guests will never suspect that nonfat yogurt (no saturated fat) was substituted for the traditional sour cream (270 sat-fat calories per cup).

Partially baked sweet pie crust (page 396)

Filling

2 tablespoons unbleached white flour
½ cup sugar
⅛ teaspoon salt
1 cup nonfat yogurt
1 egg

¼ teaspoon grated nutmeg
1 teaspoon vanilla extract
5 cups peeled pears (or tart apples), cut into bite-size pieces

Topping

3 tablespoons sugar
3 tablespoons unbleached white flour

½ teaspoon cinnamon
4 teaspoons margarine

Preheat oven to 400°F.

In a large bowl, combine flour, sugar, and salt. Mix in nonfat yogurt. Blend in egg. Add nutmeg and vanilla. Fold in pears.

Pour pear mixture into pie crust and bake at 400°F for 15 minutes. Lower heat to 350°F and continue baking for 25 minutes more.

Mix together topping ingredients.

Remove pie from oven and sprinkle topping over filling.

Raise heat to 375°F and bake until topping is brown.

Makes 12 slices
Per slice: 236 Total calories; 11 Sat-fat calories

Q COCOA BROWNIES

⅓ cup margarine	1 egg white
½ cup sugar	⅓ cup unsweetened cocoa
¼ cup light corn syrup	½ cup flour
2 teaspoons vanilla	½ teaspoon salt
1 egg	½ cup chopped walnuts

Preheat oven to 350°F. Grease an 8 × 8-inch baking pan with margarine.

In a large bowl, cream margarine and sugar.

Add corn syrup, vanilla, egg, and egg white and mix until well blended.

Combine cocoa, flour, and salt and slowly add to batter.

Fold in nuts and pour batter into baking pan.

Bake for 25–30 minutes or until a cake tester comes out clean.

Makes 16 squares
Per brownie: 115 Total calories; 9 Sat-fat calories

Q CINNAMON SWEET CAKES

A family favorite that can be made on the spur of the moment.

¼ cup olive oil	¾ cup whole-wheat flour
1 egg	¾ cup unbleached white flour
½ cup skim milk	2 teaspoons baking powder
½ cup sugar	½ teaspoon salt

Topping

½ cup brown sugar	1 tablespoon margarine
½ cup coarsely chopped walnuts	1 teaspoon cinnamon
1 tablespoon unbleached white flour	

Preheat oven to 375°F. Grease an 8 × 8-inch baking pan with margarine.

In a large mixing bowl, beat together oil, egg, and skim milk.

Add sugar, whole-wheat flour, white flour, baking powder, and salt and beat until smooth.

Spoon batter into baking pan. (Batter will be thick.)

To make the topping, combine brown sugar, walnuts, flour, and cinnamon in a small bowl.

Melt margarine and stir into mixture.

Sprinkle topping over batter.

Bake for about 25 minutes or until a cake tester comes out clean.

Makes 16 squares
Per square: 148 Total calories; 8 Sat-fat calories

GLAZED CINNAMON BUNS

1 tablespoon active dry yeast
3 tablespoons sugar
½ cup warm water
1½ cups whole-wheat flour
1½+ cups unbleached white flour
1 teaspoon salt
1½ tablespoons olive oil
½ cup nonfat skim milk

1 egg white
⅓ cup firmly packed brown sugar
2 teaspoons cinnamon
½ cup raisins
1 cup confectioners' sugar
2–3 tablespoons nonfat skim milk

Place yeast, sugar, and water in a large bowl or the bowl of a food processor. Let proof until foamy.

Add 1½ cups of whole-wheat flour, 1½ cups of white flour, salt, oil, milk, and egg white and mix or process. Keep adding flour until dough becomes fairly stiff.

Knead dough for 10 minutes or process for 15 seconds or until dough is smooth and elastic, adding more flour if necessary.

Place dough in bowl you have greased with a drop or two of olive oil, cover with a dish towel, and let rise in a warm place for 1 hour or until doubled in bulk.

When the dough has doubled in size, place it on a lightly floured surface.

Grease a 12-cup muffin tin with margarine. Set aside.

While the dough rests, combine brown sugar, cinnamon, and raisins and set aside.

Roll dough into a 9 × 12-inch rectangle.

Sprinkle cinnamon mixture evenly over the dough.

Starting with the long side of the rectangle, roll the dough *tightly* into a jelly roll. Cut it crosswise into 12 even pieces.

Place each piece, cut side up, into a muffin cup. Cover with a towel and let rise 45 minutes.

Preheat oven to 400°F. Bake buns for 15–20 minutes or until nicely browned. Transfer them to a cooling rack.

Place confectioners' sugar in bowl of an electric mixer. Add 1 tablespoon of milk and mix on low speed until smooth. Add more milk very slowly if mixture is too thick.

Spoon glaze over tops of buns.

Makes 12 buns
Per bun: 120 Total calories; 3 Sat-fat calories

Q   # MANDELBROT

These cookies are addictive. Thank you, Esther Krashes!

⅔ cup sugar   1½ cups unbleached white flour
¼ cup olive oil   1 teaspoon baking powder
3 egg whites   ½ cup coarsely ground almonds
1 egg   1 teaspoon orange extract

Preheat oven to 350°F.

Lightly grease a cookie sheet with margarine or olive oil.

In a large mixing bowl, cream sugar and olive oil.

Mix in egg whites and egg.

Add flour and baking powder and mix until smooth.

Stir in almonds and orange extract.

Pour onto cookie sheet. Spread into rectangle (8″ × 10″), about ½ inch thick.

Bake for 20 minutes or until lightly browned.

Remove cookie sheet from oven.

Cut dough into strips about 3 inches wide and then score (do not cut through) into bars about ¾ inch wide.

Turn strips over and bake 10 more minutes or until crisp.

Break into bars.

Makes 4 dozen bars
Per bar: 46 Total calories; 2 Sat-fat calories

Q

HONEY GRAHAM CRACKERS

1 cup whole-wheat flour	2 tablespoons margarine
½ cup unbleached white flour	2 tablespoons light brown sugar
½ teaspoon baking powder	2 tablespoons honey
¼ teaspoon baking soda	½ teaspoon vanilla
Pinch of salt	2 tablespoons skim milk

Preheat oven to 350°F and grease a cookie sheet with margarine.

Combine flours, baking powder, baking soda, and salt, and set aside.

Cream margarine, sugar, and honey in an electric mixer.

Mix in vanilla.

Add flour mixture and milk.

Gather dough together (add a drop of milk if too dry) and knead into a ball.

Roll dough onto cookie sheet into a rectangle, ⅛ inch thick.

If dough is too sticky, sprinkle it with flour.

Without moving dough, cut into 3-inch squares.

Lightly score a line through the center of each square and pierce each side several times with a fork.

Bake 10–15 minutes, until edges brown. Remove crackers and cool on a wire rack.

Crackers will become crisp as they cool.

Makes 18 crackers
Per cracker: 58 Total calories; 2 Sat-fat calories

Q

MARVELOUS COOKIES

A cookie made with healthy ingredients which is absolutely scrumptious. Refrain from eating too many, as each contains about 39 fat calories.

¼ cup margarine	¾ teaspoon baking powder
¼ cup olive oil	1 cup wheat germ
½ cup brown sugar	1½ cups rolled oats
1 egg	½ cup raisins
1½ teaspoons vanilla	½ cup chopped walnuts
½ cup whole-wheat flour	1–2 tablespoons water, if
½ teaspoon salt	necessary

Preheat oven to 375°F. Grease a cookie sheet with margarine.

Cream margarine, oil, and brown sugar.

Add egg and vanilla and beat well.

Add whole-wheat flour, salt, baking powder, wheat germ, rolled oats, raisins, and nuts and mix well. Add water if too dry.

Drop batter by teaspoonfuls onto cookie sheet and bake 10–12 minutes.

Makes 3 dozen cookies
Per cookie: 80 Total calories; 5 Sat-fat calories

APPLE-NUT COOKIES

⅓ cup margarine
½ cup brown sugar
1 egg
1 cup unbleached white flour
½ cup whole-wheat flour
½ teaspoon baking soda
1 teaspoon baking powder
½ teaspoon salt

1 teaspoon cinnamon
¼ teaspoon grated nutmeg
3 tablespoons milk
¼ cup raisins
½ cup chopped walnuts
2½ cups peeled, diced cooking apples

Preheat oven to 400°F. Lightly grease a cookie sheet with margarine.

In a large mixing bowl, cream margarine and brown sugar.

Add egg and beat until batter is smooth.

Combine white flour, whole-wheat flour, baking soda, baking powder, salt, cinnamon, and nutmeg.

Mix into batter alternately with milk.

Stir in raisins and nuts. Fold in apples.

Drop batter by teaspoonfuls onto cookie sheet and bake for 10–12 minutes or until golden brown.

Makes 3 dozen cookies
Per cookie: 62 Total calories; 4 Sat-fat calories

OATMEAL COOKIES

¼ cup olive oil
⅓ cup brown sugar
2 tablespoons sugar
1 egg white
¾ teaspoon vanilla
3 tablespoons water

2 cups rolled oats
⅓ cup unbleached white flour
⅓ cup whole-wheat flour
¼ teaspoon salt
½ teaspoon baking soda
1 teaspoon cinnamon

Preheat oven to 350°F. Grease a cookie sheet with margarine.
Cream oil and sugars.
Mix in egg white, vanilla, and water.
Add oats, white flour, whole-wheat flour, salt, baking soda, and cinnamon and mix until blended. Do not overmix or you will lose the texture of the oats.
Drop batter by teaspoonfuls onto cookie sheet and bake for 10–15 minutes.

Makes 2 dozen cookies
Per cookie: 65 Total calories; 3 Sat-fat calories

MERINGUE SHELLS WITH FRESH STRAWBERRIES AND WARM RASPBERRY SAUCE

Here's a delectable dessert that has no saturated fat or total fat. It is extremely simple to prepare and, later, to assemble. Make sure to budget in 1 to 2 hours baking time for the meringue.

Meringue Shells

4 egg whites at room
   temperature
⅛ teaspoon salt
⅛ teaspoon cream of tartar

¾ cup sugar
½ teaspoon vanilla
¼ teaspoon almond extract

Filling

1 pint strawberries, washed, hulled, and halved (actually any berry or cut-up fruit will do)

Sauce

1 package (10 oz) frozen raspberries	1 teaspoon cornstarch
	½ teaspoon lemon juice

The Meringue

Preheat oven to 275°F. Completely cover your baking sheet with a piece of brown paper. Set aside.

In a very clean mixing bowl, whip egg whites until foamy. Continue whipping as you add salt and cream of tartar. When egg whites form soft peaks, slowly add sugar while continuing to beat until whites are glossy and stiff. Mix in vanilla and almond extract.

On the brown paper, use a spoon or spatula to spread the meringue into 6 shells, 4–5 inches across with a raised edge about 1 inch high. You may also use a pastry tube to squeeze out concentric circles to form a base and sides. The shells should be deep enough to hold the fruit.

Bake for 2 hours. Turn off heat and let meringues sit in closed oven for 2 hours or overnight. Gently remove meringues, as they crack easily.

The Filling

Fill the shell cavity with a mound of strawberries.

The Raspberry Sauce

Thaw raspberries or, if you forgot to plan ahead, place pouch containing raspberries into a bowl of warm water for about 2 minutes to thaw. When partially thawed, purée the raspberries in a blender.

Place cornstarch in a small saucepan. Add 1 tablespoon of purée and mix with cornstarch until smooth. Stir in remaining purée and add lemon juice. Bring to a boil and simmer for 1 minute.

Spoon several tablespoons of the warm sauce over the strawberries. You may also refrigerate the sauce and serve it cold.

6 servings
Per serving: 130 Total calories; 0 Sat-fat calories

☐ ## PEARS HÉLÈNE

Pears Hélène made with cocoa and margarine are wonderful, just like their counterpart made with chocolate and butter.

The chocolate sauce is a good all-purpose dessert sauce. You can store it in the refrigerator for weeks.

Pears

4 ripe pears	¼ cup sugar
2 cups water	1 tablespoon fresh lemon juice

Chocolate Sauce

3 tablespoons sugar	1 tablespoon light corn syrup
2 tablespoons unsweetened cocoa	1 tablespoon margarine
1 tablespoon cornstarch	½ teaspoon vanilla
2 tablespoons water	

The Pears

Peel pears, cut them in half, core them, and cut off the stems.

In a pot large enough to hold pears, combine water, sugar, and lemon juice and bring to a boil.

Spoon pears into liquid, reduce heat, and simmer, covered, for 5 minutes. Pears should be tender, not mushy.

Drain poached pears and chill.

The Chocolate Sauce

In a small saucepan, combine sugar, cocoa, and cornstarch.

Mix in water and corn syrup and blend well.

Cook over medium heat until mixture comes to a boil.

Remove from heat and stir for about 1 minute.

Add margarine and vanilla and continue to stir until sauce is well blended.

On each plate, place 2 pear halves, cut-side up, and pour warm sauce over them.

4 servings
Per serving: 205 Total calories; 5 Sat-fat calories

THREE

FOOD TABLES

CONTENTS

BEVERAGES

FOOD	AMOUNT	TOTAL CALORIES	SAT-FAT CALORIES
Alcoholic			
Beer			
regular	12 fl oz	150	0
light	12 fl oz	95	0
Gin, rum, vodka, whiskey			
80 proof	1½ fl oz	95	0
Other			
brandy Alexander	5 fl oz	185	65
piña colada	5 fl oz	215	85
eggnog	8 fl oz	342	102
Wine			
dessert	3½ fl oz	140	0
table	3½ fl oz	75	0
Carbonated			
Club soda	12 fl oz	0	0
Cola			
regular	12 fl oz	160	0
diet (artificially sweetened)	12 fl oz	trace	0

BEVERAGES

FOOD	AMOUNT	TOTAL CALORIES	SAT-FAT CALORIES
Ginger ale	12 fl oz	125	0
Grape	12 fl oz	180	0
Lemon-lime	12 fl oz	155	0
Orange	12 fl oz	180	0
Pepper-type	12 fl oz	160	0
Root beer	12 fl oz	165	0

Other
FOOD	AMOUNT	TOTAL CALORIES	SAT-FAT CALORIES
Cocoa			
Hershey's made with whole milk	6 fl oz	90	35
Hershey's made with skim milk	6 fl oz	38	1
Coffee			
brewed	6 fl oz	trace	trace
instant	6 fl oz	trace	trace
Fruit drinks, noncarbonated			
Canned			
fruit punch drink	6 fl oz	85	0
grape drink	6 fl oz	100	0
pineapple-grapefruit juice drink	6 fl oz	90	0
Frozen			
lemonade (diluted)	6 fl oz	80	trace

Fruit juices: see **FRUITS AND FRUIT JUICES.**

Milk beverages: see **DAIRY PRODUCTS AND EGGS.**

DAIRY PRODUCTS AND EGGS

FOOD	AMOUNT	TOTAL CALORIES	SAT-FAT CALORIES
Butter			
Regular	1 tablespoon	100	65
	1 stick (½ cup)	813	515
Whipped	1 tablespoon	67	38
	1 stick (½ cup)	542	344

(For margarine, see **FATS AND OILS.**)

FOOD	AMOUNT	TOTAL CALORIES	SAT-FAT CALORIES
Cheese			
American	1 oz	106	50
American cheese spread	1 oz	82	34

DAIRY PRODUCTS AND EGGS

FOOD	AMOUNT	TOTAL CALORIES	SAT-FAT CALORIES
American Lite-Line (Borden)	1 oz	50	18
Blue	1 oz	100	48
Brick	1 oz	105	48
Camembert	1 oz	85	39
Caraway	1 oz	90	36
Cheddar	1 oz	114	54
Colby	1 oz	112	52
Cottage			
creamed	½ cup	117	29
dry curd	½ cup	96	3
1% fat	½ cup	82	7
2% fat	½ cup	102	12
Cream			
regular	1 oz	99	56
	1 tbsp	52	26
whipped	1 tbsp	37	19
Edam	1 oz	101	45
Farmer			
Friendship	1 oz	40	18
May-Bud	1 oz	90	41
Feta	1 oz	75	38
Fontina	1 oz	110	49
Gjetöst	1 oz	132	49
Gouda	1 oz	101	45
Gruyère	1 oz	117	48
Limburger	1 oz	93	43
Monterey Jack	1 oz	100	45
Mozzarella			
whole milk	1 oz	80	34
low moisture	1 oz	90	40
part skim	1 oz	72	26
low moisture, part skim	1 oz	79	28
Muenster	1 oz	104	49
Neufchâtel	1 oz	74	38
Ole Smokey (Land O' Lakes)	1 oz	90	36
Parmesan			
grated	1 oz	129	49
	1 tbsp	23	9
hard	1 oz	111	42
Pimiento	1 oz	106	50
Port du Salut	1 oz	100	43

DAIRY PRODUCTS AND EGGS

FOOD	AMOUNT	TOTAL CALORIES	SAT-FAT CALORIES
Provolone	1 oz	100	44
Ricotta			
whole milk	½ cup	216	93
part skim milk	½ cup	171	55
Romano	1 oz	110	43
Roquefort	1 oz	105	49
Swiss			
natural	1 oz	107	45
processed	1 oz	95	41
Tilsit	1 oz	96	43

Reduced-Fat Cheeses

FOOD	AMOUNT	TOTAL CALORIES	SAT-FAT CALORIES
Alpine Lace			
Free n' Lean			
Cheddar	1 oz	35	0
Mozzarella	1 oz	35	0
Swiss-Lo	1 oz	90	36
Churny			
Lite Reduced Fat			
Cheddar	1 oz	80	27
Colby	1 oz	80	27
Monterey Jack	1 oz	80	27
Formagg			
Process Cheese Substitute			
American flavor	1 oz	70	9
Shredded Cheddar	1 oz	70	9
Shredded Mozzarella	1 oz	70	9
Kraft			
Golden Image Cheddar Style Chunk	1 oz	110	18
Light Naturals Reduced Fat			
Colby	1 oz	80	27
Sharp Cheddar	1 oz	90	27
Shredded Part-Skim Mozzarella	1 oz	80	27
Shredded Sharp Cheddar	1 oz	90	27
Swiss	1 oz	80	27
Light Singles, American flavor	1 oz	70	27
Philadelphia Cream Cheese	1 oz	100	45
Philadelphia Light Cream Cheese	1 oz	80	36

DAIRY PRODUCTS AND EGGS

FOOD	AMOUNT	TOTAL CALORIES	SAT-FAT CALORIES
Weight Watchers			
Flavor Cheese Product			
American	1 oz	50	9
Natural Mild Cheddar	1 oz	80	27
Sharp Cheddar	1 oz	50	9
Swiss Flavor	1 oz	50	9
Cream			
Half-and-half	1 tbsp	20	10
Light, coffee or table	1 tbsp	29	16
	1 cup	469	260
(Coffee whiteners: see *Imitation Dairy Creamers.*)			
Medium (25% fat)	1 tbsp	37	21
	1 cup	583	335
Light whipping	1 tbsp	44	26
	1 cup	699	416
Heavy whipping	1 tbsp	52	31
	1 cup	821	493
Whipped cream topping	1 tbsp	8	4
(pressurized)	1 cup	154	75
Sour	1 tbsp	26	14
	1 cup	493	270
Light (Breakstone)	1 tbsp	25	9
Frozen Desserts			
Frozen yogurt			
Baskin-Robbins			
low-fat			
small	1	150–175	29 e
medium	1	211–246	41 e
large	1	270–315	53 e
nonfat			
small	1	100–125	0
medium	1	140–176	0
large	1	180–225	0

e indicates estimated sat-fat calories.

DAIRY PRODUCTS AND EGGS

FOOD	AMOUNT	TOTAL CALORIES	SAT-FAT CALORIES
Frozen yogurt			
Breyers			
Low-Fat Vanilla	½ cup	120	6 e
Colombo			
Lite	4 fl oz	102	12
nonfat	4 fl oz	90	0
Elan Premium	4 fl oz	130	18 e
Ely's Inspirations	3 fl oz	80	6 e
Everything Yogurt			
low-fat	4 fl oz	95	12
nonfat	4 fl oz	80	0
Häagen-Dazs			
Strawberry	3 fl oz	120	18 e
Vanilla	3 fl oz	130	18 e
Vanilla Almond Crunch	3 fl oz	150	29 e
ICBIY			
nonfat			
small	6¾ fl oz	135	0
medium	9⅓ fl oz	187	0
large	12 fl oz	240	0
original			
small	6¾ fl oz	182	43 e
medium	9⅓ fl oz	252	59 e
large	12 fl oz	324	76 e
sugar-free nonfat			
small	6¾ fl oz	115	0
medium	9⅓ fl oz	159	0
large	12 fl oz	204	0
Lucerne	3 fl oz	80	12 e
TCBY			
nonfat			
kiddie cup	1	88	0
small cup	1	162	0
regular cup	1	226	0
large cup	1	289	0
super cup	1	418	0
giant cup	1	869	0

e indicates estimated sat-fat calories.

DAIRY PRODUCTS AND EGGS

FOOD	AMOUNT	TOTAL CALORIES	SAT-FAT CALORIES
Frozen yogurt			
TCBY (*cont.*)			
regular			
kiddie cup	1	96	14
small cup	1	177	27
regular cup	1	246	37
large cup	1	316	48
super cup	1	456	68
giant cup	1	948	142
Yoplait Soft	3 fl oz	90	12 e
Ice Cream, Light Ice Cream, Ice Milk			
Baskin-Robbins			
ice cream			
Chocolate	1 scoop	270	81 e
Chocolate Chip	1 scoop	260	87 e
Chocolate Raspberry Truffle	1 scoop	310	99 e
French Vanilla	1 scoop	280	105 e
Jamoca Almond Fudge	1 scoop	270	81 e
Pralines 'n Cream	1 scoop	280	81 e
Rocky Road	1 scoop	300	81 e
Vanilla	1 scoop	240	81 e
Very Berry Strawberry	1 scoop	220	58 e
World Class Chocolate	1 scoop	280	81 e
light ice cream			
Chocolate Caramel Nut	½ cup	130	28
Espresso and Cream	½ cup	120	28
Praline Dream	½ cup	130	34
Strawberry Royale	½ cup	110	15
Sherbet, rainbow	1 scoop	160	12 e
Ben & Jerry's			
premium			
Chocolate	4 fl oz	290	105 e
French Vanilla	4 fl oz	270	99 e
ice milk			
Coffee Almond Fudge	4 fl oz	230	58 e
Sweet Cream & Cookies	4 fl oz	220	47 e

e indicates estimated sat-fat calories.

DAIRY PRODUCTS AND EGGS

FOOD	AMOUNT	TOTAL CALORIES	SAT-FAT CALORIES
Ice Cream, Light Ice Cream,			
Ice Milk			
Breyers			
ice cream			
Butter Pecan	½ cup	180	70 e
Chocolate	½ cup	160	47 e
Mint Chocolate Chip	½ cup	170	53 e
Vanilla	½ cup	150	47 e
Vanilla Fudge Twirl	½ cup	160	47 e
Marble Classics			
Chocolate Chip Mousse	½ cup	230	81 e
Praline Caramel	½ cup	240	87 e
Raspberry Parfait	½ cup	200	64 e
Strawberry Cream	½ cup	180	53 e
Light Ice Milk			
Fudge Toffee Parfait	½ cup	140	27
Heavenly Hash	½ cup	150	27
Praline Almond	½ cup	130	18
Vanilla	½ cup	130	18
Vanilla Chocolate Strawberry	½ cup	120	18
Häagen-Dazs			
Butter Pecan	4 fl oz	290	99 e
Chocolate	4 fl oz	250	99 e
Chocolate Chocolate Chip	4 fl oz	290	105 e
Coffee	4 fl oz	250	99 e
Coffee Toffee Crunch	4 fl oz	300	111 e
Deep Chocolate Peanut Butter	4 fl oz	330	111 e
Macadamia Brittle	4 fl oz	280	105 e
Rum Raisin	4 fl oz	250	99 e
Strawberry	4 fl oz	230	87 e
Vanilla	4 fl oz	250	99 e
Vanilla Fudge	4 fl oz	280	105 e
Vanilla Swiss Almond	4 fl oz	290	111 e
Lucerne			
ice cream			
Mint Chocolate Chip	½ cup	145	47 e

e indicates estimated sat-fat calories.

DAIRY PRODUCTS AND EGGS

FOOD	AMOUNT	TOTAL CALORIES	SAT-FAT CALORIES
Ice Cream, Light Ice Cream, Ice Milk			
Lucerne (*cont.*)			
light (ice milk)			
Chocolate	½ cup	120	18 e
Cookies and Cream	½ cup	135	23 e
Rocky Road	½ cup	130	23 e
Strawberries and Cream	½ cup	105	12 e
Toasted Almond	½ cup	125	23 e
Vanilla	½ cup	110	18 e
fat-free	½ cup	100	0
Sealtest			
Butter Pecan	½ cup	160	58 e
Chocolate Chip	½ cup	150	47 e
Vanilla	½ cup	140	41 e
Sealtest Free	½ cup	100	0
Weight Watchers			
Fudge Marble	½ cup	120	18 e
Swiss Vanilla	½ cup	100	18 e
Shakes, thick			
Chocolate	10.6 fl oz	356	45
Vanilla	11 fl oz	350	53

(For Dairy bars, see **SUGARS AND SWEETS,** *Frozen Novelties.*)

Imitation Dairy Creamers

Dry creamers			
Coffee-Mate	1 tbsp	10	<9
Lite	1 tbsp	8	<9
Cremora	1 tbsp	10	<9
Lite	1 tbsp	8	0
Frozen liquid creamers			
Poly Rich, Coffee Rich	1 tbsp	20	<9

Milk

Buttermilk	1 cup	99	0–12

e indicates estimated sat-fat calories.

DAIRY PRODUCTS AND EGGS

FOOD	AMOUNT	TOTAL CALORIES	SAT-FAT CALORIES
Canned			
condensed, sweetened	1 oz	123	19
	1 cup	982	151
evaporated, skim	1 oz	25	0
	½ cup	99	1
evaporated, whole	1 oz	42	13
	½ cup	169	52
Chocolate			
2% milk	1 cup	179	28
whole milk	1 cup	208	47
malted (1 cup milk + ¾ oz powder)	1 cup	233	50
cocoa powder with nonfat dry milk	1 oz	100	5
Low-fat, 1%	1 cup	104	14
Low-fat, 2%	1 cup	121	27
Nonfat			
dry	¼ cup	109	1
instant	3.2 oz envelope (for 1 qt)	326	4
Skim	1 cup	86	0–3
Whole	1 cup	150	45
Whole, dry	¼ cup	159	48
Yogurt			
Breyers	8 fl oz	260	18 e
Colombo			
classic			
Black Cherry	8 fl oz	230	35 e
French Vanilla	8 fl oz	215	41 e
Peach Melba	8 fl oz	230	35 e
nonfat lite			
Fruit flavors	8 fl oz	190	<9
Plain	8 fl oz	110	<9
Vanilla	8 fl oz	160	<9

e indicates estimated sat-fat calories.

DAIRY PRODUCTS AND EGGS

FOOD	AMOUNT	TOTAL CALORIES	SAT-FAT CALORIES
Dannon			
classic flavors	8 fl oz	200	18 e
fat-free	6 fl oz	150	0
fruit low-fat	8 fl oz	240	18 e
light (nonfat)	8 fl oz	100	0
La Yogurt			
nonfat	8 fl oz	190	0
100% natural	6 fl oz	190	23 e
Light 'n Lively	8 fl oz	100	0
Weight Watchers			
Ultimate 90	8 fl oz	90	0
Whitney's 100% Natural	6 fl oz	190	29 e
Yoplait			
custard style, fruit	6 fl oz	190	23 e
custard style, vanilla	6 fl oz	180	23 e
light (nonfat)	6 fl oz	80	0
original, fruit	6 fl oz	190	18 e
original, vanilla	6 fl oz	180	18 e
Eggs			
Large, fresh	1	79	15
white	1	16	0
yolk	1	63	15
Egg Substitutes			
Fleischmann's			
Egg Beaters	¼ cup	25	0
Healthy Choice			
Cholesterol-Free Egg Product	¼ cup	30	<9
Morningside Farms			
Scramblers	¼ cup	60	0
Second Nature	¼ cup	60	9
Mixed Dairy Dishes			
Fettuccine Alfredo	1 cup	880	377
Macaroni and cheese			
canned	1 cup	230	42
homemade	1 cup	430	88
Quiche Lorraine (8-inch)	1 slice (⅛ pie)	600	209

e indicates estimated sat-fat calories.

FAST FOODS*

FOOD	AMOUNT	TOTAL CALORIES	SAT-FAT CALORIES
Arby's			
Bacon platter	1	869	92
Baked potato			
Broccoli and Cheddar	1	417	62
Butter with sour cream	1	463	109
Deluxe	1	621	163
Mushroom and cheese	1	515	52
Plain	1	240	0
Beef 'n Cheddar	1 serving	451	64
Biscuit			
bacon	1	318	39
ham	1	323	35
plain	1	280	30
sausage	1	460	85
Blueberry muffin	1	200	17
Blueberry turnover	1	320	57
Cheddar fries	1 serving	399	81
Cheesecake	1 serving	306	67
Chicken			
breast sandwich	1	489	35
Cordon Bleu	1 serving	658	80
grilled barbecue	1 serving	378	38
grilled deluxe	1 serving	426	47
roast club	1	513	45
roast deluxe	1	373	29
Chocolate chip cookie	1	130	18
Cinnamon-nut Danish	1	340	17
Croissant			
bacon and egg	1	389	126
ham and cheese	1	345	109
mushroom and cheese	1	493	137
plain	1	260	94
sausage and egg	1	519	167
Curly fries	1 serving	337	67
Egg platter	1	460	65

*We would like to thank Michael Jacobson of the Center for Science in the Public Interest for providing many of the values in this section. For more nutrition information and analysis of fast foods, see *The Fast-Food Guide* by Michael Jacobson and Sarah Fritschner (Workman Publishing, 1991).

FAST FOODS

FOOD	AMOUNT	TOTAL CALORIES	SAT-FAT CALORIES
Fish fillet sandwich	1	537	55
French fries			
large	1 serving	492	54
medium	1 serving	394	43
small	1 serving	246	27
Ham 'n cheese	1	330	33
Ham platter	1	518	71
Horsey sauce	1	55	6
Hot chocolate	1	110	6
Philly beef 'n Swiss	1	498	56
Polar Swirl			
Butterfinger	1	457	76
Heath	1	543	47
Oreo	1	482	94
Peanut Butter Cup	1	517	73
Snickers	1	511	60
Potato cakes	1 serving	204	20
Roast beef			
bac'n Cheddar deluxe	1	532	72
French dip	1	345	51
French dip 'n Swiss	1	425	70
giant	1 serving	530	94
junior	1 serving	218	32
regular	1 serving	353	66
super	1 serving	529	73
Salad			
cashew chicken	1 serving	590	81
chef	1 serving	210	45
garden	1 serving	149	38
side	1 serving	25	0
Salad dressing			
blue cheese	4 tbsp	295	52
buttermilk ranch	4 tbsp	349	50
honey French	4 tbsp	322	35
light Italian	4 tbsp	23	1
Thousand Island	4 tbsp	298	39
Sausage platter	1	640	120
Shake			
chocolate	1	451	25
jamocha	1	368	22
vanilla	1	330	35

FAST FOODS

FOOD	AMOUNT	TOTAL CALORIES	SAT-FAT CALORIES
Soup			
beef with vegetables and barley	1 serving	96	10
Boston clam chowder	1 serving	207	32
cream of broccoli	1 serving	180	43
french onion	1 serving	67	5
lumberjack mixed vegetables	1 serving	89	15
old-fashioned chicken noodle	1 serving	99	5
pilgrim's corn chowder	1 serving	193	32
split pea with ham	1 serving	200	44
tomato florentine	1 serving	84	8
Wisconsin cheese	1 serving	287	73
Sub deluxe	1	482	45
Toastix	1	420	41
Turkey deluxe	1	399	32
Turnover			
apple	1	303	62
cherry	1	280	48
Burger King			
Apple pie	1	311	36
Bacon bits	1 packet	16	0
Bagel			
plain	1	272	9
with bacon, egg, and cheese	1	453	63
with cream cheese	1	370	54
with egg and cheese	1	407	45
with ham, egg, and cheese	1	438	54
with sausage, egg, and cheese	1	626	108
Biscuit			
plain	1	332	27
with bacon	1	378	45
with bacon and egg	1	467	63
with sausage	1	478	72
with sausage and egg	1	568	90
Broiler Chicken Sandwich	1	379	27
Broiler Sauce	1 serving	90	9
Bull's Eye Barbecue Sauce	1 serving	22	0
Burger Buddies	1	349	63
Burger King A.M. Express Dip	1 serving	84	0
Cheeseburger	1	318	63
deluxe	1	390	72

FAST FOODS

FOOD	AMOUNT	TOTAL CALORIES	SAT-FAT CALORIES
Cheeseburger (*cont.*)			
double	1	483	117
bacon	1	515	126
bacon deluxe	1	592	144
barbecue bacon	1	536	126
mushroom swiss	1	473	108
Chicken sandwich	1	685	72
Chicken Tenders	6 pieces	236	27
Croissan'wich			
plain	1	180	18
with bacon, egg, and cheese	1	361	72
with egg and cheese	1	315	63
with ham, egg, and cheese	1	346	63
with sausage, egg, and cheese	1	534	117
Croutons	1 packet	31	<9
Danish			
apple cinnamon	1	390	27
cheese	1	406	45
cinnamon raisin	1	449	36
Dipping sauce			
barbecue	1 serving	36	0
honey	1 serving	91	0
ranch	1 serving	171	27
sweet and sour	1 serving	45	0
French fries	1 medium	372	45
French toast sticks	1 serving	538	45
Hamburger	1	272	36
deluxe	1	344	54
Mini Muffins			
blueberry	1	292	27
lemon poppyseed	1	318	27
raisin oat bran	1	291	18
Mushroom topping	1 serving	13	0
Ocean Catch fish filet sandwich	1	495	36
Onion rings	1 serving	339	45
Salad			
chef	1	178	36
chunky chicken	1	142	9
garden	1	95	27
side	1	25	0

FAST FOODS

FOOD	AMOUNT	TOTAL CALORIES	SAT-FAT CALORIES
Salad dressing			
bleu cheese	4 tbsp	300	63
French	4 tbsp	290	27
olive oil and vinegar	4 tbsp	310	45
ranch	4 tbsp	350	63
reduced-calorie light Italian	4 tbsp	170	27
Thousand Island	4 tbsp	290	45
Scrambled egg platter	1	549	81
with bacon	1	610	99
with sausage	1	768	135
Shake, regular			
chocolate	1	326	54
chocolate, syrup added	1	409	54
strawberry, syrup added	1	394	54
vanilla	1	334	54
Tartar sauce	1 serving	134	18
Tater Tenders	1 serving	213	27
Whopper	1	614	108
with cheese	1	706	144
double	1	844	171
double with cheese	1	935	198
Carl's Jr.			
Bacon	2 strips	45	9
Breakfast burrito	1 serving	430	108
Charbroiler sandwich			
BBQ chicken	1	400	18
chicken club	1	570	72
Cheeseburger			
western bacon	1	730	180
double classic	1	710	153
double western bacon	1	1030	288
Chocolate chip cookie	1 (2.5 oz)	330	63
Cinnamon rolls	1 serving	460	9
Country-fried steak sandwich	1	720	99
Danish	1	520	9
English muffin with margarine	1	190	9
Filet of fish sandwich	1	550	99
French fries			
large	1 serving	546	63
regular	1 serving	420	45
small	1 serving	281	27

FAST FOODS

FOOD	AMOUNT	TOTAL CALORIES	SAT-FAT CALORIES
French toast dips, no syrup	1 serving	490	54
Fudge brownie	1 serving	430	45
Guacamole	1 serving	50	9
Hamburger	1	320	45
famous star	1	610	117
old time star	1	460	81
super star	1	820	216
Hash brown nuggets	1 serving	270	36
Hot cakes with margarine, no syrup	1 serving	510	45
Jr. crisp burrito	3 (1 serving)	420	81
Muffin			
blueberry	1	340	9
bran	1	310	0
Onion rings	1 serving	520	54
Potato			
bacon and cheese	1	730	135
broccoli and cheese	1	590	99
cheese	1	690	135
fiesta	1	720	126
Lite	1	290	0
sour cream and chive	1	470	63
Roast beef sandwich			
club	1	620	99
deluxe	1	540	90
Salad dressing			
blue cheese	1 packet (2 oz)	300	54
house	1 packet (2 oz)	220	54
Italian	1 packet (2 oz)	240	36
reduced-calorie French	1 packet (2 oz)	80	0
Thousand Island	1 packet (2 oz)	220	54
Salad			
chicken	1 serving	200	36
garden, large	1 serving	100	27
garden, small	1 serving	50	18
taco	1 serving	310	99
Salsa	1 serving	8	0
Sausage	1 patty	190	45
Scrambled Eggs	1 serving	120	36
Shake			
large	1	459	45
regular	1	350	36
small	1	268	27

FAST FOODS

FOOD	AMOUNT	TOTAL CALORIES	SAT-FAT CALORIES
Sunrise sandwich	1	300	54
with bacon	1	345	63
with sausage	1	490	99
Taco sauce	1 serving	8	0
Zucchini	1 serving	390	54
Dairy Queen			
BBQ nugget sauces	1 serving	41	0
Buster bar	1 bar	448	169 e
Chicken breast fillet sandwich	1	450	36
with cheese	1	500	63
Chipper sandwich	1	318	41 e
Cone			
large	1	340	58 e
regular	1	240	41 e
small	1	140	23 e
dipped, chocolate			
large	1	510	139 e
regular	1	340	93 e
small	1	190	53 e
DQ sandwich	1	140	23 e
Dilly bar	1	210	76 e
Fish fillet sandwich	1	390	27
with cheese	1	440	54
Float	1	410	41 e
Freeze	1	500	70 e
French fries			
large	1 serving	340	27
regular	1 serving	210	18
Frozen yogurt, vanilla	4 oz	100	0
Fudge nut bar	1	406	145 e
Grilled chicken sandwich	1	300	18
Hamburger			
double	1	480	108
double with cheese	1	590	162
single	1	330	54
single with cheese	1	380	81
Heath Blizzard	1	800	139 e

e indicates estimated sat-fat calories.

FAST FOODS

FOOD	AMOUNT	TOTAL CALORIES	SAT-FAT CALORIES
Hot dog	1	240	27
with cheese	1	300	54
with cheese and chili	1	340	63
with chili	1	290	36
quarter-pound	1	480	122 e
with cheese	1	533	180 e
with cheese and chili	1	575	172 e
Malt			
large	1	889	122 e
regular	1	760	105 e
small	1	438	58 e
Mr. Misty Float	1	390	41 e
Mr. Misty Freeze	1	500	70 e
Mr. Misty Kiss	1	70	0
Mr. Misty			
large	1	340	0
regular	1	250	0
small	1	190	0
Onion rings, regular	1 serving	240	27
Parfait	1	430	47 e
Peanut Buster parfait	1	740	197 e
Shake			
large	1	831	128 e
regular	1	710	111 e
small	1	409	64 e
Sundae, chocolate			
large	1	440	58 e
regular	1	310	47 e
small	1	190	23 e
Ultimate burger	1	730	189
Domino's Pizza (16″ diameter)			
Cheese	2 slices	376	50
Deluxe	2 slices	498	84
Double cheese/pepperoni	2 slices	545	120
Ham	2 slices	417	53
Pepperoni	2 slices	460	76
Sausage/mushroom	2 slices	430	69
Veggie	2 slices	498	92

e indicates estimated sat-fat calories.

FAST FOODS

FOOD	AMOUNT	TOTAL CALORIES	SAT-FAT CALORIES
Hardee's			
Apple turnover	1	270	36
Barbecue sauce	1 packet (½ oz)	14	0
Big cookie	1 serving	250	36
Big Twin	1	450	99
Big Twin sauce	½ oz	50	0
Biscuit 'N' Gravy	1	440	54
Biscuit			
bacon	1	360	36
bacon and egg	1	410	45
bacon, egg, and cheese	1	460	72
Canadian Rise 'N' Shine	1	470	72
chicken	1	430	36
cinnamon 'N' raisin	1	320	45
country ham	1	350	27
country ham and egg	1	400	36
ham	1	320	18
ham and egg	1	370	36
ham, egg, and cheese	1	420	54
Rise 'N' Shine	1	320	27
sausage	1	440	63
sausage and egg	1	490	72
steak	1	500	63
steak and egg	1	550	72
Cheeseburger	1	320	63
bacon	1	610	144
quarter-pound	1	500	126
Chicken			
Fiesta salad	1	280	81
fillet sandwich	1	370	18
grilled sandwich	1	310	9
Stix	6 pieces	210	18
Cool Twist cone			
chocolate	1	200	36
vanilla	1	190	36
vanilla/chocolate	1	190	36
Cool Twist Sundae			
caramel	1	330	45
hot fudge	1	320	54
strawberry	1	260	45

FAST FOODS

FOOD	AMOUNT	TOTAL CALORIES	SAT-FAT CALORIES
Crispy Curls	1 serving	300	27
Dipping sauce			
BBQ	1 packet	30	0
honey	1 packet	45	0
sweet 'n' sour	1 packet	40	0
sweet mustard	1 packet	50	0
Fisherman's fillet sandwich	1	500	54
French fries			
"Big Fry"	5.5 oz	500	45
large	4 oz	360	27
regular	2.5 oz	230	18
Hamburger	1	270	36
Big Deluxe	1	500	108
Deluxe (The Lean 1)	1	420	72
Mushroom 'n' swiss	1	490	117
Hash rounds	1 serving	230	27
Horseradish	1 packet (¼ oz)	25	0
Hot dog, all-beef	1	300	72
Hot ham 'n' cheese sandwich	1	330	45
Pancakes	3 pancakes	280	9
with 1 sausage patty	3 pancakes	430	54
with 2 bacon strips	3 pancakes	350	27
Roast beef			
big	1 serving	360	54
regular	1 serving	310	45
Salad dressing			
blue cheese	4 tbsp	210	27
house	4 tbsp	290	36
reduced-calorie French	4 tbsp	130	9
reduced-calorie Italian	4 tbsp	90	9
Thousand Island	4 tbsp	250	27
Salad			
chef	1	240	81
garden	1	210	72
side	1	20	0
Shake			
chocolate	1	460	45
strawberry	1	440	45
vanilla	1	400	45
Tartar sauce	⅔ oz	90	9

FAST FOODS

FOOD	AMOUNT	TOTAL CALORIES	SAT-FAT CALORIES
Turkey club sandwich	1	390	36
Jack in the Box			
Apple turnover	1 serving	410	61
Breakfast Jack®	1	307	47
Cheeseburger	1	315	51
bacon	1	705	135
double	1	467	111
ultimate	1	942	238
Cheesecake	1 serving	309	81
Chicken			
fajita pita	1 sandwich	292	26
grilled fillet sandwich	1	408	37
strips	4 pieces	349	31
	6 pieces	523	43
supreme	1 serving	575	75
Crescent, sausage	1	584	140
Crescent, supreme	1	547	119
Egg rolls	3 pieces	405	70
	5 pieces	675	117
Fish supreme	1 serving	554	66
French fries			
jumbo	1 serving	442	54
regular	1 serving	353	41
small	1 serving	221	26
Guacamole	1 serving	55	NA
Ham and turkey melt	1 sandwich	592	99
Hamburger	1	267	37
Grilled sourdough	1	712	143
Swiss and bacon burger	1	678	180
Hash browns	1 serving	116	15
Jumbo Jack®	1	584	99
with cheese	1	677	126
Milk shakes			
chocolate	1	330	39
strawberry	1	320	39
vanilla	1	320	32
Onion rings	1 serving	382	50
Pancake platter	1	612	77
Salad dressing			
bleu cheese	4 tbsp	262	36
buttermilk	4 tbsp	362	52

FAST FOODS

FOOD	AMOUNT	TOTAL CALORIES	SAT-FAT CALORIES
Salad dressing (cont.)			
reduced-calorie French	4 tbsp	176	11
Thousand Island	4 tbsp	312	45
Salad			
chef	1	325	76
side	1	51	18
taco	1	503	121
Salsa	1 serving	8	0
Sauce			
BBQ	1 serving	44	0
seafood cocktail	1 serving	32	0
sweet and sour	1 serving	40	0
Scrambled egg platter	1	662	137
Scrambled egg pocket	1	431	68
Sesame breadsticks	1 serving	70	NA
Shrimp	10 pieces	270	65
	15 pieces	404	97
Taco	1 serving	191	34
super	1 serving	288	53
Taquitos	5 pieces	363	45
	7 pieces	508	62
Tortilla chips	1 serving	139	13
KFC (Kentucky Fried Chicken)			
Baked beans	1 serving	133	5
Buttermilk biscuit	1	235	29
Chicken			
Chargrill			
breast	1 serving	239	32
drumstick	1 serving	106	14
thigh	1 serving	171	29
wing	1 serving	119	19
Colonel's Sandwich	1	482	51
deluxe	1	547	72
Extra Tasty Crisp			
center breast	1 serving	342	43
drumstick	1 serving	204	31
side breast	1 serving	343	50
thigh	1 serving	406	69
wing	1 serving	254	40
Hot wings	6 pieces	376	48
Kentucky nuggets	6 pieces	276	38

FAST FOODS

FOOD	AMOUNT	TOTAL CALORIES	SAT-FAT CALORIES
Chicken (*cont.*)			
Lite 'n Crispy			
center breast	1 serving	220	26
drumstick	1 serving	121	15
side breast	1 serving	204	29
thigh	1 serving	246	3
Original Recipe			
center breast	1 serving	283	34
drumstick	1 serving	146	20
side breast	1 serving	267	38
thigh	1 serving	294	48
wing	1 serving	178	27
Chicken Littles sandwich	1	169	18
Chocolate pudding	1 serving	156	52
Coleslaw	1 serving	119	9
Corn on the cob	1 serving	176	4
French fries	1 serving	244	23
Mashed potatoes and gravy	1 serving	71	4
Nugget sauce			
barbecue	1 serving	35	1
honey	1 serving	49	0
mustard	1 serving	36	1
sweet 'n sour	1 serving	58	1
Parfait			
apple shortcake	1	276	47
chocolate creme	1	360	97
fudge brownie	1	331	44
lemon cream	1	513	78
strawberry shortcake	1	230	50
Potato salad	1 serving	177	16
Vanilla pudding	1 serving	159	53
Long John Silver's			
Baked potato, no toppings	1	150	0
Catfish fillet	1 piece	180	23
Chicken, baked	1 serving	140	11
Chicken plank	1 piece	110	13
Clam chowder with cod	1 serving	140	16
Clams, breaded	1 serving	240	23
Cod, baked	1 serving	130	0
Coleslaw, drained on fork	1 serving	140	9
Corn on the Cob with Whirl	1 ear	270	23

FAST FOODS

FOOD	AMOUNT	TOTAL CALORIES	SAT-FAT CALORIES
Fish			
Battered	1 piece	150	16
Homestyle	1 piece	125	14
Sandwich, Homestyle	1 serving	510	44
Fryes	1 serving	220	23
Gumbo with cod and shrimp bobs	1 serving	120	19
Hushpuppies	1 piece	70	4
Pie			
lemon meringue	1 serving	260	22
pecan	1 serving	530	65
Salad			
ocean chef	1 serving	250	6
seafood	1 scoop	210	7
side, no dressing	1 serving	20	0
Salad dressing			
bleu cheese	1 packet	120	4
ranch	1 packet	140	4
reduced-calorie Italian	1 packet	18	4
sea salad	1 packet	140	25
Sauce			
honey-mustard	1 packet	60	0
seafood	1 packet	45	3
sweet-n-sour	1 packet	60	0
tartar	1 packet	80	5
Shrimp			
battered	1 piece	40	6
breaded	1 order	190	21
McDonald's			
Apple bran muffin	1 serving	190	0
Apple pie	1 serving	260	43
Bacon bits	1 serving	16	0
Big Mac	1	560	91
Biscuit	1	260	31
with bacon, egg, and cheese	1	440	74
with sausage	1	440	84
with sausage and egg	1	520	101
Cheeseburger	1	310	47
Chicken			
grilled breast sandwich	1	252	9
McChicken	1 serving	490	49
McNuggets	6 pieces	290	37

FAST FOODS

FOOD	AMOUNT	TOTAL CALORIES	SAT-FAT CALORIES
Cookies			
Chocolatey Chip	1 serving	330	45
McDonaldland	1 serving	290	17
Croutons	1 serving	50	4
Danish			
apple	1	390	32
cinnamon	1	440	38
iced cheese	1	390	54
raspberry	1	410	28
English muffin with butter	1	170	22
Filet-O-Fish	1 serving	440	47
French fries			
large	1 serving	400	40
medium	1 serving	310	32
small	1 serving	220	27
Frozen yogurt, low-fat			
cone	1	100	4
sundae, hot caramel	1	270	14
sundae, hot fudge	1	240	22
sundae, strawberry	1	210	5
Hamburger	1	260	32
Hash brown potatoes	1 serving	130	14
Hotcakes with butter and syrup	1 serving	410	33
McD.L.T.	1	580	104
McMuffin			
egg	1	290	34
sausage	1	370	70
sausage with egg	1	440	86
Milkshake, low-fat			
chocolate	1	320	7
strawberry	1	320	5
vanilla	1	290	5
Orange sorbet ice			
cone	1	106	0
sundae	1	142	0
Pork sausage	1	180	53
Quarter Pounder	1	410	73
with cheese	1	520	101
Salad			
chef	1	230	53
chunky chicken	1	140	8

FAST FOODS

FOOD	AMOUNT	TOTAL CALORIES	SAT-FAT CALORIES
Salad (*cont.*)			
garden	1	110	26
side	1	60	14
Salad dressing			
bleu cheese	4 tbsp	350	58
Lite vinaigrette	4 tbsp	60	4
peppercorn	4 tbsp	400	62
ranch	4 tbsp	330	49
red French reduced-calorie	4 tbsp	160	10
Thousand Island	4 tbsp	390	54
Sauce			
Barbecue	1 serving	50	1
Hot mustard	1 serving	70	4
Sweet and sour	1 serving	60	0
Scrambled eggs	1 serving	140	30
Pizza Hut			
Pan pizza (medium)			
cheese	2 slices	492	81
pepperoni	2 slices	540	83
super supreme	2 slices	563	108
supreme	2 slices	589	124
Thin 'n Crispy pizza (medium)			
cheese	2 slices	398	94
pepperoni	2 slices	413	95
super supreme	2 slices	463	93
supreme	2 slices	459	99
Traditional Hand-tossed pizza (medium)			
cheese	2 slices	518	122
pepperoni	2 slices	500	116
super supreme	2 slices	556	117
supreme	2 slices	540	124
Personal Pan pizza			
pepperoni	Whole	675	112
supreme	Whole	647	101
Taco Bell			
Burrito			
bean with red sauce	1 serving	447	18
beef with red sauce	1 serving	493	72
supreme with red sauce	1 serving	503	72

FAST FOODS

FOOD	AMOUNT	TOTAL CALORIES	SAT-FAT CALORIES
Chilito	1 serving	383	72
Cinnamon Twists	1 order	171	27
Combination burrito	1 serving	407	45
Enchirito with red sauce	1 serving	382	81
Guacamole	1 serving	34	0
Mexican pizza	1 serving	575	99
Meximelt	1 serving	266	72
Nachos	1 serving	346	54
Bellgrande	1 serving	649	108
supreme	1 serving	367	45
Nachos cheese	1 serving	103	27
Pico de Gallo	1 packet	8	0
Pintos and cheese with red sauce	1 serving	190	36
Salad dressing			
ranch	4 tbsp	236	45
Sauce			
green	1 packet	4	0
hot taco	1 packet	3	0
red sauce	1 packet	10	0
taco	1 packet	2	0
Taco	1 serving	183	45
Bellgrande	1 serving	335	99
Taco, soft			
beef	1 serving	225	45
chicken	1 serving	210	36
steak	1 serving	218	45
Taco Salad	1	905	171
no shell	1	484	126
Taco Supreme	1 serving	230	72
soft	1 serving	272	72
Tostada with red sauce	1 serving	243	36
Wendy's			
Bacon bits	1 serving	40	6
Baked potato, plain	1	270	0
bacon and cheese	1	520	46
broccoli and cheese	1	400	26
cheese	1	420	36
chili and cheese	1	500	36
sour cream and chives	1	500	84

FAST FOODS

FOOD	AMOUNT	TOTAL CALORIES	SAT-FAT CALORIES
Big Classic	1	570	53
with cheese	1	640	85
double	1	750	98
with cheese	1	820	130
Breadsticks	2	30	0
Cheese			
imitation Parmesan	1 oz	80	27
Parmesan, grated	1 oz	130	49
shredded, salad bar, imitation	1 oz	90	36
Cheeseburger	1	410	83
double	1	590	128
Jr.	1	310	45
Jr. bacon	1	430	50
Jr. Swiss deluxe	1	360	30
Chicken			
club sandwich	1	506	45
Crispy Nuggets	6 pieces	280	40
salad	1 serving	120	14
sandwich			
fried	1	430	25
grilled	1	340	22
Chili	9 oz serving	220	23
Chocolate chip cookie	1 order	275	38
Chocolate milk	8 fl oz	160	25
Chow mein noodles	½ oz	74	5
Coleslaw	2 oz	70	8
Cottage cheese	½ cup	108	27
Fettuccine	1 serving	190	5
Fish fillet sandwich	1	460	45
French fries			
biggie	1 serving	449	42
large	1 serving	312	29
small	1 serving	240	22
Frosty dairy dessert			
large	1	680	73
medium	1	520	56
small	1	400	43
Garbanzo beans	1 serving	46	1
Garlic toast	1 serving	70	5

FAST FOODS

FOOD	AMOUNT	TOTAL CALORIES	SAT-FAT CALORIES
Hamburger			
double	1	520	96
Jr.	1	260	30
single	1	340	51
Pasta medley	1 serving	60	3
Potato salad	¼ cup	125	7
Refried beans	1 serving	70	8
Rotini	1 serving	90	3
Salad dressing			
blue cheese	4 tbsp	360	68
celery seed	4 tbsp	280	32
French	4 tbsp	240	31
golden Italian	4 tbsp	180	18
Hidden Valley Ranch	4 tbsp	200	9
Italian Caesar	4 tbsp	320	50
reduced-calorie bacon and tomato	4 tbsp	180	22
sweet red French	4 tbsp	280	29
Thousand Island	4 tbsp	280	38
Sauce			
alfredo	2 oz	35	7
barbecue sauce for chicken nuggets	2 oz	50	0
cheese	2 oz	39	9
picante	2 oz	18	0
spaghetti	2 oz	28	0
spaghetti meat	2 oz	60	6
sweet and sour for chicken nuggets	1 oz	45	0
sweet mustard for chicken nuggets	1 oz	50	0
taco	1 oz	16	0
tartar	1 tbsp	120	19
Seafood salad	1	110	2
Sour topping	1 oz	58	45
Spanish rice	1 serving	70	2
Sunflower seeds and raisins	1 oz	140	67
Taco chips	2 oz	260	6
Taco meat	1 serving	110	15
Taco shells	1	45	6
Three-bean salad	¼ cup	60	<9

FAST FOODS

FOOD	AMOUNT	TOTAL CALORIES	SAT-FAT CALORIES
Tortilla	1	110	4
Tuna salad	1 serving	100	8
Turkey ham	¼ cup	35	4

FATS AND OILS

FOOD	AMOUNT	TOTAL CALORIES	SAT-FAT CALORIES
Animal Fats			
Beef tallow	1 tbsp	116	58
Butter			
regular	1 pat	36	23
	1 tbsp	100	65
	1 stick	813	515
whipped	1 tsp	23	12
	1 tbsp	67	38
Butter oil, anhydrous	1 tbsp	112	71
Chicken fat	1 tbsp	115	34
Duck fat	1 tbsp	115	39
Goose fat	1 tbsp	115	32
Lard (pork)	1 tbsp	116	45
Mutton tallow	1 tbsp	116	55
Turkey fat	1 tbsp	115	34
Margarines, Spreads, and Substitutes			
Blue Bonnet	1 tbsp	100	18
Butter blend	1 tbsp	90	18
Butter Buds			
flavored sprinkles	½ tsp	4	0
prepared liquid	2 tbsp	12	<9
Chiffon	1 tbsp	90	18
Country Morning Blend			
Light, soft	1 tbsp	60	27
soft	1 tbsp	90	27
stick	1 tbsp	100	27
Fleischmann's			
extra-light corn oil spread	1 tbsp	50	9
light corn oil spread (stick)	1 tbsp	80	9
soft	1 tbsp	100	18

FATS AND OILS

FOOD	AMOUNT	TOTAL CALORIES	SAT-FAT CALORIES
Fleischmann's (*cont.*)			
squeeze spread	1 tbsp	90	9
stick	1 tbsp	100	18
I Can't Believe It's Not Butter	1 tbsp	90	18
Imperial Diet Reduced	1 tbsp	50	9
Kraft			
Diet reduced-calorie	1 tbsp	50	9
Touch of Butter	1 tbsp	90	18
Touch of Butter spread	1 tbsp	50	9
Land O' Lakes			
Country Morning Blend (stick)	1 tbsp	105	27
Country Morning Blend Light (tub)	1 tbsp	60	27
margarine	1 tbsp	105	27
Mazola	1 tbsp	100	18
McCormick Best O'Butter	½ tsp	4	<9
Molly McButter	½ tsp	4	0
Mother's	1 tbsp	100	18
Mrs. Filbert's			
corn oil, soft	1 tbsp	100	18
corn oil spread	1 tbsp	70	9
Spread 25	1 tbsp	70	9
Nucoa Heart Beat	1 tbsp	25	<9
Parkay			
soft	1 tbsp	100	18
soft diet reduced-calorie	1 tbsp	50	9
squeeze spread	1 tbsp	90	18
Promise			
extra-light (tub)	1 tbsp	50	<9
stick	1 tbsp	90	18
sweet unsalted tub	1 tbsp	90	18
tub	1 tbsp	90	9
Shedd's Spread			
Country Crock	1 tbsp	70	9
squeezable	1 tbsp	80	9
stick	1 tbsp	80	18
Weight Watchers	1 tbsp	50	9
Oils			
Canola	1 tbsp	120	9
Cocoa butter	1 tbsp	120	73

FATS AND OILS

FOOD	AMOUNT	TOTAL CALORIES	SAT-FAT CALORIES
Coconut	1 tbsp	120	106
Corn	1 tbsp	120	15
Cottonseed	1 tbsp	120	32
Olive	1 tbsp	119	16
Palm	1 tbsp	120	60
Palm kernel	1 tbsp	120	100
Peanut	1 tbsp	119	21
Safflower	1 tbsp	120	11
Sesame	1 tbsp	120	17
Soybean	1 tbsp	120	18
Sunflower	1 tbsp	120	13
Walnut	1 tbsp	120	11

Salad Dressings and Mayonnaises

FOOD	AMOUNT	TOTAL CALORIES	SAT-FAT CALORIES
Blue cheese	1 tbsp	77	14
French			
low-calorie	1 tbsp	22	1
regular	1 tbsp	67	14
Italian			
low calorie	1 tbsp	16	2
regular	1 tbsp	69	9
Mayonnaise and Salad Dressing			
Bright Day	1 tbsp	60	9
Hain Safflower	1 tbsp	110	9
Hellman's			
cholesterol-free reduced-calorie	1 tbsp	50	9
light	1 tbsp	50	9
real	1 tbsp	100	18
Hollywood Safflower	1 tbsp	110	9
Kraft			
cholesterol-free	1 tbsp	90	9
light, reduced-calorie	1 tbsp	50	9
real	1 tbsp	100	18
Miracle Whip Salad Dressing			
cholesterol-free reduced-calorie	1 tbsp	70	9
light, reduced-calorie	1 tbsp	45	9
regular	1 tbsp	70	9
Russian			
low-calorie	1 tbsp	23	1
regular	1 tbsp	76	10
Sesame seed	1 tbsp	68	8

FATS AND OILS

FOOD	AMOUNT	TOTAL CALORIES	SAT-FAT CALORIES
Thousand Island			
low-calorie	1 tbsp	24	2
regular	1 tbsp	59	8
Shortenings			
Crisco	1 tbsp	113	30
Household			
hydrogenated soybean and hydrogenated cottonseed	1 tbsp	113	29
hydrogenated soybean and palm	1 tbsp	113	35
lard and vegetable oil	1 tbsp	115	47

FISH AND SHELLFISH

(See also **FROZEN AND MICROWAVE FOODS.**)

FOOD	AMOUNT	TOTAL CALORIES	SAT-FAT CALORIES
Abalone, raw	1 oz	98	3
Anchovy, canned	1 oz	49	12
Anchovy, canned and drained	1 oz	60	6
Bass, freshwater, steamed or baked	1 oz	33	1
Bass, striped, oven-fried	1 oz	56	5
Bluefish, baked w/margarine	1 oz	45	3
Catfish, freshwater, steamed or baked	1 oz	35	3
Caviar	1 tbsp	42	15
Cisco (lake herring), steamed or baked	1 oz	33	1
Clams			
raw, cherrystones or littlenecks	4–5	56	trace
	1 oz	23	trace
canned, drained, chopped	1 cup	157	13
canned, solids and liquid	1 oz	15	1
Cod, broiled without added fat	1 oz	29	trace
Crab			
steamed, pieces	1 cup	144	9
steamed	1 oz	26	trace
canned, white or king, not packed	1 cup	135	7

FISH AND SHELLFISH

FOOD	AMOUNT	TOTAL CALORIES	SAT-FAT CALORIES
Croaker, Atlantic, baked	1 oz	38	3
Crayfish, steamed	1 oz	25	1
Dogfish, spiny (grayfish), baked or steamed	1 oz	53	7
Drum, freshwater, steamed or baked	1 oz	41	3
Eel, baked or steamed	1 oz	79	11
Flounder			
baked or steamed w/o added fat	1 oz	28	1
Gefilte fish	1 piece (1.5 oz)	35	2
Grouper (red, black, speckled hind), baked or steamed	1 oz	30	trace
Haddock			
baked or steamed	1 oz	27	trace
oven-fried	1 fillet	182	12
Hake, steamed or baked	1 oz	25	1
Halibut			
baked or steamed	1 oz	34	1
broiled w/margarine	1 fillet	214	17
Herring			
canned	1 piece	221	25
pickled	1 piece	33	4
Lobster			
canned	1 oz	26	1
cooked	1 cup	138	7
	1 lb	431	21
Newburg	1 cup	485	160
Lox (smoked salmon)	1 oz	33	2
Mackerel			
baked or steamed	1 oz	65	11
broiled with butter	1 fillet	248	60
canned	1 oz	52	10
fried in vegetable fat	1 oz	53	10
Mullet, striped, baked or steamed	1 oz	50	4
Mussels, cooked	1 oz	49	2
Ocean perch			
baked or steamed	1 oz	32	1
Oysters			
raw	1 cup (13–19)	160	12
fried	4	108	17
oyster stew (2 parts milk, 1 part oyster)	1 cup	233	80

FISH AND SHELLFISH

FOOD	AMOUNT	TOTAL CALORIES	SAT-FAT CALORIES
Perch, white, baked or steamed	1 oz	40	2
Perch, yellow, baked or steamed	1 oz	31	1
Pike, northern, baked or steamed	1 oz	30	trace
Pike, walleye, baked or steamed	1 oz	32	1
Pollock, baked or steamed	1 oz	32	trace
Pompano, baked or steamed	1 oz	57	11
Rockfish, baked or steamed	1 oz	33	1
Sablefish, baked or steamed	1 oz	65	10
Salmon, Atlantic, baked or steamed	1 oz	74	3
Salmon, chinook (king), baked or steamed	1 oz	76	8
Salmon			
chum, canned	1 oz	39	5
coho (silver), canned	1 oz	43	3
pink, baked or steamed	1 oz	41	2
pink, canned	1 oz	40	3
sockeye (red), baked or steamed	1 oz	47	5
Sardines, drained	1 can (3¼ oz)	187	31
Scallops			
steamed	1 oz	32	1
Shrimp			
raw, large	1	7	trace
raw, medium	1	4	trace
raw, small	1	2	trace
canned	1 oz	36	trace
	1 cup	148	2
french-fried	1 oz	63	7
Smelt, baked or steamed	1 oz	33	2
Snapper, red, baked or steamed	1 oz	33	1
Sole, baked or steamed	1 oz	28	1
Squid			
floured and fried	1 oz	50	5
raw	1 oz	26	1
Sturgeon, baked or steamed	1 oz	45	4
Swordfish, baked or steamed	1 oz	40	2
Trout, steamed			
brook	1 oz	38	3
lake	1 oz	57	5
Tuna			
chunk light, oil packed, drained	1 oz	56	5
solid white, water-packed, drained	1 oz	45	1

FISH AND SHELLFISH

FOOD	AMOUNT	TOTAL CALORIES	SAT-FAT CALORIES
Tuna salad	½ cup	190	15
Whitefish, lake, baked or steamed	1 oz	53	3
Whitefish, smoked	1 oz	30	.5
Imitation Fish			
Crab, Alaska King	1 oz	29	1
Shrimp	1 oz	31	1
Surimi	1 oz	28	trace

FROZEN AND MICROWAVE FOODS

FOOD	AMOUNT	TOTAL CALORIES	SAT-FAT CALORIES
Breakfast Foods			
Aunt Jemima			
French Toast	2 slices	220	41 e
Pancakes	3	210	23 e
Blueberry	3	220	23 e
Buttermilk	3	210	18 e
Waffles			
Homestyle	1	90	8 e
Lite Healthy	1	60	0
Kellogg's			
Eggo Waffles			
Blueberry	1	130	14 e
Buttermilk	1	120	14 e
Homestyle	1	120	14 e
Nutri-Grain (Eggo)			
Multi-Bran	1	120	9
Raisin and Bran	1	130	9
Waffle	1	130	9
Morningside Farms			
Breakfast Links	2	120	9
Breakfast Patties	2	190	18
Grillers	1	180	18

e indicates estimated sat-fat calories.

FROZEN AND MICROWAVE FOODS

FOOD	AMOUNT	TOTAL CALORIES	SAT-FAT CALORIES
Pillsbury Hungry Jack			
Microwave Pancakes	3	260	11 e
Swanson			
Great Starts Budget			
Scrambled Eggs and Home Fries	1 box	260	51 e
6 Silver Dollar Pancakes with Sausage	1 box	310	42 e
Great Starts Breakfast			
Belgian Waffle with Bacon	1 box	230	81 e
Cinnamon Swirl French Toast with Sausages	1 box	390	122 e
Pancakes			
with 3 Bacon Slices	1 box	400	54 e
with Sausages	1 box	460	66 e
Reduced-Cholesterol Scrambled Eggs with			
3 Mini Oat Bran Muffins	1 box	250	18
Sausage, Egg, and Cheese on a Biscuit	1 box	440	108 e
Scrambled Eggs			
and Sausage with Hashed Brown Potatoes	1 box	420	102 e
Home Fried Potatoes, 3 Bacon Slices	1 box	340	70
Weight Watchers Microwave Breakfast			
Belgian Waffles	1 waffle	120	18
Cheese Sweet Rolls	1 roll	180	<9
Coffee Cakes with Cinnamon Streusel	1 cake	190	9
English Muffin Sandwich with Egg, Ham, and Cheese	1	230	27
French toast	1 slice	170	9
Muffins			
Banana Nut	1 muffin	170	9
Blueberry	1 muffin	170	9

e indicates estimated sat-fat calories.

FROZEN AND MICROWAVE FOODS

FOOD	AMOUNT	TOTAL CALORIES	SAT-FAT CALORIES
Lunches and Sandwiches			
The Budget Gourmet Hot Lunch			
Baked Potato			
with Cheddar Cheese Sauce and Bacon	1 package	320	70 e
with Cheese Sauce and Broccoli	1 package	290	58 e
Chicken and Cheese Tortellini	1 package	350	42 e
Chicken Oriental and Vegetables	1 package	290	24 e
Fettuccine Alfredo with Broccoli	1 package	320	99 e
Fish and Chips	1 package	370	52 e
Open Faced			
Chicken Parmesan	1 package	320	30 e
Italian-Style Meatballs	1 package	470	129 e
Roast Beef with Mashed Potatoes and Gravy	1 package	340	98 e
Turkey with Mashed Potatoes and Gravy	1 package	290	55 e
Oriental Beef and Rice	1 package	230	9 e
Lean Pockets			
Chicken Fajitas	1 package	260	34 e
Pizza Deluxe	1 package	290	53 e
Turkey, Broccoli, and Cheese	1 package	230	30 e
Dinners			
The Budget Gourmet			
Light & Healthy Dinners			
Beef Pot Roast	10.5 oz	210	18
Chicken Breast Parmigiana	11.0 oz	260	27
Herbed Chicken Breast with Fettuccine	11.0 oz	240	27
Italian Style Meatloaf	11.0 oz	270	36
Sirloin of Beef in Wine Sauce	11.0 oz	230	18
Sirloin Salisbury Steak	11.0 oz	260	36
Special Recipe Sirloin of Beef	11.0 oz	250	36
Stuffed Turkey Breast	11.0 oz	230	18
Teriyaki Chicken Breast	11.0 oz	270	9

e indicates estimated sat-fat calories.

FROZEN AND MICROWAVE FOODS

FOOD	AMOUNT	TOTAL CALORIES	SAT-FAT CALORIES
Eating Right			
Beef Pepper Steak	10.0 oz	290	27
Beef Sirloin Tips and Noodles	9.0 oz	250	27
Chicken Breast			
and Vegetables	9.0 oz	200	9
Glazed	10.0 oz	240	9
Parmesan	9.0 oz	300	27
Fettuccine Alfredo	10.0 oz	220	27
Lasagna with Meat Sauce	10.0 oz	270	27
Macaroni and Cheese	9.0 oz	270	27
Shrimp Vegetable Stir-Fry	9.0 oz	220	9
Sirloin Salisbury Steak	9.5 oz	230	27
Sliced Turkey Breast	10.0 oz	250	18
Swedish Meatballs	10.0 oz	290	18
Gorton's			
Natural Cut			
breaded fish fillets	2 fillets	230	27
breaded fish sticks	4 sticks	200	27
Crispy Batter Fish Fillets			
haddock	2 fillets	300	81
flounder	2 fillets	280	72
Larger Cut Ranch	1 fillet	330	59 e
Microwave Fish Fillets	2 fillets	340	108
Healthy Choice			
Baked Cheese Ravioli	9.0 oz	240	9
Beef Fajitas	7.0 oz	210	18
Beef Pepper Steak and Rice with Broccoli	9.5 oz	250	18
Cheese Manicotti	9.25 oz	230	18
Chicken			
a l'Orange	9.0 oz	260	<9
and Vegetables	11.5 oz	210	<9
Chow Mein	8.5 oz	220	9
Fajitas	7.0 oz	200	9
Fettuccine	8.5 oz	240	18
Glazed	8.5 oz	230	9
Fettuccine Alfredo	8.0 oz	240	18
Lasagna with Meat Sauce	9.0 oz	260	18

e indicates estimated sat-fat calories.

FROZEN AND MICROWAVE FOODS

FOOD	AMOUNT	TOTAL CALORIES	SAT-FAT CALORIES
Healthy Choice (*cont.*)			
Linguini with Shrimp and Tomato Sauce	9.5 oz	230	9
Macaroni and Cheese	9.0 oz	280	27
Mandarin Chicken with Rice and Broccoli	11.0 oz	260	<9
Rigatoni in Meat Sauce	9.5 oz	240	18
Roasted Turkey and Mushrooms in Gravy	8.5 oz	200	9
Seafood Newburg	8.0 oz	200	9
Sole with Lemon Butter Sauce	8.25 oz	230	18
Spaghetti with Meat Sauce	10.0 oz	280	18
Zucchini Lasagna	11.5 oz	240	18
Healthy Choice Dinners			
Beef			
Enchilada	12.75 oz	360	27
Pepper Steak	11.0 oz	290	27
Sirloin Tips	11.75 oz	290	27
Breast of Turkey	10.5 oz	290	18
Chicken			
and Pasta Divan	11.5 oz	310	18
Dijon	11.0 oz	260	9
Enchilada	12.75 oz	330	27
Herb Roasted	11.0 oz	260	9
Mesquite	10.5 oz	310	<9
Oriental	11.25 oz	230	<9
Parmigiana	11.5 oz	280	18
Salsa	11.25 oz	240	9
Sweet and Sour	11.5 oz	280	<9
Salisbury Steak	11.5 oz	300	27
Shrimp Creole	11.25 oz	210	<9
Shrimp Marinara	10.5 oz	260	<9
Yankee Pot Roast	11.0 oz	260	18
Le Menu			
Beef Sirloin Tips	11.5 oz	400	77 e
Chicken Parmigiana	11.75 oz	410	85 e
Ham Steak	11 oz	300	38 e
Salisbury Steak	10.5 oz	370	90 e
Yankee Pot Roast	10 oz	330	59 e

e indicates estimated sat-fat calories.

FROZEN AND MICROWAVE FOODS

FOOD	AMOUNT	TOTAL CALORIES	SAT-FAT CALORIES
Le Menu Healthy			
Chicken Breast			
Glazed	10.0 oz	230	9
Herb-Roasted	7.75 oz	260	18
Salisbury Steak	10.0 oz	280	36
Traditional Turkey	8.25 oz	200	9
Le Menu Light Style			
Glazed Chicken Breast	10.0 oz	270	18
Herb Roasted Chicken	9.25 oz	240	18
Herb-Roasted Chicken Breast	7.75 oz	260	18
Salisbury Steak	10.5 oz	230	36
Traditional Turkey	8.25 oz	200	9
Lean Cuisine			
Breast of Chicken			
in Herb Cream Sauce	9½ oz	260	27
Parmesan	10 oz	240	18
Cheese Cannelloni	9⅛ oz	260	45
Cheese French Bread Pizza	5⅛ oz	320	27
Chicken			
a l'Orange	8 oz	250	9
and Vegetables	11¾ oz	260	18
Cacciatore	10⅞ oz	250	9
Chow Mein	11¼ oz	250	9
Enchanadas	9⅞ oz	270	18
Fiesta	8½ oz	250	9
Glazed	8½ oz	270	9
French Bread Pizza			
Deluxe Sausage, Pepperoni, and Mushroom	6⅛ oz	340	27
Pepperoni	5¼ oz	340	36
Lasagna	10¼ oz	260	27
Oriental Beef	8⅝ oz	250	18
Rigatoni Bake	9¾ oz	260	27
Salisbury Steak	9½ oz	260	18
Sliced Turkey Breast	7⅞ oz	240	9
Spaghetti with Beef and Mushroom Sauce	11½ oz	280	18
Tuna Lasagna	9¾ oz	270	18
Turkey Dijon	9½ oz	270	27
Zucchini Lasagna	11 oz	260	27

FROZEN AND MICROWAVE FOODS

FOOD	AMOUNT	TOTAL CALORIES	SAT-FAT CALORIES
Mrs. Paul's			
Budget Line			
Battered Fish Portions	2 portions	300	27
Breaded Fish Portions	2 portions	230	18
Breaded Fish Sticks	4 sticks	140	9
Regular			
Batter Dipped Fish Fillets	2 fillets	430	36
Crispy Breaded Fish Fillets	2 fillets	220	18
Crispy Breaded Fish Sticks	4 sticks	190	9
Light Fillets			
flounder	4.25 oz	240	18
haddock	4.25 oz	220	9
n' Sauce	4.1 oz	140	9
Snoopy's Choice (Healthy Choice)			
Chicken and Pasta with Cream Sauce	8.5 oz	230	9
Chunky Beef Stew	8.5 oz	140	9
Chunky Chicken Stew	8.5 oz	130	<9
Lasagna with Meat Sauce	8.5 oz	280	27
Macaroni and Cheese with Sliced Turkey Franks	8.5 oz	280	18
Mini Beef Ravioli in Tomato Sauce	8.5 oz	300	27
Spaghetti with Meatballs and Sauce	8.5 oz	180	9
Swanson			
Beef Pot Pie	1 package (7 oz)	370	85 e
Chicken Pot Pie	1 package (7 oz)	380	59 e
Turkey Pot Pie	1 package (7 oz)	380	57 e
Taste O'Sea			
Flounder Dinner	8 oz	480	73 e
Seafood Platter	7.5 oz	530	81 e
Ultra Slim Fast			
Beef Pepper Steak	12 oz	270	18
Chicken			
and Vegetables	12 oz	290	<9
Fettuccine	12 oz	380	36
Mesquite Chicken	12 oz	360	<9
Roasted in Mushroom Sauce	12 oz	280	18
Sweet and Sour	12 oz	330	<9

e indicates estimated sat-fat calories.

FROZEN AND MICROWAVE FOODS

FOOD	AMOUNT	TOTAL CALORIES	SAT-FAT CALORIES
Ultra Slim Fast (*cont.*)			
Country Style Vegetables and Beef Tips	12 oz	230	18
Pasta Primavera	12 oz	340	36
Shrimp Creole	12 oz	240	9
Shrimp Marinara	12 oz	290	9
Spaghetti with Beef and Mushroom Sauce	12 oz	370	27
Turkey Medallions in Herb Sauce	12 oz	280	18
Van de Kamp's			
Light Fillets			
Flounder Lightly Breaded	1 fillet	240	18
Haddock Lightly Breaded	1 fillet	240	18
Sole Lightly Breaded	1 fillet	240	18
Regular			
Breaded Fish Fillets	2 fillets	280	27
Breaded Fish Sticks	4 sticks	200	18
Crispy Breaded Large Fish Fillets	1 fillet	290	27
Weight Watchers			
Angel Hair Pasta	10 oz	210	9
Baked Cheese Ravioli	9 oz	290	45
Baked Potato			
Broccoli and Cheese	10.5 oz	250	36
Ham Lorraine	11 oz	250	18
Homestyle Turkey	12 oz	300	27
Beef Enchiladas Ranchero	9.12 oz	300	36
Cheese Tortellini	9 oz	310	9
Chicken			
Cordon Bleu	8 oz	230	36
Divan Baked Potato	11 oz	270	18
Enchiladas Suiza	9.37 oz	330	54
Fajitas	6.75 oz	230	18
Fettuccine	8.25 oz	280	27
Homestyle and Noodles	9 oz	240	18
Imperial	9.25 oz	220	9
Kiev	7 oz	230	27
Deluxe Combination Pizza	7.15 oz	330	27
Fettuccine Alfredo	9 oz	260	36
Lasagna			
Garden	11 oz	290	18

FROZEN AND MICROWAVE FOODS

FOOD	AMOUNT	TOTAL CALORIES	SAT-FAT CALORIES
Weight Watchers (*cont.*)			
Lasagna (*cont.*)			
Italian Cheese	11 oz	350	36
with Meat Sauce	11 oz	330	45
London Broil in Mushroom Sauce	7.37 oz	140	9
Oven Fried Fish	7.08 oz	240	<9
Pepperoni Pizza	6.09 oz	320	27
Spaghetti with Meat Sauce	10.5 oz	280	27
Stuffed Turkey Breast	8.5 oz	260	36

(For more frozen grains, see **GRAIN PRODUCTS,** *Bread, Pastries.* For more frozen sweets and desserts, see **DAIRY PRODUCTS AND EGGS,** *Frozen Desserts;* **SUGARS AND SWEETS,** *Frozen Novelties.*)

FRUITS AND FRUIT JUICES

FOOD	AMOUNT	TOTAL CALORIES	SAT-FAT CALORIES
Apples, raw			
unpeeled, cored (2¾-inch)	1	80	1
unpeeled, cored (3¼-inch)	1	125	1
unpeeled, sliced	1 cup	64	1
peeled, cored	1	72	1
peeled, sliced	1 cup	65	1
Apple juice	1 cup	115	trace
Applesauce, canned			
sweetened	1 cup	195	1
unsweetened	1 cup	105	trace
Apricots			
raw, pitted	3	50	trace
canned in heavy syrup	1 cup	215	trace
	3 halves	70	trace
canned in juice	1 cup	120	trace
	3 halves	40	trace
Apricots, dried			
uncooked	1 cup	310	trace
cooked, unsweetened	1 cup	210	trace

FRUITS AND FRUIT JUICES

FOOD	AMOUNT	TOTAL CALORIES	SAT-FAT CALORIES
Avocados			
California	1	305	41
Florida	1	340	48
Bananas			
whole	1	105	2
sliced	1 cup	140	3
Blackberries	1 cup	75	2
Blueberries			
raw	1 cup	80	trace
frozen, sweetened	10 oz	230	trace
	1 cup	185	trace
frozen, unsweetened	1 cup	78	trace
	20 oz	287	trace
Cantaloupe	½ melon	95	1
Cherries			
sour red, pitted, canned in water	1 cup	90	1
sweet, pitted	10	50	1
Cranberry juice cocktail, sweetened	1 cup	145	trace
Cranberry sauce, sweetened, canned, strained	1 cup	420	trace
Dates			
whole, pitted	10	230	1
chopped	1 cup	490	3
Figs, dried	10	475	4
Fruit cocktail			
canned in heavy syrup	1 cup	185	trace
canned in juice	1 cup	115	trace
Grapefruit			
fresh	½	40	trace
canned, sections	1 cup	150	trace
Grapefruit juice			
fresh	1 cup	95	trace
canned, unsweetened	1 cup	95	trace
canned, sweetened	1 cup	115	trace
Grapes			
Thompson seedless	10	35	1
	1 cup	97	1
Tokay and Emperor	10	40	1
Grape juice, canned or bottled	1 cup	155	1
Honeydew melon	¹⁄₁₀ melon	45	trace
Kiwi fruit	1	45	trace

FRUITS AND FRUIT JUICES

FOOD	AMOUNT	TOTAL CALORIES	SAT-FAT CALORIES
Lemons	1	15	trace
Lemon juice			
fresh	1 cup	60	trace
	1 tbsp	4	trace
canned or bottled	1 cup	50	1
	1 tbsp	3	trace
Lime juice			
fresh	1 cup	65	trace
	1 tbsp	4	trace
canned, unsweetened	1 cup	50	1
Mangos	1	135	1
Nectarines	1	65	1
Oranges			
whole	1	60	trace
sections	1 cup	85	trace
Orange juice			
fresh	1 cup	110	0
canned, unsweetened	1 cup	105	trace
diluted concentrate	1 cup	110	trace
Orange and grapefruit juice, canned	1 cup	105	trace
Papaya, fresh, cubed	1 cup	65	1
Peaches			
fresh, whole	1 peach	35	trace
fresh, sliced	1 cup	75	trace
canned in heavy syrup	1 cup	190	trace
	1 half	60	trace
canned in juice	1 cup	110	trace
	1 half	35	trace
dried, uncooked	1 cup	380	1
dried, cooked, unsweetened	1 cup	200	1
Pears			
Bartlett, cored	1	100	trace
Bosc, cored	1	85	trace
D'Anjou, cored	1	120	trace
canned in heavy syrup	1 cup	190	trace
	1 half	60	trace
canned in juice	1 cup	125	trace
	1 half	40	trace
Pineapple			
fresh, diced	1 cup	75	trace

FRUITS AND FRUIT JUICES

FOOD	AMOUNT	TOTAL CALORIES	SAT-FAT CALORIES
Pineapple (*cont.*)			
canned in heavy syrup			
crushed, chunks, tidbits	1 cup	200	trace
slices	1 slice	45	trace
canned in juice			
chunks or tidbits	1 cup	150	trace
slices	1 slice	35	trace
Pineapple juice, unsweetened, canned	1 cup	140	trace
Plantains			
fresh	1	220	3
cooked, boiled, sliced	1 cup	180	1
Plums			
fresh, pitted	1 (6.5/lb)	35	trace
	1 (15/lb)	15	trace
canned in heavy syrup	1 cup	230	trace
	3 plums	120	trace
canned in juice	1 cup	145	trace
	3 plums	55	trace
Prunes, dried			
uncooked	10	201	trace
	1 cup	385	1
cooked, unsweetened	1 cup	225	trace
Prune juice	1 cup	180	trace
Raisins, seedless	1 cup	435	2
	1 packet (½ oz)	40	trace
Raspberries			
fresh	1 cup	60	trace
frozen, sweetened	10 oz	295	trace
	1 cup	255	trace
Rhubarb, cooked, sweetened	1 cup	280	trace
Strawberries			
fresh, whole	1 cup	45	trace
frozen, sweetened, sliced	10 oz	275	trace
	1 cup	245	trace
Tangerines			
fresh	1	35	trace
canned in light syrup	1 cup	155	trace
Watermelon	1 slice (4 × 8 inches)	155	3
diced	1 cup	50	1

GRAIN PRODUCTS

FOOD	AMOUNT	TOTAL CALORIES	SAT-FAT CALORIES
Bread			
Bagels			
plain or water	1	200	3
Biscuits			
plain or water, enriched	1	95	7
frozen (Pillsbury)			
1869 Brand	1 biscuit	100	9
Big Country	1 biscuit	100	<9
Grands! Cinnamon Raisin	1 biscuit	190	18
Hungry Jack No Cholesterol	1 biscuit	90	<9
Boston brown, canned	½-inch slice	95	7
Cracked wheat	1 loaf (1 lb)	1190	28
	1 slice (18/loaf)	65	2
Croissants	1 (2 oz)	260	93
Frozen (Sara Lee)			
Original Butter	1 croissant	170	53 e
Petite Butter	1 croissant	120	35 e
Croutons (Brownberry)	½ oz	60	<9
Crumbs, dry	1 cup	390	14
Devonshire plain	½ oz	50	<9
Shake 'n Bake	¼ envelope	80	<9
English muffins, plain	1	140	3
French			
baguette	1 ½-inch slice	70	trace
mini baguette	2 oz	140	<9
French toast	1 slice	155	14
Frozen Breads (Pillsbury)			
Cornbread Twists	1 twist	70	<9
Crusty French Loaf	1-inch slice	60	0
Soft Breadsticks	1 stick	100	<9
White Pipin' Hot Loaf	1-inch slice	70	0
Italian	¾-inch slice	85	trace
Mixed grain	1 slice (18/loaf)	65	2
Muffins			
made with butter			
Oat Bran	1 (5½ oz)	430	90
made with soy oil			
Blueberry	1 (2 oz)	140	13
	1 (4 oz)	280	20
Bran	1 (2 oz)	150	13
	1 (4 oz)	300	20

e indicates estimated sat-fat calories.

GRAIN PRODUCTS

FOOD	AMOUNT	TOTAL CALORIES	SAT-FAT CALORIES
Muffins (*cont.*)			
Made with soy oil			
Corn	1 (2 oz)	180	13
	1 (4 oz)	360	20
Oat Bran	1 (4 oz)	300	20
frozen			
Pepperidge Farm			
Blueberry	1 muffin	170	9
Corn	1 muffin	180	9
Sara Lee			
Apple Spice	1 muffin	220	22 e
Blueberry	1 muffin	200	22 e
Free and Light Blueberry	1 muffin	120	0
Snack Muffins			
Cheese Streusel	1 muffin	220	64 e
Chunky Chocolate	1 muffin	220	22 e
Oatmeal	1 slice (18/loaf)	65	2
Pita			
White	1 (6½ in)	120	1
	1 mini	80	trace
Whole Wheat	1 (6½ in)	110	1
	1 mini	70	trace
Pumpernickel	1 slice (15/loaf)	80	2
Raisin	1 slice (18/loaf)	70	2
Rolls			
dinner	1	85	5
frankfurter and hamburger	1	115	5
hard	1	155	4
hoagie or sub	1	400	16
Rye	1 slice (18/loaf)	65	2
Stuffing mix			
dry	1 cup	500	55
moist	1 cup	420	48
Wheat	1 slice (18/loaf)	65	2
White	1 slice (18/loaf)	65	3
	1 slice (22/loaf)	55	2
Whole-wheat	1 slice (16/loaf)	70	4

e indicates estimated sat-fat calories.

GRAIN PRODUCTS

FOOD	AMOUNT	TOTAL CALORIES	SAT-FAT CALORIES
Breakfast Bars, Tarts, and Granola Bars			
Breakfast Bars and Tarts			
Carnation			
Chocolate Chip	1 bar	200	49 e
Peanut Butter with Chocolate Chips	1 bar	200	49 e
Fibar			
Cocoa Peanut Crunch	1 bar (1.2 oz)	130	6 e
Raspberry or Strawberry	1 bar (1 oz)	100	4 e
Kellogg's			
Bars			
Nutri-Grain Cereal	1 bar	150	9
Rice Krispie bars, chocolate chip	1 bar	120	22 e
Pop-Tarts			
Brown Sugar Cinnamon	1 pastry	210	18
all other flavors	1 pastry	200–210	9
Kudos			
Chocolate Chip	1 bar	180	79 e
Cookies and Creme	1 bar	190	95 e
Nutty Fudge	1 bar	200	95 e
Peanut Butter	1 bar	200	95 e
Granola Bars			
Nature Valley Oat Bran			
Honey Graham Flavor	1 bar	110	<9
Oats 'n Honey	1 bar	120	9
Nature's Choice Fresh & Chewy			
Peanut Butter	1 bar	90	4 e
all other flavors	1 bar	90	2 e
Quaker Oats Chewy			
Apple	1 bar (1 oz)	120	16 e
Chocolate Chip	1 bar (1 oz)	130	27 e
Maple Oatmeal	1 bar (1 oz)	130	22 e
Peanut Butter and Chocolate Chip	1 bar (1 oz)	130	27 e

e indicates estimated sat-fat calories.

GRAIN PRODUCTS

FOOD	AMOUNT	TOTAL CALORIES	SAT-FAT CALORIES
Breakfast Cereals, Cold			
All-Bran	1 oz (⅓ cup)	70	1
Bran flakes (40%)			
Kellogg's	1 oz (¾ cup	90	1
Post	1 oz (⅔ cup)	90	1
Cap'n Crunch	1 oz (¾ cup)	120	15
Cheerios	1 oz (1¼ cups)	110	3
Honey Nut	1 oz (¾ cup)	105	1
Corn flakes	1 oz (1¼ cups)	110	0
Cracklin' Oat Bran	1 oz (½ cup)	110	9
Froot Loops	1 oz (1 cup)	110	2
Golden Grahams	1 oz (¾ cup)	110	6
Grape Nuts	1 oz (¼ cup)	100	trace
Heartland Natural	1 oz (¼ cup)	130	11
Lucky Charms	1 oz (1 cup)	110	2
Nature Valley Granola	1 oz (⅓ cup)	125	30
Oat Bake	1 oz (⅓ cup)	110	14
100% Natural Cereal			
plain	1 oz (¼ cup)	133	37
with raisins and nuts	1 oz (¼ cup)	128	32
Product 19	1 oz (¾ cup)	110	trace
Raisin Bran			
Kellogg's	1 oz (¾ cup)	90	1
Post	1 oz (½ cup)	85	1
Rice Krispies	1 oz (1 cup)	110	trace
Shredded Wheat	1 oz (⅔ cup)	110	trace
Special K	1 oz (1⅓ cups)	110	trace
Super Sugar Crisp	1 oz (⅞ cup)	105	trace
Sugar Frosted Flakes	1 oz (¾ cup)	110	trace
Total	1 oz (1 cup)	100	1
Trix	1 oz (1 cup)	110	2
Wheaties	1 oz (1 cup)	100	1
Breakfast Cereals, Hot			
Corn (hominy) grits, cooked			
regular and quick	1 cup	145	trace
instant, plain	1 packet	80	trace
Cream of Wheat regular, quick, instant, cooked	1 cup	140	1

e indicates estimated sat-fat calories.

GRAIN PRODUCTS

FOOD	AMOUNT	TOTAL CALORIES	SAT-FAT CALORIES
Mix'n Eat, plain, cooked	1 packet	100	trace
Malt-O-Meal, cooked	1 cup	120	trace
Oat bran			
cooked	1 cup	110	4
uncooked	1 cup	330	12
Oatmeal or rolled oats regular, quick, instant			
cooked	1 cup	110	4
plain	1 packet	105	3
flavored	1 packet	160	3
uncooked	⅓ cup	104	3
Crackers			
Devonsheer			
Melba Rounds			
Garlic or Sesame	½ oz (~5)	60	<9
Vegetable	½ oz (~5)	60	0
all other	½ oz (~5)	50	0
Melba Toast	½ oz (~3)	50	0
Keebler			
Cinnamon Crisp Grahams	4	70	<9
Club	4	60	<9
Club and Cheddar Cracker Sandwich	1	70	<9
Clubettes	22	70	<9
Harvest Wheats	4	60	<9
Honey Grahams	4	70	<9
Munch'ems	½ oz	70	<9
Thin Bits	12	70	<9
Town House	4	70	<9
Toasteds	4	60	<9
Wheatables	11	70	<9
Zesta Saltines	5	60	<9
Nabisco			
American Classic	½ oz (4)	70	<9
Better Cheddars	½ oz (10)	70	<9
Cheddar Wedges	½ oz (~31)	70	<9
Chicken in a Bisket	½ oz (7)	80	9
Harvest Crisps	½ oz (6)	60	<9
Honey Maid Grahams	½ oz (~2)	60	<9
Nips Cheese Snack	½ oz (13)	70	<9

GRAIN PRODUCTS

FOOD	AMOUNT	TOTAL CALORIES	SAT-FAT CALORIES
Nabisco (*cont.*)			
Oat Thins	½ oz (8)	70	<9
Oysterettes	½ oz (18)	60	<9
Premium			
Bits	½ oz (16)	70	<9
all other varieties	½ oz (5)	60	<9
Ritz Bits			
Mini Ritz	½ oz (22)	70	<9
Sandwiches with Cheese	½ oz (~6)	80	9
Ritz	½ oz (4)	70	<9
Sociables	½ oz (6)	70	<9
Swiss Cheese	½ oz (7)	70	<9
Teddy Grahams	½ oz (11)	60	<9
Toasted Bran Thins	½ oz (7)	60	<9
Triscuit	½ oz (3)	60	<9
Bits	½ oz (8)	60	<9
Rye	½ oz (3)	60	<9
Wheat 'n Bran	½ oz (3)	60	<9
Vegetable Thins	½ oz (7)	70	<9
Waverly	½ oz (4)	70	<9
Wheat Thins	½ oz (8)	70	<9
Wheatsworth	½ oz (4)	70	<9
Pepperidge Farm			
Butter Thins	4	70	9
Crispy Graham	½ oz (~4)	70	<9
English Water Biscuits	4	70	0
Garden Vegetable	½ oz (~5)	70	<9
Hearty Wheat	4	100	9
Low-Salt Symphony Assortment			
Butter-Flavored Thins	4	70	9
Sesame	4	80	9
Toasted Wheat	4	80	9
Multi-Grain	½ oz (~4)	70	<9
Toasted Rice	½ oz (~4)	70	<9
Sunshine			
American Heritage			
Sesame	4	80	9
Wheat Bran	4	60	9
Cheese Shuffles	18	70	9
Cheez-It	12	70	9

GRAIN PRODUCTS

FOOD	AMOUNT	TOTAL CALORIES	SAT-FAT CALORIES
Sunshine (*cont.*)			
Grahams			
Cinnamon	1	70	9
Grahamy Bears	9	130	9
Honey	1	60	<9
Hi Ho Deluxe	4	80	9
Low-Salt	4	80	9
Whole-Wheat	4	65	9
Krispy	5	60	<9
Oat Bran, heart-shaped	8	80	9
Oyster and Soup	16	60	<9
Wheats, heart-shaped	8	70	9
Flour			
Buckwheat flour, light	1 cup	340	2
Cornmeal			
whole-ground, dry	1 cup	442	6
Cornstarch	1 tbsp	29	0
Rice, white	1 cup	578	5
Rye			
light	1 cup	374	1
medium	1 cup	361	2
dark	1 cup	415	4
Semolina	1 cup	605	2
Wheat flour			
cake or pastry, sifted	1 cup	350	1
self-rising, unsifted	1 cup	440	2
white (unbleached)			
sifted	1 cup	420	2
unsifted	1 tbsp	26	0
	1 cup	455	2
whole-wheat	1 cup	400	3
Grains (Cereal Grasses)			
Barley, pearl, light, uncooked	1 cup	704	4
Buckwheat groats			
dry	1 cup	567	9
cooked	1 cup	182	2

GRAIN PRODUCTS

FOOD	AMOUNT	TOTAL CALORIES	SAT-FAT CALORIES
Bulgur			
dry	1 cup	478	3
cooked	1 cup	152	1
Couscous			
dry	1 cup	692	2
cooked	1 cup	201	trace
Farina			
dry	1 cup	649	1
cooked	1 cup	116	trace
Millet			
raw	1 cup	756	13
cooked	1 cup	287	4
Rice			
Brown			
raw	1 cup	687	9
cooked	1 cup	218	3
White			
Glutinous			
raw	1 cup	685	2
cooked	1 cup	234	1
Long-grain			
raw	1 cup	676	3
cooked	1 cup	264	1
Instant, prepared	1 cup	161	1
Parboiled			
dry	1 cup	688	3
cooked	1 cup	199	1
Wild			
raw	1 cup	571	2
cooked	1 cup	166	1
Rice bran, crude	1 cup	262	31
Sorghum	1 cup	650	8
Wheat bran, crude	½ cup	65	2
Wheat germ			
crude	1 tbsp	23	1
	1 cup	414	17
toasted	1 oz	108	5
	1 cup	431	19

GRAIN PRODUCTS

FOOD	AMOUNT	TOTAL CALORIES	SAT-FAT CALORIES
Miscellaneous			
(See also ***Breakfast Foods***, **FROZEN AND MICROWAVE FOODS**.)			
Pancakes			
buckwheat	1 (4-inch)	55	8
plain, from mix	1 (4-inch)	60	5
Tortillas, corn	1	65	1
Waffles, from mix	1 (7-inch)	205	24
Pastas			
Fresh refrigerated			
as purchased	4½ oz	368	4
cooked	2 oz	75	1
Macaroni, cooked			
firm	1 cup	190	1
tender	1 cup	155	1
Noodles			
Chinese cellophane	1 cup	492	trace
chow mein, canned	1 cup	220	19
egg, cooked	1 cup	200	5
Spaghetti			
dry	8 oz	838	4
cooked	1 cup	190	1
Pastries			
(See also ***Breakfast Bars, Tarts, and Granola Bars*** and **SUGARS AND SWEETS**.)			
Danish pastry			
packaged ring	1 (12 oz)	1305	196
round, plain	1	20	32
round, fruit	1	235	35
Doughnuts			
cake-type, plain	1 medium	210	25
yeast-leavened, glazed	1	235	47
Frozen			
Pepperidge Farm			
Apple Turnover	1 turnover	300	46 e
Cinnamon Rolls	1 roll	280	38 e

GRAIN PRODUCTS

FOOD	AMOUNT	TOTAL CALORIES	SAT-FAT CALORIES
Pillsbury			
Cinnamon Rolls with Icing	1 roll	110	9
Coffee Cake			
Cinnamon Streusel with Icing	1 slice	180	18
Streusel Pecan Crumb	1 slice	180	18
Danish Rolls	1 roll	150	18
Toaster Strudels			
apple	1 pastry	200	18
blueberry	1 pastry	190	18
cinnamon	1 pastry	200	18
strawberry	1 pastry	190	18
Sara Lee			
Deluxe Cinnamon Rolls	1 roll	230	64 e
Free & Light			
Apple Danish	⅛ cake	130	0
Toaster pastries	1	210	15

*Snack Foods (*See also **SNACK FOODS.***)*

Pretzels			
sourdough	1 (1 oz)	100	0
sticks	10 (2¼ in)	65	1
twisted			
Dutch	1	240	1
thin	10	240	2

e indicates estimated sat-fat calories.

MEATS (BEEF, GAME, LAMB, PORK, AND VEAL)

(See also **FAST FOODS, FROZEN AND MICROWAVE FOODS,** and
SAUSAGES AND LUNCHEON MEATS.)

FOOD	AMOUNT	TOTAL CALORIES	SAT-FAT CALORIES
Beef			
*Remember that the following calorie figures are for **only 1 ounce** of beef!*			
Arm pot roast, braised			
lean and fat	1 oz	99	27
lean only	1 oz	68	11
Bottom round steak, braised			
lean and fat	1 oz	74	14
lean only	1 oz	67	9
Brisket flat half, braised			
lean and fat	1 oz	116	37
lean only	1 oz	77	17
Chuck steak, braised			
lean and fat	1 oz	108	32
lean only	1 oz	78	18
Club steak, broiled			
lean and fat	1 oz	129	50
lean only	1 oz	69	16
Flank steak, broiled			
lean and fat	1 oz	72	18
lean only	1 oz	69	16
Ground beef			
raw			
extra lean	1 oz	66	17
lean	1 oz	75	21
regular	1 oz	88	28
broiled, medium			
extra lean	1 oz	72	16
lean	1 oz	77	18
regular	1 oz	82	21
pan-fried, medium			
extra lean	1 oz	72	16
lean	1 oz	78	19
regular	1 oz	87	23
Porterhouse steak, broiled			
lean and fat	1 oz	85	22
lean only	1 oz	64	13
Rib roast			
lean and fat	1 oz	108	34
lean only	1 oz	70	17

MEATS (BEEF, GAME, LAMB, PORK, AND VEAL)

FOOD	AMOUNT	TOTAL CALORIES	SAT-FAT CALORIES
Round steak, broiled			
lean and fat	1 oz	78	19
lean only	1 oz	54	7
Rump roast			
lean and fat	1 oz	98	33
lean only	1 oz	59	11
Shortribs, braised			
lean and fat	1 oz	133	45
lean only	1 oz	84	20
Sirloin steak, broiled			
lean and fat	1 oz	79	19
lean only	1 oz	62	12
T-bone steak, broiled			
lean and fat	1 oz	92	26
lean only	1 oz	61	11
Tenderloin steak, broiled			
lean and fat	1 oz	75	18
lean only	1 oz	58	9
Top round steak, broiled			
lean and fat	1 oz	60	8
lean only	1 oz	55	6

Mixed Beef Dishes
(See also **FROZEN AND MICROWAVE FOODS.**)

FOOD	AMOUNT	TOTAL CALORIES	SAT-FAT CALORIES
Beef and vegetable stew	1 cup	220	40
Beef potpie (9-inch)	1 slice (3/pie)	515	71
Chili con carne, canned	1 cup	340	52
Chop suey with beef and pork	1 cup	300	39
Lasagna	1/12 casserole	570	142
Spaghetti with meatballs and tomato sauce			
canned	1 cup	260	22
homemade	1 cup	330	35

Variety Meats and By-products

FOOD	AMOUNT	TOTAL CALORIES	SAT-FAT CALORIES
Liver, braised	1 oz	46	5
Fine liver pâté	1/2 cup	289	104
Tongue, simmered	1 oz	81	23

MEATS (BEEF, GAME, LAMB, PORK, AND VEAL)

FOOD	AMOUNT	TOTAL CALORIES	SAT-FAT CALORIES
Game			
*Remember that the following calorie figures are for **only 1 ounce** of game!*			
Antelope, roasted	1 oz	42	2
Beefalo, roasted	1 oz	53	7
Bison, roasted	1 oz	41	2
Boar, wild, roasted	1 oz	45	3
Buffalo, water, roasted	1 oz	37	2
Caribou, roasted	1 oz	47	4
Deer, roasted	1 oz	45	3
Elk, roasted	1 oz	41	2
Goat, roasted	1 oz	41	2
Horse, roasted	1 oz	50	5
Moose, roasted	1 oz	38	1
Rabbit			
domesticated			
roasted	1 oz	44	5
stewed	1 oz	58	6
wild, stewed	1 oz	49	3
Squirrel, roasted	1 oz	39	1
Lamb			
*Remember that the following calorie figures are for **only 1 ounce** of lamb!*			
Foreshank			
lean and fat, braised	1 oz	69	14
lean only, braised	1 oz	53	6
Lean, whole (shank and sirloin)			
lean and fat, roasted	1 oz	73	18
lean only, roasted	1 oz	54	7
Leg, shank half			
lean and fat, roasted	1 oz	64	13
lean only, roasted	1 oz	51	6
Leg, sirloin half			
lean and fat, roasted	1 oz	83	23
lean only, roasted	1 oz	58	8
Loin			
lean and fat, broiled	1 oz	89	25
lean only, broiled	1 oz	61	9
Rib			
lean and fat, roasted	1 oz	102	33
lean only, roasted	1 oz	66	12

MEATS (BEEF, GAME, LAMB, PORK, AND VEAL)

FOOD	AMOUNT	TOTAL CALORIES	SAT-FAT CALORIES
Shoulder, whole (arm and blade)			
lean and fat, braised	1 oz	97	27
lean only, braised	1 oz	80	16
Cubed lamb for stew or kabob			
(leg and shoulder), lean only			
braised	1 oz	63	8
broiled	1 oz	53	7
Ground lamb	1 oz	81	26

Pork

*Remember that most of the following calorie figures are for **only 1 ounce** of pork!*

Loin			
whole, broiled			
lean and fat	1 oz	98	25
	1 chop	284	73
lean only	1 oz	73	13
	1 chop	169	31
blade			
broiled			
lean and fat	1 oz	111	31
	1 chop	303	84
lean only	1 oz	80	17
	1 chop	175	38
pan-fried			
lean and fat	1 oz	117	34
	1 chop	368	107
lean only	1 oz	85	19
	1 chop	177	39
center loin			
broiled			
lean and fat	1 oz	90	20
	1 chop	275	63
lean only	1 oz	65	9
	1 chop	166	23
pan-fried			
lean and fat	1 oz	106	28
	1 chop	333	88
lean only	1 oz	75	14
	1 chop	178	33

MEATS (BEEF, GAME, LAMB, PORK, AND VEAL)

FOOD	AMOUNT	TOTAL CALORIES	SAT-FAT CALORIES
Loin (*cont.*)			
center rib			
broiled			
lean and fat	1 oz	97	24
	1 chop	264	66
lean only	1 oz	73	13
	1 chop	162	29
pan-fried			
lean and fat	1 oz	110	30
	1 chop	343	94
lean only	1 oz	73	13
	1 chop	160	29
sirloin, broiled			
lean and fat	1 oz	94	23
	1 chop	278	69
lean only	1 oz	69	12
	1 chop	165	29
tenderloin, lean only, roasted	1 oz	47	4
top loin			
broiled			
lean and fat	1 oz	102	26
	1 chop	295	76
lean only	1 oz	73	13
	1 chop	165	30
pan-fried			
lean and fat	1 oz	111	31
	1 chop	337	93
lean only	1 oz	73	13
	1 chop	157	29
Shoulder			
whole, roasted			
lean and fat	1 oz	92	24
lean only	1 oz	69	13
arm, picnic, braised			
lean and fat	1 oz	98	24
lean only	1 oz	70	11
blade, Boston, braised			
lean and fat	1 oz	105	26
lean only	1 oz	83	15

MEATS (BEEF, GAME, LAMB, PORK, AND VEAL)

FOOD	AMOUNT	TOTAL CALORIES	SAT-FAT CALORIES
Spareribs, braised			
lean and fat	1 oz	113	30
Pork Products, Cured			
(See also **SAUSAGES AND LUNCHEON MEATS.**)			
Bacon, cooked	1 oz	163	44
	3 slices	109	30
Breakfast strips, cooked	1 oz	130	33
	3 slices	156	39
Canadian-style bacon, grilled	1 oz	52	7
	2 slices	86	12
Feet, pickled	1 oz	58	14
Salt pork, raw	1 oz	205	75
Variety Meats and By-products			
Chitterlings, simmered	1 oz	86	26
Feet, simmered	1 oz	55	11
Liver			
Country pâté	½ cup	430	140
Scrapple	1 oz	61	14
Veal			
*Remember that the following calorie figures are for **only 1 ounce** of veal!*			
Breast, lean and fat, braised	1 oz	86	26
Cutlet, lean and fat, braised	1 oz	62	12
Ground, broiled	1 oz	49	8
Leg			
top round, lean and fat, braised	1 oz	65	7
top round, lean, braised	1 oz	58	5
Loin			
lean and fat, braised	1 oz	84	17
lean, roasted	1 oz	50	7
Rib			
lean and fat, roasted	1 oz	65	14
lean, braised	1 oz	62	7
Shoulder			
arm, lean and fat, braised	1 oz	67	10
arm, lean, roasted	1 oz	47	6
blade, lean and fat, braised	1 oz	64	9
blade, lean, roasted	1 oz	49	7

MEATS (BEEF, GAME, LAMB, PORK, AND VEAL)

FOOD	AMOUNT	TOTAL CALORIES	SAT-FAT CALORIES
Sirloin			
lean and fat, braised	1 oz	72	13
lean, roasted	1 oz	48	6

NUTS AND SEEDS

FOOD	AMOUNT	TOTAL CALORIES	SAT-FAT CALORIES
Nuts			
Almonds, shelled			
slivered	1 cup	795	60
whole	1 oz (24 nuts)	165	13
Almond butter			
plain	1 tbsp	101	8
honey-cinnamon	1 tbsp	96	7
Almond paste	1 oz	127	7
Brazil nuts, shelled	1 oz (8 medium)	186	41
Butternuts, dried	1 oz	174	3
Cashew nuts			
dry-roasted	1 oz (18 medium)	163	23
	1 cup	785	113
oil-roasted	1 oz (18 medium)	163	24
	1 cup	750	112
	1 cup	750	112
Cashew butter, plain	1 oz	167	25
	1 tbsp	94	14
Chestnuts, Chinese			
raw	1 oz	64	0
dried	1 oz	103	1
boiled or steamed	1 oz	44	0
roasted	1 oz	68	0
Chestnuts, European			
boiled or steamed	1 oz	37	1
roasted	1 oz (3 nuts)	70	1
	1 cup	270	4
Chestnuts, Japanese			
raw	1 oz	44	0
dried	1 oz	102	0

NUTS AND SEEDS

FOOD	AMOUNT	TOTAL CALORIES	SAT-FAT CALORIES
Chestnuts, Japanese (*cont.*)			
boiled or steamed	1 oz	16	0
roasted	1 oz	57	0
Coconut meat			
raw, shredded or grated	1 cup	283	214
dried, creamed	1 oz	194	157
dried, sweetened, flaked, canned	1 oz	126	72
	1 cup	341	195
dried, sweetened, flaked	1 oz	135	72
	1 cup	351	190
dried, sweetened, shredded	1 oz	142	81
	1 cup	466	263
dried, toasted	1 oz	168	107
Coconut cream			
fresh	1 tbsp	49	42
	1 cup	792	664
canned	1 tbsp	36	27
	1 cup	568	419
Coconut milk			
fresh	1 tbsp	35	29
	1 cup	552	457
canned	1 tbsp	30	26
	1 cup	445	385
frozen	1 tbsp	30	25
	1 cup	486	398
Filberts or hazelnuts, chopped	1 oz	180	12
	1 cup	725	48
Formulated, wheat-based			
unflavored	1 oz	177	22
flavored	1 oz	184	24
Hickory nuts, dried	1 oz	187	18
Macadamia nuts			
dried	1 oz	199	28
oil-roasted	1 oz (24 halves)	204	29
	1 cup	960	139
Mixed nuts			
dry-roasted, w/peanuts	1 oz	169	18
oil-roasted, w/peanuts	1 oz	175	22
oil-roasted, w/o peanuts	1 oz	175	23
Peanuts, shelled			
dry-roasted	1 oz (35 kernels)	161	17
	1 cup	827	90

NUTS AND SEEDS

FOOD	AMOUNT	TOTAL CALORIES	SAT-FAT CALORIES
Peanuts, shelled (*cont.*)			
oil-roasted	1 oz	165	18
	1 cup	840	89
Peanut butter, smooth	1 tbsp	95	12
Peanut flour	1 tbsp	13	0
Pecans			
dried	1 oz	190	14
	1 cup	720	53
dry-roasted	1 oz	187	13
oil-roasted	1 oz	195	15
Pecan flour	1 oz	93	0
Pine nuts, dried	1 oz	146	20
	1 tbsp	51	7
Pistachio nuts			
dried	1 oz	164	16
dry-roasted	1 oz (47 kernels)	172	17
Soybean kernels, roasted or toasted	1 oz	129	8
Walnuts, black, dried	1 oz (14 halves)	172	9
	1 cup	760	41
Walnuts, English or Persian, dried	1 oz (14 halves)	182	14
	1 cup	770	60
Seeds			
Pumpkin and squash			
whole, roasted	1 tbsp	18	1
kernels, dried	1 tbsp	47	7
kernels, roasted	1 tbsp	74	10
Sesame, kernels, dried	1 cup	882	104
	1 tbsp	47	6
Sunflower			
in shell, roasted, salted	1 oz	86	8
shelled, dry-roasted, salted	1 tbsp	46	4
shelled, oil-roasted, salted	1 tbsp	51	5
Tahini	1 tbsp	90	10
Miscellaneous			
Trail mix	1 oz	165	25

POULTRY

(See also **FAST FOODS, FROZEN AND MICROWAVE FOODS,** and **SAUSAGES AND LUNCHEON MEATS.**)

FOOD	AMOUNT	TOTAL CALORIES	SAT-FAT CALORIES
Chicken			
Back			
meat and skin			
fried, batter-dipped	1 oz	94	15
	½ back	397	63
fried, flour-coated	1 oz	94	14
	½ back	238	36
roasted	1 oz	85	15
	½ back	159	28
meat only			
raw	1 oz	39	4
	½ back	70	7
fried, flour-coated, cooked	1 oz	53	5
without skin	½ back	110	16
Breast			
meat and skin			
fried, batter-dipped	1 oz	74	9
	½ breast	364	44
fried, flour-coated	1 oz	63	6
	½ breast	218	22
roasted	1 oz	56	6
	½ breast	193	19
meat only			
raw	1 oz	31	1
	½ breast	129	4
fried, flour-coated cooked	1 oz	37	2
without skin	½ breast	148	6
Drumstick			
meat and skin			
fried, batter-dipped	1 oz	76	11
	1 drumstick	193	27
fried, flour-coated	1 oz	70	9
	1 drumstick	120	16
roasted	1 oz	61	8
	1 drumstick	112	14
meat only			
raw	1 oz	34	2
	1 drumstick	74	5
fried, flour-coated, cooked	1 oz	40	3
without skin	1 drumstick	80	7

POULTRY

FOOD	AMOUNT	TOTAL CALORIES	SAT-FAT CALORIES
Leg			
meat and skin			
fried, batter-dipped	1 oz	77	11
	1 leg	431	61
fried, flour-coated	1 oz	72	10
	1 leg	285	39
roasted	1 oz	66	9
	1 leg	265	38
meat only			
raw	1 oz	34	3
	1 leg	156	11
fried, flour-coated, cooked	1 oz	39	3
without skin	1 leg	169	12
Liver, simmered	1 oz	53	5
chopped chicken livers	1 tbsp	28	4
Neck			
meat and skin			
fried, batter-dipped	1 oz	94	16
	1 neck	172	29
fried, flour-coated	1 oz	94	16
	1 neck	119	21
simmered	1 oz	70	13
	1 neck	94	17
meat only			
raw	1 oz	44	6
	1 neck	31	4
fried, flour-coated, cooked	1 oz	58	7
without skin	1 neck	49	5
Thigh			
meat and skin			
fried, batter-dipped	1 oz	79	11
	1 thigh	238	34
fried, flour-coated	1 oz	74	10
	1 thigh	162	23
roasted	1 oz	70	11
	1 thigh	153	24
meat only			
raw	1 oz	34	3
	1 thigh	82	6
fried, flour-coated, cooked	1 oz	37	4
without skin	1 thigh	86	7

POULTRY

FOOD	AMOUNT	TOTAL CALORIES	SAT-FAT CALORIES
Wing			
meat and skin			
fried, batter-dipped	1 oz	92	15
	1 wing	159	26
fried, flour-coated	1 oz	91	15
	1 wing	103	17
roasted	1 oz	82	14
	1 wing	99	17
meat only			
raw	1 oz	36	2
	1 wing	36	2
fried, flour-coated, cooked	1 oz	38	2
without skin	1 wing	37	2

Mixed Chicken Dishes
(See also **FROZEN AND MICROWAVE FOODS**.)

Chicken à la king	1 cup	470	116
Chicken and noodles	1 cup	365	46
Chicken chow mein			
canned	1 cup	95	1
homemade	1 cup	255	37
Chicken potpie (9-inch)	1 slice (3/pie)	545	93
Chicken salad	½ cup	340	30

Duck
Domestic, roasted

meat and skin	1 oz	96	25
	½ duck	1287	332
meat only	1 oz	57	11
	½ duck	445	83
Wild, raw			
meat and skin	1 oz	60	13
	½ duck	571	125
breast meat only	1 oz	35	3
	½ duck	102	10

Goose, (domestic)

Meat and skin, roasted	1 oz	86	18
Meat only, roasted	1 oz	67	12
Liver, simmered	1 oz	38	4

POULTRY

FOOD	AMOUNT	TOTAL CALORIES	SAT-FAT CALORIES
Pheasant			
Meat and skin, raw	1 oz	51	7
Meat only, raw	1 oz	38	3
Breast, meat only, raw	1 oz	38	3
Leg, meat only, raw	1 oz	38	4
Quail			
Meat and skin, raw	1 oz	54	9
Meat only, raw	1 oz	38	3
Breast, meat only, raw	1 oz	35	2
Squab (pigeon)			
Meat and skin, raw	1 oz	83	21
Meat only, raw	1 oz	40	5
Breast, meat only, raw	1 oz	38	3
Turkey			
Back, roasted			
meat and skin	1 oz	58	8
	½ back	265	35
meat only	1 oz	48	5
	½ back	164	16
Breast, roasted			
meat and skin	1 oz	43	2
	½ breast	526	27
meat only	1 oz	38	½
	½ breast	413	6
Cutlets	1 oz	38	½
Leg, roasted			
meat and skin	1 oz	48	4
	1 leg	418	37
meat only	1 oz	45	3
	1 leg	355	26
Wing, roasted			
meat and skin	1 oz	59	7
	1 wing	186	22
meat only	1 oz	46	3
	1 wing	98	6

(For chicken and turkey frankfurters and chicken and turkey cold cuts, see
SAUSAGES AND LUNCHEON MEATS.)

RESTAURANT FOOD

FOOD	AMOUNT	TOTAL CALORIES	SAT-FAT CALORIES
*Chinese**			
Barbecued pork (not fried)	1 whole dish	1374	355
Barbecued spareribs	1 whole dish	1863	480
Beef with any vegetable	1 whole dish	1572	263
Chicken with any vegetable	1 whole dish	1224	102
Chicken with cashews	1 whole dish	1765	186
Egg rolls (each)	1 whole dish	152	30
Hunan shrimp (not deep-fried)	1 whole dish	1068	100
Kung Pao beef	1 whole dish	2458	444
Kung Pao chicken	1 whole dish	1806	158
Kung Pao shrimp	1 whole dish	1068	115
Lemon chicken	1 whole dish	1003	103
Moo Shu beef	1 whole dish	1310	258
Moo Shu pork	1 whole dish	1383	292
Orange beef	1 whole dish	1710	342
Pork with vegetables	1 whole dish	1574	338
Sweet-and-sour pork	1 whole dish	1845	389
Sweet-and-sour shrimp	1 whole dish	1069	130
Szechuan pork	1 whole dish	1694	356

SAUCES AND GRAVIES

FOOD	AMOUNT	TOTAL CALORIES	SAT-FAT CALORIES
Sauces			
Barbecue, ready-to-serve	1 cup	188	6
Béarnaise	1 tbsp	53	29
	½ cup	423	232
Cheese	1 tbsp	28	14
	½ cup	225	110
Curry, dehydrated, prepared with milk	1 cup	270	54
Curry cream	1 tbsp	40	20
	½ cup	317	160
Hollandaise	1 tbsp	82	47
	½ cup	670	377

*These are estimates. Actual values vary from restaurant to restaurant.

SAUCES AND GRAVIES

FOOD	AMOUNT	TOTAL CALORIES	SAT-FAT CALORIES
Mushroom, dehydrated, prepared with milk	1 cup	228	49
Sour cream, dehydrated, prepared with milk	1 cup	509	145
Soy	1 tbsp	11	0
Spaghetti, dehydrated	1 packet (1.5 oz)	118	2
	1 serving (¼ packet)	28	1
Spaghetti with mushrooms, dehydrated	1 packet (1.4 oz)	118	20
Stroganoff, dehydrated, prepared with milk and water	1 cup	271	61
Sweet and sour, dehydrated, prepared with water and vinegar	1 cup	294	0
Teriyaki, dehydrated, prepared with water	1 cup	131	1
Teriyaki, ready-to-serve	1 tbsp	15	0
Tomato sauce			
canned	1 cup	74	0
with herbs and cheese	1 cup	144	14
Prego			
Tomato and Basil	4 oz	110	12 e
3 Cheeses	4 oz	100	12 e
Sausage and Green Pepper	4 oz	160	28 e
White	1 tbsp	24	11
	½ cup	195	88
Gravies			
Au jus, canned	1 cup	38	2
Au jus, dehydrated, prepared with water	1 cup	19	4
Beef, canned	1 cup	124	25
Brown, dehydrated, prepared with water	1 cup	9	1
Chicken, canned	1 cup	189	30
Chicken, dehydrated, prepared with water	1 cup	83	5
Mushroom			
canned	1 cup	120	9
dehydrated, prepared with water	1 cup	70	5

e indicates estimated sat-fat calories.

SAUCES AND GRAVIES

FOOD	AMOUNT	TOTAL CALORIES	SAT-FAT CALORIES
Onion, dehydrated, prepared with water	1 cup	80	4
Pork, dehydrated, prepared with water	1 cup	76	7
Turkey, canned	1 cup	122	13

SAUSAGES AND LUNCHEON MEATS

FOOD	AMOUNT	TOTAL CALORIES	SAT-FAT CALORIES
Barbecue loaf, pork, beef	1 oz	49	8
	1 slice (.8 oz)	40	7
Beerwurst, beer salami			
beef	1 oz	92	31
	1 slice (.8 oz)	75	25
	1 slice (.25 oz)	19	6
pork	1 oz	68	16
	1 slice (.8 oz)	55	13
	1 slice (.25 oz)	14	3
Berliner, pork, beef	1 oz	65	15
	1 slice (.8 oz)	53	13
Blood sausage	1 oz	107	34
	1 slice (.8 oz)	95	30
Bockwurst, raw	1 oz	87	26
	1 link (2.3 oz)	200	59
Bologna			
beef	1 oz = 1 slice	89	30
	1 slice (.8 oz)	72	24
beef and pork	1 oz = 1 slice	89	27
	1 slice (.8 oz)	73	22
pork	1 oz = 1 slice	70	18
	1 slice (.8 oz)	57	14
Bratwurst, pork, beef	1 oz	92	25
	1 link (2.5 oz)	226	63
Bratwurst, pork, cooked	1 oz	85	24
	1 link (3 oz)	256	71

SAUSAGES AND LUNCHEON MEATS

FOOD	AMOUNT	TOTAL CALORIES	SAT-FAT CALORIES
Braunschweiger, pork	1 oz	102	28
	1 slice (.6 oz)	65	18
Breakfast strips, beef	1 slice	51	15
	1 oz	127	37
Cheesefurter, cheese smokie, pork, beef	1 oz	93	27
	1 frank	141	40
Chicken roll, light meat	1 oz = 1 slice	45	5
Corned beef			
brisket	1 oz	71	16
canned	1 oz	71	16
loaf, jellied	1 oz = 1 slice	46	7
Dried beef, cured	1 oz	47	4
Dutch brand loaf, pork, beef	1 oz = 1 slice	68	16
Frankfurter			
beef	1 oz	91	31
	1 frank (2 oz)	184	61
	1 frank (1.6 oz)	145	48
beef and pork	1 oz	91	27
	1 frank (2 oz)	183	55
	1 frank (1.6 oz)	144	44
chicken	1 oz	73	14
	1 frank (1.6 oz)	116	22
turkey	1 oz	70	15
	1 frank (2 oz)	140	30
Ham			
chopped	1 oz	68	16
	1 slice (.74 oz)	50	12
minced	1 oz	75	18
	1 slice (.74 oz)	55	14
sliced, extra lean	1 oz = 1 slice	37	4
sliced, regular	1 oz = 1 slice	52	9
Ham and cheese loaf	1 oz = 1 slice	73	19
Ham and cheese spread	1 oz	69	22
	1 tbsp	37	12
Ham salad spread	1 oz	61	13
	1 tbsp	32	7
Headcheese, pork	1 oz = 1 slice	60	13
Honey loaf, pork, beef	1 oz = 1 slice	36	4
Honey roll sausage, beef	1 oz	52	10
	1 slice (.8 oz)	42	8

SAUSAGES AND LUNCHEON MEATS

FOOD	AMOUNT	TOTAL CALORIES	SAT-FAT CALORIES
Italian sausage, cooked, pork	1 oz	92	23
	1 link (5/lb)	216	55
	1 link (4/lb)	268	68
Kielbasa, kolbassy, pork, beef	1 oz	88	25
	1 slice (.9 oz)	81	23
Knackwurst, knockwurst, pork, beef	1 oz	87	26
	1 link (2.4 oz)	209	62
Lebanon bologna, beef	1 oz	64	16
	1 slice (.8 oz)	52	13
Liver cheese, pork	1.3 oz	86	23
	1 slice	115	31
Liver sausage, liverwurst, pork	1 oz	93	27
	1 slice (.6 oz)	59	17
Luncheon meat			
beef, loaved	1 oz = 1 slice	87	29
beef, thin sliced	1 oz	35	3
	5 slices (.74 oz)	26	2
pork, beef	1 oz	100	30
pork, canned	1 oz	95	28
	1 slice (.74 oz)	70	20
Luncheon sausage, pork and beef	1 oz	74	19
	1 slice (.8 oz)	60	16
Luxury loaf, pork	1 oz = 1 slice	40	4
Mortadella, beef, pork	1 oz	88	24
	1 slice (.5 oz)	47	13
Mother's loaf, pork	1 oz	80	20
	1 slice (.74 oz)	59	15
New England brand sausage, pork, beef	1 oz	46	6
	1 slice (.8 oz)	37	5
Olive loaf, pork	1 oz = 1 slice	67	15
Pastrami			
beef	1 oz	99	27
turkey	1 oz = 1 slice	40	9
Peppered loaf, pork, beef	1 oz = 1 slice	42	6
Pepperoni, pork, beef	1 oz	141	41
	1 slice (.2 oz)	27	8
	1 sausage (9 oz)	1248	364
Pickle and pimiento loaf, pork	1 oz = 1 slice	74	20
Picnic loaf, pork, beef	1 oz = 1 slice	66	15

SAUSAGES AND LUNCHEON MEATS

FOOD	AMOUNT	TOTAL CALORIES	SAT-FAT CALORIES
Polish sausage, pork	1 oz	92	26
	1 sausage (8 oz)	739	211
Pork and beef sausage, cooked	1 oz = 1 patty	112	33
	1 link (.46 oz)	52	15
Pork sausage, cooked	1 oz = 1 patty	105	38
	1 link (.46 oz)	48	13
Poultry salad sandwich spread	1 oz	57	9
	1 tbsp	26	4
Salami			
beef, cooked	1 oz	72	22
	1 slice (.8 oz)	58	17
beef and pork, cooked	1 oz	71	21
	1 slice (.8 oz)	57	17
pork, dry or hard	1 oz	115	30
	1 slice (.35 oz)	41	11
pork, beef, dry or hard	1 oz	118	31
	1 slice (.35 oz)	42	11
Sandwich spread, pork, beef	1 oz	67	15
	1 tbsp	35	8
Smoked link sausage			
pork	1 oz	110	29
	1 link (2.4 oz)	265	69
	1 link (.56 oz)	62	16
pork and beef	1 oz	95	27
	1 link (2.4 oz)	229	65
	1 link (.56 oz)	54	15
Thuringer, cervelat, summer	1 oz	98	31
sausage, beef, pork	1 slice (.8 oz)	80	25
Turkey breast meat	1 oz	31	1
	1 slice (.74 oz)	23	1
Turkey ham, cured turkey thigh meat	1 oz = 1 slice	36	4
Turkey roll			
light and dark meat	1 oz = 1 slice	42	5
light meat	1 oz = 1 slice	42	5
Vienna sausage, beef and pork, canned	1 oz	79	24
	1 sausage (.56 oz)	45	13

SNACK FOODS

(See also **GRAIN PRODUCTS,** *Breakfast Bars, Tarts* and *Granola Bars* and *Crackers.*)

FOOD	AMOUNT	TOTAL CALORIES	SAT-FAT CALORIES
Cape Cod			
Popcorn with Cheddar Cheese	½ oz	80	21 e
Potato Chips	1 oz	150	19 e
Cracker Jack	1 oz (~⅔ cup)	120	4 e
Eagle			
Potato Chips			
Hawaiian Kettle	1 oz	150	19 e
Idaho Russett	1 oz	150	19 e
Ridged	1 oz	150	24 e
Thins	1 oz	150	24 e
Frito-Lay			
Cheetos			
Crunchy	1 oz	150	39 e
Curls	1 oz	160	39 e
Crunch Tators	1 oz	140	19 e
Doritos	1 oz (~15 chips)	140	30 e
Light	1 oz (~15 chips)	110	17 e
Fritos	1 oz	150	25 e
Munchos Potato Crisps	1 oz	160	27 e
Potato Chips (Lays)	1 oz	150	27 e
Bar-B-Q Flavored	1 oz	150	25 e
Sour Cream and Onion	1 oz	160	27 e
Pretzels (Rold Gold)			
Bavarian	1 oz	110	5 e
Thins	1 oz	110	3 e
Ruffles Potato Chips	1 oz	150	25 e
Light	1 oz (~17 chips)	120	16 e
Sun Chips	1 oz	140	19 e
Tositos	1 oz (~11 chips)	140	22 e
General Mills			
Bugles	1 oz	150	64 e
Keebler			
Butter Pretzel Knots and Braids	1 oz	110	<9
Hooplas!	1 oz	140	9
O'Boisies			
Potato Chips	1 oz	150	18
Sour Cream and Onion	1 oz	150	18

e indicates estimated sat-fat calories.

SNACK FOODS

FOOD	AMOUNT	TOTAL CALORIES	SAT-FAT CALORIES
Keebler (*cont.*)			
Pop Deluxe			
Honey Caramel Glazed	1 oz	120	9
White Cheddar	1 oz	140	18
Ripplin's Potato Chips	1 oz	150	18
Tato Skins	1 oz	150	9
M&M Mars			
Pretzel Combos			
Cheddar Cheese Filling	1 oz	130	26 e
Cheese Pizza	1 oz	130	22 e
Orville Redenbacher's			
Microwave Popping Corn			
Butter	3 cups popped	100	16 e
Light	3 cups popped	60	5 e
Cheddar Cheese	3 cups popped	150	57 e
Natural	3 cups popped	100	16 e
Pepperidge Farm			
Goldfish			
Cheddar Cheese	½ oz	60	<9
Low-Salt Cheddar Cheese	1 oz	120	9
Original	½ oz	60	<9
Parmesan Cheese	½ oz	60	<9
Pizza Flavored	½ oz	60	<9
Pretzel	½ oz	60	<9
Snack Mix			
Classic	1 oz	140	9
Lightly Smoked Flavor	1 oz	150	9
Spicy	1 oz	140	18
Snack Sticks			
Sesame	8	140	9
Three-Cheese	8	130	18
Pop·Secret			
Microwave Popcorn			
Butter Flavor	3 cups popped	120	18 e
Light	3 cups popped	90	9 e
Natural	3 cups popped	120	18 e
Procter & Gamble			
Pringles	1 oz	170	27
Light	0.9 oz (~14 chips)	130	9

e indicates estimated sat-fat calories.

SNACK FOODS

FOOD	AMOUNT	TOTAL CALORIES	SAT-FAT CALORIES
Ralston			
Chex Mix			
Barbeque	1 oz (⅔ cup)	130	14 e
Traditional	1 oz (⅔ cup)	120	14 e
Smartfood			
Popcorn			
Cheddar Cheese	½ oz (1⅔ cup)	80	18 e
Light Butter	½ oz (1⅔ cup)	70	11 e
Snyder's of Hanover			
Chips			
Potato	1 oz	150	27
Ripple	1 oz	150	27
Sour Cream and Onion	1 oz	150	27
Pretzels			
Hard Sourdough	1 oz	100	0
Mini	1 oz	110	3 e
Oat Bran	1 oz	100	0
Rods	1 oz	110	3 e
Stix	1 oz	110	3 e
Very Thin	1 oz	110	3 e
Snack Mix	1 oz	130	9
Utz			
Potato Chips	1 oz	150	18
Ripples	1 oz	150	18
Sour Cream and Onion	1 oz	160	27
Tortilla Chips			
Restaurant-style	1 oz	150	9
Tortilla Chips, Ranch	1 oz	150	19 e

e indicates estimated sat-fat calories.

SOUPS

FOOD	AMOUNT	TOTAL CALORIES	SAT-FAT CALORIES
Canned			
Asparagus, cream of, condensed			
prepared with milk	1 cup	161	30
prepared with water	1 cup	87	9
Bean, black, condensed, prepared with water	1 cup	116	4
Bean with bacon, condensed, prepared with water	1 cup	173	14
Bean with frankfurters, condensed, prepared with water	1 cup	187	19
Bean with ham, chunky, ready-to-serve	1 cup	231	30
Beef broth or bouillon, ready-to-serve	1 cup	6	2
Beef, chunky, ready-to-serve	1 cup	171	23
Beef noodle, condensed, prepared with water	1 cup	84	10
Celery, cream of, condensed			
prepared with milk	1 cup	165	36
prepared with water	1 cup	90	13
Cheese, condensed			
prepared with milk	1 cup	230	82
prepared with water	1 cup	155	60
Chicken and dumplings, condensed, prepared with water	1 cup	97	12
Chicken broth			
condensed	1 cup	78	7
prepared with water	1 cup	39	4
Chicken, chunky, ready-to-serve	1 cup	178	18
Chicken, cream of, condensed			
prepared with milk	1 cup	191	42
prepared with water	1 cup	116	19
Chicken gumbo, condensed, prepared with water	1 cup	56	3
Chicken noodle, condensed, prepared with water	1 cup	75	6
Chicken noodle with meatballs, ready-to-serve	1 cup	99	10
Chicken rice, chunky, ready-to-serve	1 cup	127	9

SOUPS

FOOD	AMOUNT	TOTAL CALORIES	SAT-FAT CALORIES
Chicken rice, condensed, prepared with water	1 cup	60	4
Chicken vegetable, chunky, ready-to-serve	1 cup	167	13
Chicken vegetable, condensed, prepared with water	1 cup	74	8
Chili beef, condensed, prepared with water	1 cup	169	30
Clam chowder, Manhattan, chunky, ready-to-serve	1 cup	133	19
Clam chowder, Manhattan, condensed, prepared with water	1 cup	78	4
Clam chowder, New England, condensed			
prepared with milk	1 cup	163	27
Consommé with gelatin, condensed, prepared with water	1 cup	29	0
Crab, ready-to-serve	1 cup	76	3
Gazpacho, ready-to-serve	1 cup	57	3
Lentil with ham, ready-to-serve	1 cup	140	10
Minestrone, chunky, ready-to-serve	1 cup	127	13
Minestrone, condensed, prepared with water	1 cup	83	5
Mushroom, cream of, condensed			
prepared with milk	1 cup	203	46
prepared with water	1 cup	129	22
Mushroom with beef stock, condensed, prepared with water	1 cup	85	14
Onion, condensed, prepared with water	1 cup	57	2
Onion, French	1 cup	275	70
Oyster stew, condensed			
prepared with milk	1 cup	134	45
prepared with water	1 cup	59	23
Pea, green, condensed			
prepared with milk	1 cup	239	36
prepared with water	1 cup	164	13

SOUPS

FOOD	AMOUNT	TOTAL CALORIES	SAT-FAT CALORIES
Pea, split, with ham, chunky, ready-to-serve	1 cup	184	14
Pea, split, with ham, condensed, prepared with water	1 cup	189	16
Pepperpot, condensed, prepared with water	1 cup	103	19
Potato, cream of, condensed			
prepared with milk	1 cup	148	34
prepared with water	1 cup	73	11
Scotch broth, condensed, prepared with water	1 cup	80	10
Shrimp, cream of, condensed			
prepared with milk	1 cup	165	52
prepared with water	1 cup	90	29
Stockpot, condensed, prepared with water	1 cup	100	8
Tomato beef with noodle, condensed, prepared with water	1 cup	140	14
Tomato bisque, condensed			
prepared with milk	1 cup	198	28
prepared with water	1 cup	123	5
Tomato, condensed			
prepared with milk	1 cup	160	26
prepared with water	1 cup	86	3
Tomato rice, condensed, prepared with water	1 cup	120	5
Turkey, chunky, ready-to-serve	1 cup	136	11
Turkey noodle, condensed, prepared with water	1 cup	69	5
Turkey vegetable, condensed, prepared with water	1 cup	74	8
Vegetable chunky, ready-to-serve	1 cup	122	5
Vegetable, vegetarian, condensed, prepared with water	1 cup	72	3
Vegetable with beef, condensed, prepared with water	1 cup	79	8
Vegetable with beef broth, condensed, prepared with water	1 cup	81	4

SOUPS

FOOD	AMOUNT	TOTAL CALORIES	SAT-FAT CALORIES
Dehydrated			
Asparagus, cream of, prepared with water .	1 cup	59	2
Bean with bacon, prepared with water	1 cup	106	9
Beef broth or bouillon, prepared with water	1 cup	19	3
Beef broth, cubed, prepared with water	1 cup	8	1
Beef noodle, prepared with water	1 cup	41	2
Cauliflower, prepared with water	1 cup	68	2
Celery, cream of, prepared with water	1 cup	63	2
Chicken broth or bouillon, prepared with water	1 cup	21	2
Chicken broth, cubed, prepared with water	1 cup	13	1
Chicken, cream of, prepared with water	1 cup	107	31
Chicken noodle, prepared with water	1 cup	53	2
Chicken rice, prepared with water	1 cup	60	3
Chicken vegetable, prepared with water	1 cup	49	2
Clam chowder, Manhattan	1 cup	65	2
Clam chowder, New England	1 cup	95	6
Consommé, with gelatin added, prepared with water	1 cup	17	trace
Leek, prepared with water	1 cup	71	9
Minestrone, prepared with water	1 cup	79	7
Mushroom, prepared with water	1 cup	96	7
Onion, prepared with water	1 cup	28	1
Oxtail, prepared with water	1 cup	71	11
Pea, green or split, prepared with water	1 cup	133	4
Tomato, prepared with water	1 cup	102	10
Tomato vegetable, prepared with water	1 cup	55	4
Vegetable beef, prepared with water	1 cup	53	5
Vegetable, cream of, prepared with water	1 cup	105	13

SOUPS

FOOD	AMOUNT	TOTAL CALORIES	SAT-FAT CALORIES
Restaurant (prepared with cream, butter, etc.)			
Clam chowder, New England	1 cup	230	65
Mushroom, cream of	1 cup	170	98
Onion, French	1 cup	350	65
Vichyssoise	1 cup	315	140

SUGARS AND SWEETS

FOOD	AMOUNT	TOTAL CALORIES	SAT-FAT CALORIES
Cakes			
Frozen			
Pepperidge Farm (individual)			
Carrot Cake	1 cake	260	54
Coconut Cake	1 cake	230	36
Dessert Light			
Chocolate Mousse Cake	1 cake	190	27
Strawberry Shortcake	1 cake	170	9
Strawberry Cheesecake	1 cake	300	45
3-Layer Cake			
Chocolate Fudge Stripe	1⅝ oz	170	27
Coconut	1⅝ oz	180	27
Devil's Food	1⅝ oz	180	27
Strawberry Stripe	1½ oz	160	27
Pillsbury			
Coffee Cake			
Cinnamon Streusel with Icing	1 slice	180	18
Streusel Pecan Crumb	1 slice	180	18
Sara Lee			
Free & Light			
Chocolate Cake	⅛ cake	110	0
Pound Cake	⅒ cake	70	0
Lights (individual)			
Black Forest Cake	1 cake	170	29 e
Carrot Cake	1 cake	170	23 e

e indicates estimated sat-fat calories.

SUGARS AND SWEETS

FOOD	AMOUNT	TOTAL CALORIES	SAT-FAT CALORIES
Sara Lee (*cont.*)			
Lights (individual)			
Double Chocolate Cake	1 cake	150	14 e
Lemon Cream Cake	1 cake	180	35 e
Strawberry French Cheesecake	1 cake	150	5 e
Pound Cake	1.1 oz	130	41 e
Weight Watchers			
Cherries and Cream Cake	1 cake	190	9
Strawberry Cheesecake	1 cake	180	9
Commercial or restaurant			
Baked Alaska	¹⁄₁₂ cake	263	60
Angel food	¹⁄₁₂ cake	125	trace
Cheesecake (9-inch-round)	¹⁄₁₂ cake	280	89
Decadent chocolate cake	¹⁄₁₂ cake	450	110
Devil's food, with cream filling	1 small cake	105	15
German chocolate cake	¹⁄₁₆ cake	521	145
Hazelnut torte	¹⁄₁₆ cake	315	56
Pound (9 × 5 × 3 inches)	¹⁄₁₂ cake	318	95
Sponge, with cream filling	1 small cake	155	15
White, with white frosting (9-inch-round)	¹⁄₁₆ cake	230	35
Yellow, with chocolate frosting (9-inch-round)	¹⁄₁₆ cake	260	75
Home			
Made from mixes			
Angel food (9¾-inch round)	1 piece (12/cake)	125	trace
Coffeecake, crumb (7¾ × 5⅝ × 1¼ inches)	1 piece (6/cake)	230	18
Devil's food, with chocolate frosting (9-inch round)	1 piece (16/cake)	235	32
Cupcakes	1	120	16
Gingerbread (8-inch square)	1 piece (9/cake)	175	10

*Cake mix made with vegetable shortening; frosting made with margarine
e indicates estimated sat-fat calories.

SUGARS AND SWEETS

FOOD	AMOUNT	TOTAL CALORIES	SAT-FAT CALORIES
Yellow, with chocolate frosting (9-inch round)	1 piece (16/cake)	235	27
Made from scratch (with vegetable oil)			
Carrot, with cream cheese frosting (10-inch tube cake)	1 piece (16/cake)	385	37
Fruitcake, dark (7½-inch round)	1 piece (32/cake)	165	14
Plain sheet cake (9-inch square)			
without frosting	1 piece (9/cake)	315	30
with uncooked white frosting	1 piece (9/cake)	445	41

Snack Cakes
Hostess

Light Cakes			
Apple Spice	1 cake (1.5 oz)	130	0
Vanilla-Pudding-Filled Chocolate Cakes	1 cake (1.5 oz)	130	0
Regular creme-filled	1 cake (1.75 oz)	180	27
Cupcakes			
Lights	1 (1.5 oz)	130	0
Regular	1 (1.75 oz)	180	27
Twinkies			
Lights	1 (1.25 oz)	110	0
Regular	1 (1.5 oz)	160	27

Candy
(See also **GRAIN PRODUCTS**, *Breakfast Bars, Tarts, and Granola Bars.*)

Caramels, plain or chocolate	1 oz	115	20
Carob chips	1 oz or 2⅔ tbsp	140	52
Chocolate			
baking	1 oz	145	81
chips	1 oz or 2⅔ tbsp	140	45
milk, plain	1 oz	145	49
milk, w/almonds	1 oz	150	43
semisweet	1 cup (6 oz)	860	326
sweet, dark	1 oz	150	53

SUGARS AND SWEETS

FOOD	AMOUNT	TOTAL CALORIES	SAT-FAT CALORIES
Fondant, uncoated (mints, candy corn, other)	1 oz	105	0
Fudge, chocolate, plain	1 oz	115	19
Hard candies	1 oz	110	0
Jellybeans	1 oz	105	trace
Marshmallows	1 oz	90	0
Candy Bars			
Almond Joy	1 bar (1.76 oz)	250	77 e
Bounty			
Dark Chocolate with Coconut	1 bar	150	54 e
Milk Chocolate with Coconut	1 bar	140	47 e
Butterfinger Chips	1 oz	130	18
5th Avenue	1 bar (2 oz)	280	66 e
Hershey's			
with Almond	1 bar (1.45 oz)	230	77 e
Bar None	1 bar	240	91 e
Milk Chocolate	1 bar (1.55 oz)	240	77 e
Kit Kat	1 bar (1.5 oz)	230	78 e
M&M's	1.69 oz	240	55 e
M&M's Peanut	1.74 oz	250	60 e
Mars Almond	1 bar	240	60 e
Milky Way	1 bar (2.15 oz)	280	60 e
	1 bar (fun size)	110	22 e
Mr. Goodbar	1 bar (1.65 oz)	270	99 e
Mounds	1 bar (1.9 oz)	260	94 e
Nestlé Crunch	1 oz	150	38 e
PB Max	1 piece (1.48 oz)	240	82 e
Raisinets	1 oz	130	27 e
Reese's Milk Chocolate Peanut Butter Cups	6 cups (1.65 oz)	260	82 e
Snickers	1 bar	280	71 e
	1 snack bar	180	44 e
Symphony	1.75 oz (5 blocks)	270	88 e
Almonds and Toffee Chips	1.75 oz (5 blocks)	280	93 e

e indicates estimated sat-fat calories.

SUGARS AND SWEETS

FOOD	AMOUNT	TOTAL CALORIES	SAT-FAT CALORIES
3 Musketeers	1 bar (fun size)	80	16 e
Twix	1 bar (2 oz)	140	38 e
Cookies and Bars			
Delicious			
Teenage Mutant Ninja Turtles	9	64	5
Duncan Hines			
Chocolate Chip	2	110	18
Milk Chocolate Chip	2	110	18
Oatmeal Raisin	2	110	9
Keebler			
Chocolate Fudge	1	80	9
Chips Deluxe			
Bite-size	4	80	18
Improved Recipe	1	80	18
Deluxe Grahams	2	90	27
E. L. Fudge	1	60	<9
Elfkins (all varieties)	4	70	9
French Vanilla Creme	1	80	<9
Fudge Sticks	2	100	27
Fudge Stripes	1	50	18
Grasshopper	2	70	27
Magic Middles			
Chocolate Chip	1	80	9
Shortbread	1	80	9
Mini Middles (all varieties)	4	80	9
Pecan Sandies	1	80	9
Bite-size	4	90	9
Rainbow Chips Deluxe	1	80	9
Improved Recipe	1	70	18
Soft Batch			
Oatmeal Raisin	1	70	<9
all other varieties	1	80	9
Nabisco			
Chips Ahoy!	1	50	<9
Chewy	1	60	9
Chocolate Chunk Pecan	1	100	18
Chunky Chocolate Chip	1	90	18
Mini (bite-size)	½ oz (~6)	70	9

*e indicates estimated sat-fat calories.

SUGARS AND SWEETS

FOOD	AMOUNT	TOTAL CALORIES	SAT-FAT CALORIES
Nabisco (*cont.*)			
Mallomars	1	60	9
Newtons			
Apple	1	80	<9
Cinnamon Raisin	1	60	<9
Fig	1	60	<9
Raspberry	1	80	<9
Nilla Cinnamon Wafers	3	60	<9
Nilla Wafers	3	60	<9
Nutter Butter	1	70	<9
Oreo Chocolate Sandwich	1	50	<9
Oreo Double Stuf	1	70	9
Pinwheels	1	130	18
Suddenly S'Mores	1	90	9
Pepperidge Farm			
Apricot Raspberry Fruit	2	100	18
Beacon Hill Chocolate Chocolate Walnut	1	120	18
Bordeaux	2	70	0
Brownie Chocolate Nut	2	110	18
Brussels	2	110	18
Capri	1	80	9
Cardiff	4	80	9
Chantilly	1	80	9
Chesapeake Chocolate Chunk Pecan	1	120	18
Chessman Butter	2	90	18
Chocolate Chantilly	1	90	9
Chocolate Chip	2	100	18
Chocolate Toffee Chip	2	100	18
Chocolate Laced Pirouette	3	80	9
Dakota Milk Chocolate Oatmeal	1	110	18
Geneva	2	130	18
Ginger Man	2	70	0
Lemon Nut Crunch	2	110	18
Lido	1	90	9
Linzer	1	120	9
Milano	2	120	18
Mint Milano	2	150	18
Nantucket Chocolate Chunk	1	120	18
Naples	2	90	18

SUGARS AND SWEETS

FOOD	AMOUNT	TOTAL CALORIES	SAT-FAT CALORIES
Pepperidge Farm (*cont.*)			
Nassau	1	80	9
Orange Milano	2	150	18
Orleans	3	90	18
Pecan Shortbread	1	70	18
Santa Fe Oatmeal Raisin	1	100	9
Sausalito Milk Chocolate Macadamia	1	120	18
Shortbread	2	150	18
Sugar	2	100	18
Tahiti	1	90	18
Venice	2	120	18
Windsor	3	90	18
Winter Orleans	3	90	18
Zurich	1	60	9
Rachel's			
Brownies	1 (2 oz)	280	36
Rippin' Good			
Brite Bites Chocolate Chip	1	60	<9
Chocolate Chip	1	50	<9
Chocolate Chip Sandwich	1	80	9
Coconut Bars	1	40	<9
Cookie Jar Assortment	1	50	<9
Creme Wafers, assorted	1	50	<9
Granola & Peanut Butter Sandwich	1	70	<9
Iced Oatmeal	1	45	<9
Iced Spice	1	40	<9
Lemon Crisp	1	50	<9
Macaroon	1	50	9
Oatmeal	1	50	<9
Rippie Cremes			
Duplex Sandwich	1	50	<9
Vanilla Sandwich	1	50	<9
Striped Dainties	1	50	9
Striped Oatmeal	1	70	18
Sugar	1	50	<9
R. W. Frookie			
Animal Frackers	½ oz (~6)	60	0
Apple Cinnamon Oat Bran	1	45	4.5
Oatmeal Raisin	1	45	9

SUGARS AND SWEETS

FOOD	AMOUNT	TOTAL CALORIES	SAT-FAT CALORIES
Sunshine			
Chip-A-Roos	2	120	27
Fig Bars	2	100	<9
Fudge-Dipped Graham Crackers	3	130	18
Fudge Family Bears			
Creme-Filled	2	130	18
Peanut Butter–Filled	2	140	18
Ginger Snaps	5	100	9
Golden Fruit Raisin Biscuits	2	150	<9
Hydrox	3	160	18
Lemon Coolers	5	150	18
Oat Bran with Nuts and Raisins	2	120	9
Oatmeal	2	110	9
Chocolate Chip	2	120	18
School House	15	120	9
Sugar Wafers	3	130	9
Chocolate	3	130	9
Peanut Butter	3	120	9
Vanilla Wafers	6	130	18
Vienna Fingers	2	140	9

Frozen Novelties

(See also **DAIRY PRODUCTS AND EGGS,** *Frozen Desserts.*)

FOOD	AMOUNT	TOTAL CALORIES	SAT-FAT CALORIES
Dairy Bars			
Eskimo Pie Sugar-Free	1 bar	140	70 e
Sandwich	1 sandwich	170	35 e
Fudgsicle			
Fat-Free Fudge Pops	1 bar	70	0
Good Humor Bar	1 bar	215	81 e
Lite	1 bar	170	53 e
Häagen-Dazs			
Vanilla and Almond	1 bar (3.9 fl oz)	370	157 e
Vanilla and Milk Chocolate	1 bar (3.9 fl oz)	360	157 e
Vanilla Caramel and Peanut Brittle	1 bar (3.9 fl oz)	370	145 e
Chocolate Dark Chocolate	1 bar (3.9 fl oz)	390	145 e
Klondike			
Chocolate Chocolate	1 bar (5 fl oz)	270	111 e
Krispy	1 bar (5 fl oz)	290	111 e
Original	1 bar (5 fl oz)	280	111 e

e indicates estimated sat-fat calories.

SUGARS AND SWEETS

FOOD	AMOUNT	TOTAL CALORIES	SAT-FAT CALORIES
Dairy Bars (*cont.*)			
Rondos	1 piece	70	58 e
3 Musketeer Snack Bar (sugar-free)	1 bar (.6 fl oz)	50	23 e
Weight Watchers			
Double Fudge	1 bar	60	9
English Toffee Crunch	1 bar	120	36
Orange Vanilla Sugar-Free	1 bar	30	<9
Ices			
Baskin-Robbins			
Ice, Daiquiri	1 scoop	140	0
Sorbet			
Fruit Whip	1 scoop	80	0
Red Raspberry	1 scoop	140	0
Dole			
Fruit 'n Cream bars	1 (2.3 fl oz)	90	8
Fruit 'n Juice bars	1 (2.5 fl oz)	70	8
Jell-O			
Gelatin Pops	1 bar	35	0
Pudding Pops	1 bar	80	18
Kool-Aid			
Kool-Pops	1 bar	40	0
Minute Maid			
Fruit Juicee Bar	1 bar	60	0
Popsicle	1	50	0
Miscellaneous			
Baskin-Robbins			
Sherbet, Rainbow	1 scoop	160	12 e
Sugar-Free Dairy Dessert, Chunky	1 scoop	100	6 e
Ely's			
Grand Light Dairy Dessert			
Banana Politan, Vanilla, Chocolate, Strawberry	4 fl oz	110	23 e
Candy Bar, Almond Praline, Butter Pecan, Malt Ball 'n Fudge	4 fl oz	140	29 e
Cookies 'n Cream	4 fl oz	120	29 e

e indicates estimated sat-fat calories.

SUGARS AND SWEETS

FOOD	AMOUNT	TOTAL CALORIES	SAT-FAT CALORIES
Miscellaneous			
Grand Light Dairy Dessert (*cont.*)			
Rocky Road or Chocolate Fudge Mousse	4 fl oz	130	29 e
Vanilla	4 fl oz	100	23 e
Pastries			
Cream puff (with custard filling)	1	303	50
Danish pastry			
round piece	1	220	32
fruit, round	1	215	35
Doughnuts			
cake-type, plain	1	210	25
yeast-leavened, glazed	1	235	47
Eclair	1	240	40
Pies (9-inch-round)			
Apple	1 piece (6/pie)	405	41
fried	1 pie	255	52
Blueberry	1 piece (6/pie)	380	39
Cherry	1 piece (6/pie)	410	42
fried	1 pie	250	52
Cream	1 piece (6/pie)	455	135
Custard	1 piece (6/pie)	330	50
Lemon meringue	1 piece (6/pie)	355	39
Peach	1 piece (6/pie)	405	37
Pecan	1 piece (6/pie)	575	42
Pumpkin	1 piece (6/pie)	320	58
Strawberry tart	1 piece (8/tart)	325	60
Pie crust, from mix (9-inch-round)	for 2-crust pie	1485	204
Pies, frozen			
Mrs. Smith's Pies			
Apple	⅛ pie	220	18
Cherry	⅛ pie	220	18
Coconut Custard	⅛ pie	180	36
Dutch Apple Crumb	⅛ pie	250	18
Sara Lee			
Apple	⅒ pie	280	32 e
Dutch Apple	⅒ pie	300	32 e

e indicates estimated sat-fat calories.

SUGARS AND SWEETS

FOOD	AMOUNT	TOTAL CALORIES	SAT-FAT CALORIES
Puddings, Custards, and Mousses			
Chocolate mousse	½ cup	300	115
Crème caramel	½ cup	220	27
Custard, baked	1 cup	305	61
Gelatin	½ cup	70	0
Puddings			
canned			
chocolate	5-oz can	205	86
tapioca	5-oz can	160	43
vanilla	5-oz can	220	86
dry mix, as purchased, 4 servings/package	1 serving	100	0
Dry mix, prepared with whole milk			
chocolate, instant	½ cup	155	21
chocolate, regular	½ cup	150	22
rice	½ cup	155	21
tapioca	½ cup	145	21
vanilla, instant	½ cup	150	20
vanilla, regular	½ cup	145	21
Sugars, Syrups, etc.			
Honey	1 tbsp	65	0
Jams and preserves	1 tbsp	55	0
Molasses, blackstrap	1 tbsp	43	0
Sugars			
Brown, firmly packed	½ cup	410	0
White			
Granulated	1 cup	770	0
	1 tbsp	45	0
	1 packet	25	0
Powdered, sifted	1 cup	385	0
Syrups			
Chocolate syrup or topping			
fudge-type	1 tbsp	63	14
thin-type	1 tbsp	43	1
Corn	1 tbsp	61	0
Maple	1 tbsp	61	0

e indicates estimated sat-fat calories.

SUGARS AND SWEETS

FOOD	AMOUNT	TOTAL CALORIES	SAT-FAT CALORIES
Miscellaneous			
Ice cream cones			
cake cup	1	16	<9
sugar cone	1	60	<9

VEGETABLES AND LEGUMES

FOOD	AMOUNT	TOTAL CALORIES	SAT-FAT CALORIES
Alfalfa seeds, sprouted, raw	1 cup	10	0
Artichokes			
raw	1 medium	65	0
	1 large	83	0
cooked	1 medium	53	0
	½ cup hearts	37	0
Asparagus			
raw	½ cup	15	0
	4 spears	13	0
cooked	½ cup	22	0
	4 spears	15	0
Bamboo shoots,			
raw	1 cup	41	0
cooked	1 cup	15	0
canned	1 cup	25	0
Beans			
baked, canned			
plain or vegetarian	1 cup	235	3
with beef	1 cup	321	40
with franks	1 cup	366	54
with pork	1 cup	268	14
and sweet sauce	1 cup	282	13
and tomato sauce	1 cup	247	9
black			
raw	1 cup	661	6
boiled	1 cup	227	2

VEGETABLES AND LEGUMES

FOOD	AMOUNT	TOTAL CALORIES	SAT-FAT CALORIES
Beans (*cont.*)			
great northern			
raw	1 cup	621	6
boiled	1 cup	210	2
canned	1 cup	300	3
kidney			
raw	1 cup	613	2
boiled	1 cup	225	1
canned	1 cup	208	1
kidney, California red			
raw	1 cup	607	0
boiled	1 cup	219	0
kidney, red			
raw	1 cup	619	3
boiled	1 cup	225	1
canned	1 cup	216	1
kidney, royal red			
raw	1 cup	605	1
boiled	1 cup	218	0
lima			
raw	1 cup	176	3
boiled	1 cup	208	1
canned	1 cup	186	1
mung beans, sprouted			
raw	1 cup	32	0
navy			
raw	1 cup	697	6
boiled	1 cup	259	2
canned	1 cup	296	3
pink			
raw	1 cup	721	6
boiled	1 cup	252	2
pinto			
raw	1 cup	656	4
boiled	1 cup	235	2
canned	1 cup	186	1
refried, canned	½ cup	134	5
small white			
raw	1 cup	723	6
boiled	1 cup	253	3

VEGETABLES AND LEGUMES

FOOD	AMOUNT	TOTAL CALORIES	SAT-FAT CALORIES
Beans (*cont.*)			
snap			
raw	1 cup	34	0
cooked	1 cup	44	0
canned	1 cup	36	0
white			
raw	1 cup	674	4
boiled	1 cup	249	1
canned	1 cup	306	2
Yard-long			
raw	1 cup	580	5
boiled	1 cup	202	2
yellow			
raw	1 cup	676	12
boiled	1 cup	254	4
Beets			
raw	1 cup sliced	60	0
	2	71	0
cooked	1 cup sliced	52	0
	2	31	0
canned, drained	1 cup	54	0
Black-eyed or cowpeas			
cooked	1 cup	190	0
Broadbeans			
raw	1 cup	511	3
boiled	1 cup	186	1
canned	1 cup	183	5
Broccoli			
raw	1 cup chopped	24	0
	1 spear	42	0
cooked, chopped	1 cup chopped	46	0
	1 spear	53	0
Brussels sprouts			
raw	1 cup	38	0
	1 sprout	8	0
cooked	1 cup	60	1
	1 sprout	8	0
Cabbage			
raw	1 cup shredded	16	0
	1 head	215	15
cooked	1 cup shredded	32	0
	1 head	270	28

VEGETABLES AND LEGUMES

FOOD	AMOUNT	TOTAL CALORIES	SAT-FAT CALORIES
Cabbage, Chinese			
raw	1 cup shredded	9	0
cooked	1 cup shredded	20	0
Cabbage, red			
raw	1 cup shredded	19	0
cooked	1 cup shredded	32	0
Cabbage, Savoy			
raw	1 cup	19	0
cooked	1 cup	35	0
Carob flour	1 tbsp	14	0
	1 cup	185	1
Carrots			
raw	1	31	0
	1 cup shredded	48	0
cooked	1 cup sliced	70	0
juice	1 cup	98	0
Cauliflower, cooked or raw	3 flowerets	13	0
	1 cup	24	0
Celery, raw	1 stalk	6	0
	1 cup diced	18	0
Chard, Swiss			
raw	1 cup chopped	6	0
	1 leaf	9	0
cooked	1 cup chopped	35	0
Chickpeas or garbanzos			
raw	1 cup	729	11
boiled	1 cup	269	4
canned	1 cup	285	3
Chili with beans, canned	1 cup	286	54
Coleslaw (made with cream)	½ cup	42	2
Collard greens	1 cup chopped	27	0
Corn			
cooked	1 ear	85	1
	1 cup kernels	178	3
canned, cream-style	1 cup	186	1
popcorn (See **SNACK FOODS**.)			
pudding	1 cup	271	57
Cucumber, raw	1 cucumber	39	0
	1 cup sliced	14	0
Dandelion greens			
raw	1 cup chopped	25	0

VEGETABLES AND LEGUMES

FOOD	AMOUNT	TOTAL CALORIES	SAT-FAT CALORIES
Eggplant			
raw	1 eggplant	27	0
cooked	1 cup cubes	27	0
Endive			
raw	1 cup chopped	8	0
	1 head	86	9
Falafel	1 patty	57	4
Garlic, raw	1 clove	4	0
Hummus	⅓ cup	140	9
Kale			
raw	1 cup chopped	33	0
cooked	1 cup chopped	41	0
Leeks			
raw	1	76	0
	¼ cup chopped	16	0
cooked	1	38	0
	¼ cup chopped	8	0
Lentils			
raw	1 cup	649	2
boiled	1 cup	231	1
Lettuce, raw			
butterhead, Boston	1 head (5-inch)	21	0
	2 leaves	2	0
crisphead, iceberg	1 head (6-inch)	70	0
	1 cup shredded	5	0
looseleaf, romaine	1 cup chopped	10	0
Mushrooms			
raw	1 cup sliced	20	0
cooked	1 cup	42	1
canned	1 cup	38	0
Mushrooms, shiitake			
dried	4	44	0
cooked	4	40	0
	1 cup chopped	80	0
Okra			
raw	8 pods	36	0
	1 cup sliced	38	0
cooked	8 pods	27	0
	1 cup sliced	50	0
Onion rings, frozen, prepared	7	285	54

VEGETABLES AND LEGUMES

FOOD	AMOUNT	TOTAL CALORIES	SAT-FAT CALORIES
Onions			
raw	1 cup chopped	54	0
cooked	1 cup chopped	58	0
Onions, green, raw	1 cup chopped	26	0
Parsley, raw	10 sprigs	3	0
Parsnips			
raw	1 cup sliced	100	0
cooked	1 cup sliced	126	0
Peas, green			
raw	1 cup	118	0
cooked	1 cup	134	0
with carrots, canned	1 cup	96	6
with onions, canned	1 cup	122	8
Peas, split, boiled	1 cup	231	1
Peppers			
hot chili, raw	1	18	0
	½ cup chopped	30	0
jalapeño	½ cup chopped	17	0
sweet, raw	1	18	0
	½ cup chopped	12	0
sweet, cooked	1	13	0
	½ cup chopped	12	0
Potatoes			
baked in skin	½ lb	145	0
	1 lb	325	0
boiled in skin	1 (2 × 5 inches)	173	0
	⅓ lb	104	0
	1 cup sliced	118	0
	1 lb	345	0
boiled without skin	½ lb	146	0
	⅓ lb	88	0
	1 cup sliced	101	0
	1 lb	295	0
au gratin	1 cup	322	104
French fries (See also **FAST FOODS.**)			
frozen, oven-heated	10 strips	163	34
restaurant			
fried in vegetable oil	10 strips	158	22
fried in animal and vegetable oil	10 strips	158	31

VEGETABLES AND LEGUMES

FOOD	AMOUNT	TOTAL CALORIES	SAT-FAT CALORIES
Potatoes (*cont.*)			
hash brown	½ cup	163	38
potato chips (See **SNACK FOODS.**)			
potato pancakes			
made with eggs and margarine	1 pancake	495	31
potato puffs, frozen	1 puff	16	3
	½ cup	138	28
potato salad	½ cup	180	16
potato sticks	1 oz	148	23
scalloped	½ cup	105	25
Pumpkin, cooked	1 cup mashed	49	0
Pumpkin pie mix, canned	1 cup	282	0
Radishes, raw	10	7	0
	½ cup slices	10	0
Refried beans, canned	½ cup	134	5
Sauerkraut, canned	1 cup	44	0
Shallots, raw	1 tbsp chopped	7	0
Soybeans			
raw	1 cup	774	48
boiled	1 cup	298	20
Soy products			
miso	1 cup	565	22
tofu	1 piece (2 × 2 × 1 inch)	88	7
Spinach			
raw	1 cup chopped	6	0
	10 oz	46	0
cooked	1 cup	41	0
Spinach soufflé (whole milk, eggs, cheese, butter)	1 cup	218	64
Squash			
summer (crookneck, zucchini)			
raw	1 cup sliced	26	0
cooked	1 cup sliced	36	0
winter (acorn, butternut)			
raw	1 squash	172	0
	1 cup cubed	43	0
cooked	1 cup cubed	79	0
Succotash, cooked	1 cup	222	1

VEGETABLES AND LEGUMES

FOOD	AMOUNT	TOTAL CALORIES	SAT-FAT CALORIES
Sweet potatoes			
baked in skin	1 (2 × 5-inch)	118	0
	½ cup mashed	103	0
boiled without skin	1 cup mashed	344	0
cooked, candied (with butter)	1 piece (2½ × 2-inch)	144	31
Tomatoes			
raw	1	24	0
	1 cup chopped	35	0
cooked	1 cup	60	0
canned in tomato juice	1 cup	67	0
Tomato juice, canned	1 cup	42	0
Tomato products, canned			
marinara sauce	1 cup	171	11
paste	½ cup	110	1
purée	1 cup	102	0
sauce, canned	1 cup	74	0
with herbs and cheese	1 cup	144	14
Prego			
Sausage and Green Pepper	4 oz	160	28 e
3 cheeses	4 oz	100	12 e
Tomato and Basil	4 oz	110	12 e
spaghetti	1 cup	272	15
Turnips, cooked	1 cup cubed	28	0
Vegetable juice cocktail, canned	1 cup	44	0
Water chestnuts, canned	1 cup sliced	70	0
Yam, cooked	1 cup cubed	158	0
Zucchini			
raw	1 cup sliced	26	0
cooked	1 cup sliced	36	0

e indicates estimated sat-fat calories.

MISCELLANEOUS

FOOD	AMOUNT	TOTAL CALORIES	SAT-FAT CALORIES
Baking powder	1 tsp	5	0
Chili powder	1 tsp	10	1
Chocolate, baking	1 oz	145	81
Cinnamon	1 tsp	5	trace
Cocoa powder	¾ oz	75	3
	1 tbsp	14	trace
with nonfat dry milk	1 oz	100	5
Curry powder	1 tsp	5	trace
Garlic powder	1 tsp	10	trace
Gelatin, dry	1 envelope	25	trace
Ketchup	1 cup	290	2
	1 tbsp	15	0
Mustard	1 tsp	5	trace
Olives, canned			
green	4 medium or 3 extra large	15	2
ripe, pitted	3 small or 2 large	15	3
Oregano	1 tsp	5	trace
Paprika	1 tsp	5	trace
Pepper, black	1 tsp	5	trace
Pickles			
dill, medium	1	5	trace
fresh-pack, slices	2	10	trace
sweet, gherkin	1	20	trace
Relish, sweet	1 tbsp	20	trace
Salt	1 tsp	0	0
Vinegar, cider	1 tbsp	trace	0
Yeast			
baker's, dry, active	1 packet	20	trace

FOOD TABLES INDEX

The Food Tables Index was designed to help you find some of the harder-to-locate foods in these tables, as well as those foods that appear in several different categories.

APPENDICES

APPENDICES

THE NITTY-GRITTY OF HOW TO KEEP A FOOD RECORD

The absolutely most effective way to lower your risk of heart disease is to eat a diet low in saturated fat. To lower your cholesterol you have to know *exactly* how much saturated fat you are eating. That is why you are keeping food records. These records are for YOUR coronary arteries and YOU, not your spouse, your mother, your brother, your doctor, your dietitian — just for you, and they must be exact and accurate. They must reflect *exactly* what you eat, not what you think you *should* have eaten. Beautiful imaginary food records have no effect on cholesterol levels. If you eat 1 cup of Häagen-Dazs ice cream, record 1 cup of Häagen-Dazs ice cream. Okay. You regret your overindulgence, but being sorry won't put the ice cream back in the carton. If you don't record what you eat, you fool only yourself, not your arteries. If you exceed your sat-fat budget, your cholesterol count will be elevated whether or not you record all your sat-fat splurges. On the other hand, if you write down the 200 sat-fat calories you consumed, you can balance your sat-fat intake for the rest of the day or the next by eating less saturated fat.

Don't become frantic about your food diary. Your first records will reflect what got you into this mess in the first place. Don't feel guilty. Everyone used to wolf down hot dogs and french fries with gusto and no thought. We called whole milk pure and steak a high-protein food. Who knew? As the days and weeks progress, your records will reflect a diet lower in saturated fat and higher in complex carbohydrates. But it takes time.

> You may be interested in purchasing an inexpensive Passbook to keep track of your food intake. See the order form on the last pages of *Eater's Choice*.

KEEPING GOOD RECORDS

Time

Record What You Eat When You Eat It. Write down what you eat when you eat it. Don't fill in your record at the end of the day. You're bound to forget what you don't want to remember. Recording the time helps you see patterns in your eating. The fact that there are eight hours between your first and second entry may give you a clue as to why you were famished for lunch and gobbled down that bag of greasy potato chips.

Food and Amount

List All Foods Separately and List Amounts Accurately. Measure everything. Be accurate. Don't write down *just* "cream cheese." Write down the amount you ate as well — "cream cheese, 2 tablespoons." Don't write down *simply* "chicken breast." Write down "chicken breast with skin, batter-fried." Don't write down *merely* "roast beef sub." Ask the sandwich man how much roast beef and how much mayonnaise he gave you. (He'll know — his boss makes sure he gives everyone an exact amount.) Write down "6-inch sub roll, 4 ounces roast beef, 1 tablespoon mayonnaise." These details are important. If you eat out, ask the waiter what's in the cream sauce and how much butter is on the swordfish or rice.

Sample Food Record

	FOOD	AMOUNT		
	cream cheese	2 tbsp		
	chicken breast with skin, batter-fried	1 breast		
	Roast beef	4 oz		
	6-inch sub roll	1		
	mayonnaise	1 tbsp		

For "Hints on Measuring and Recording Foods," see page 527.

Total Calories

When people cut down on saturated fat, they often cut down on all calories. This is unhealthy. When you reduce your saturated fat intake, you must be sure to increase your intake of complex carbohydrates, fruit, and low- or nonfat dairy products. If you don't eat enough of these low-fat foods, you will miss the vitamins, minerals, and fiber they provide. You also need to eat enough calories to keep up your basal metabolic rate.

On the other hand, grossly exceeding your ideal total caloric intake indicates that you may also be overshooting your sat-fat budget. You know if you are eating too many or too few total calories only if you keep track.

Your total caloric intake should hover around the number you determined on page 55. If eating more complex carbohydrates raises the total, that's okay. Fat makes fat, not complex carbohydrates.

Use the Food Tables (look under the heading "Total Calories") and labels on packages to determine the total calories of the food you have eaten. Make sure that you adjust the total calories for the amount you eat relative to the amount listed. For example, the amount listed for Cheddar cheese is 1 ounce. The total calories for 1 ounce of Cheddar cheese are 114. If you ate 3 ounces of Cheddar cheese you would record 3 × 114 = 342 total calories.

Sat-Fat Calories

Use the Food Tables (look under the heading "Sat-Fat Calories") and labels on packages to determine the sat-fat calories of the food you have eaten. Be sure to adjust the sat-fat calories for the amount you eat relative to the amount listed. For example, the amount listed for club steak is 1 ounce. The sat-fat calories for 1 ounce of club steak are 50. No one eats 1 ounce of meat. If you ate 5 ounces of club steak, you would record 5 × 50 = 250 sat-fat calories.

If you cannot find the exact food you have eaten in the Food Tables (use the Food Tables Index on page 517), find a similar food and record its sat-fat calories. For example, if you ate veal parmigiana in a restaurant, check out the veal parmigiana entries (not low-fat) in the "Frozen and Microwave Foods" section of the Food Tables.

If you ate a mixed dish such as chicken stir-fry, estimate the sat-fat calories for the individual ingredients. For example, chicken stir-fry might contain a chicken breast without skin (4 sat-fat calories), a tablespoon of corn oil (15 sat-fat calories), green pepper, onion, and garlic (0 sat-fat calories).

When saturated fat is listed on a label, it is listed in grams. There are 9 grams per calorie of saturated fat. To find the number of sat-fat calories per gram, multiply by 9. For example, according to a label, 1 ounce of light cream cheese contains 4 grams of saturated fat: 4 grams × 9 calories/gram = 36 sat-fat calories. If you eat 1 ounce of the cream cheese, you would record 36 sat-fat calories. If you eat 1½ ounces, you would record 54 (1.5 × 36 = 54).

Your food record for breakfast might look like this:

FOOD	AMOUNT	TOTAL CALORIES	SAT-FAT CALORIES	SAT-FAT SUBTOTAL
Cheerios	1 oz	110	3	
2% milk	1 cup	121	27	
grapefruit	½	95	0	

Sat-Fat Subtotal

You should keep a running tally of your sat-fat intake. This makes you aware of how much you have "spent" and how much you have left to spend. If, by noon, you have eaten two-thirds of your sat-fat budget, you will know to budget a dinner that is low in saturated fat.

FOOD	AMOUNT	TOTAL CALORIES	SAT-FAT CALORIES	SAT-FAT SUBTOTAL
Cheerios	1 oz	110	3	3
2% milk	1 cup	121	27	30
grapefruit	½	95	0	30

Sat-Fat Total

At the end of the day, compare your sat-fat intake for the day with your sat-fat budget. Is your sat-fat consumption closer to budget than it was yesterday? Be sure to evaluate your food diary for complex carbohydrates, fruit, and dairy. Did you eat according to the recommendations in Chapter 11, "Ensuring a Balanced Diet"? Did you eat 2 to 3 fruits and 3 to 5 vegetables; 6 to 11 servings of potatoes, rice, whole-wheat bread, or cereal; 2 to 3 servings of nonfat flavored yogurt, 1% cottage cheese, or skim milk? Not only do these foods supply the vitamins, minerals, and fiber you need, they make you feel full and thus less likely to binge on high-sat-fat foods.

Get Started

Granted, keeping food records is a pain in the neck. However, the benefits greatly override the inconvenience. You'll gain insight. No longer will your elevated cholesterol level be a mystery. You'll know why your cholesterol is high, because you'll know exactly what you are eating. Those cheese and crackers you nibbled at the office cost you 150 sat-fat calories. Surprised? Is that half your sat-fat budget?

You will discover where the sat-fat lurks in the foods you eat so you can make changes. You can make changes only if you know what to change. Maybe you don't even *like* cheese and crackers 150-sat-fat-calories-worth. Maybe you'd rather spend your sat-fat calories some other way. Keeping food records is worth the bother. People who keep honest and accurate food records and eat below their sat-fat budget get the most cholesterol lowering (up to 33 percent).

Of course, you will not have to keep food records forever. Eventually, you will know the sat-fat calories of most of the foods you eat and will be able to make wise food choices that fit within your budget without recording your every bite.

HINTS ON MEASURING AND RECORDING FOODS

Liquids

Most Liquids. Use measuring cups to measure liquids.

Milk products, coffee whiteners, and cooking oils should be recorded in measuring-cup and -spoon amounts. Most other liquids should be recorded in fluid ounce amounts.

FOOD	AMOUNT		
2% Milk	1 cup		
Half-and-half	1 tbsp		
Coke	12 fl oz		
Eggnog	8 fl oz		

This table of equivalent measures will help you record liquids:

$$1 \text{ cup} = 8 \text{ fluid ounces}$$
$$\tfrac{1}{2} \text{ cup} = 4 \text{ fluid ounces}$$
$$\tfrac{1}{4} \text{ cup} = 2 \text{ fluid ounces}$$
$$2 \text{ tablespoons} = 1 \text{ fluid ounce}$$

Solid food

Meat. Read the meat package label or use a kitchen scale to measure the weight (in ounces) of *beef, lamb, pork, veal, poultry,* and *fish.* Record the weight of meat in ounces. Indicate whether the meat was raw or cooked when you weighed it and whether the fat is included or has been trimmed. If necessary, use the following estimates:

$\tfrac{1}{4}$ cup meat $= 1$ ounce meat
Chicken breast half $= 3$ ounces
4 ounces raw meat without bone $= 3$ ounces cooked
6 ounces raw meat with bone $= 3$ ounces cooked

FOOD	AMOUNT		
Flank steak, meat and fat, raw	5 oz		
Salmon, baked	6 oz		

Cereals,* Cottage Cheese, Creams, Fats, Frozen Desserts, Canned Fish, Sliced Fruit, Grains, Milks, Nuts,** Pasta, Puddings (Not Canned), Rice, Salad Dressings, Sauces and Gravies, Snacks, Soups, and Vegetables. Use measuring cups and spoons to measure and record these foods.

FOOD	AMOUNT		
Bran Chex	1 oz or ⅔ cup		
Sour Cream	3 tbsp		
Egg noodles, cooked	¾ cup		
Tomato soup, prepared with milk	1½ cups		
Cashews	12 nuts		

*If you have a scale, you may also weigh and record cereal in ounces.
**You may also weigh and record nuts in ounces or count and record the number of nuts you eat.

Fast Foods. Record by unit, piece, serving, order, or slice, except for shakes, which are measured in fluid ounces.

FOOD	AMOUNT		
McDonald's Quarter Pounder	1		
KFC (Kentucky Fried Chicken) breast	1 piece		
Jack in the Box Onion Fries	1 serving		
Long John Silver's Breaded Shrimp	1 order		
Domino's Pizza	2 slices		
Roy Rogers Chocolate Shake	11.25 fl oz		

Candy, Cheese,* Cold Cuts, Nuts, Yogurt, and Frozen Yogurt. Read the label on the package or use a scale to measure the weight (in ounces). Save packages with nutrition labeling for use later. Record weight of food in ounces.

FOOD	AMOUNT		
Swiss cheese	2 oz		
Salami, beef	0.8 oz (1 slice)		
Whitney's lemon yogurt	6 fl oz		

Bread should be recorded by slice.
Cakes and pies should be recorded by fraction of whole dessert (i.e., 1/10 cake).
Crackers and cookies should be recorded by unit (i.e., 5 crackers).
Frozen food should be recorded by package or fraction of the package you ate.
If possible, save packages with labels for future reference.

FOOD	AMOUNT		
Oatmeal bread	2 slices		
Cheesecake	1/12 cake		
Blueberry Newtons	4 cookies		
Lean Cuisine, Chicken à l'Orange	1 package		

---

*Cottage cheese and ricotta should be measured by measuring cup rather than weighed.

Here's a summary chart that lists foods and the unit used to measure them.

Summary Chart

FOOD	UNIT	EXAMPLES
Dairy/Eggs		
Butter	pat, tsp/tbsp, cup	
Cheese, hard, soft	oz	2 oz Cheddar
Cheese, curd type	cup	½ cup ricotta
Cream	tbsp	1 tbsp light cream
Milk	cup	1 cup skim
Yogurt	fl oz	8 fl oz nonfat yogurt
	cup	1 cup low-fat yogurt
Egg	1 egg	
	1 egg white	
	1 egg yolk	
Fast Foods		
	unit	1 cheeseburger
	order	1 order fried shrimp
	oz	12-oz shake
	piece	1 chicken breast
	serving	1 serving coleslaw
	slice or fraction of whole*	3 slices, 12-inch pepperoni pizza
Fats and Oils		
Margarine	tsp, tbsp, cup	2 tsp diet margarine
Oils	tsp, tbsp, cup	3 tbsp olive oil
Salad dressings	tbsp, cup	2 tbsp Russian dressing
Fish and Shellfish	oz	4 oz orange roughy
	¼ cup = 1 ounce	
	4 oz, raw = 3 oz, cooked	
Frozen and Microwave	Depends on product	Use information on food label.
Fruit	piece	1 apple
	cup	½ cup applesauce

---

*Specify diameter of whole (i.e., pizza, 14-inch diameter).

FOOD	UNIT	EXAMPLES
Grain and Pasta		
Bagels	number	1 bagel
Bread	slice	2 slices rye
Cereals	cup	⅔ cup Wheatena
	oz	1 oz Cheerios
Crackers	number	2 Wheat Thins
Pasta/rice	cup	¾ cup macaroni, dry
Popcorn	cup	5½ cups, air-popped
Rolls	number	1 poppy seed roll
Meats	oz	5 oz sirloin steak
	¼ cup = 1 ounce	
	4 oz, raw (without bone) = 3 oz, cooked	
	6 oz, raw (with bone) = 3 oz, cooked	
Nuts and Seeds	oz	1 oz pecans
	tbsp	2 tbsp peanut butter
	number	12 cashews
	cup	½ cup sunflower seeds
Poultry	piece	½ chicken breast
	oz	3 oz white meat turkey
Sauces and Gravies	tbsp	3 tbsp mushroom gravy
	cup	½ cup cream sauce
Sausages and Cold Cuts	oz	4 oz turkey bologna
	slices	3 slices salami
	links	1 link smoked sausage
Soups	cup	1½ cups tomato soup
Sweets		
Cakes	fraction of whole	1/12 chocolate cake
Cookies, bars	unit	1 sugar cookie
Pie	fraction of whole	⅙ pumpkin pie
Sugar, jelly	tsp/tbsp	1 tsp grape jam
Vegetables	cup	½ cup spinach
	unit	1 carrot

Remember to record every detail of what you eat so you have enough information to determine the fat calories later.

From the National Institutes of Health
Adult Treatment Guidelines
National Cholesterol Education Program
(See Explanatory Notes on page 534.)

CONTINUE DIETARY TREATMENT FOR AT LEAST 6 MONTHS BEFORE
CONSIDERING ADDING DRUGS. IF GOALS NOT MET BY DIET ALONE,
CONSIDER ADDING DRUGS.

From the National Institutes of Health
National Cholesterol Education Program
Cholesterol Screening and Treatment Guidelines
for Children and Adolescents (Ages 2–19)
(See Explanatory Notes on page 534.)

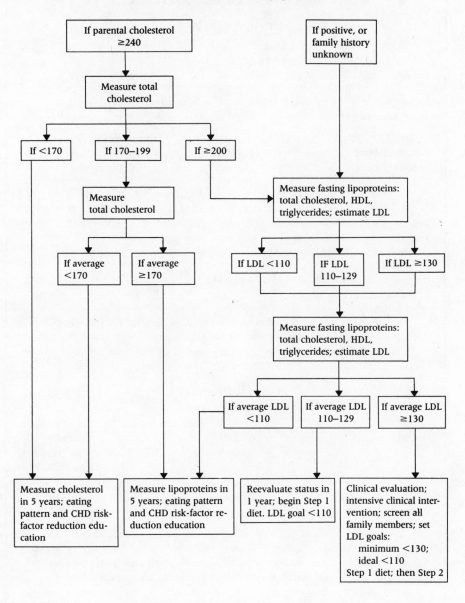

EXPLANATORY NOTES FOR ADULT TREATMENT GUIDELINES AND CHOLESTEROL SCREENING AND TREATMENT GUIDELINES FOR CHILDREN AND ADOLESCENTS

TERMINOLOGY

- CHD = coronary heart disease
- LDL = low density lipoprotein
- HDL = high density lipoprotein

LIPOPROTEIN VALUES

- All values are given in mg/dL.

DIETS	SATURATED FAT	DIETARY CHOLESTEROL
• STEP 1 DIET	<10% of calories	<300 mg/day
• STEP 2 DIET	<7% of calories	<200 mg/day

RISK FACTORS FOR CORONARY HEART DISEASE (CHD)

- Male sex • High blood pressure • Diabetes mellitus • Family history • HDL <35 mg/dL • Physical inactivity • Cigarette smoking • Severe obesity
- Cerebrovascular disease or occlusive peripheral vascular disease (PVD)

POSITIVE FAMILY HISTORY

Parents or grandparents, at 55 years of age or less, who have experienced one of the following:
- a documented heart attack, angina pectoris, peripheral vascular disease, cerebrovascular disease, or sudden cardiac death;
- diagnostic coronary arteriography and were found to have atherosclerosis;
- balloon angioplasty or coronary artery by-pass surgery

DRUGS

FIRST LINE DRUGS*	DAILY DOSAGE RANGE	MAJOR SIDE EFFECTS	PRECAUTIONS
Cholestyramine	2–6 packets 8–24 grams	GI upset, constipation	Can decrease absorption of other drugs; sudden cessation may cause toxicity from other drugs
Colestipol	2–6 packets 10–30 grams	GI upset, constipation	
Nicotinic acid	1.5–6.0 grams	Flushing	

*Probucol, gemfibrozil, clofibrate, and lovastatin may be considered for use when bile acid sequestrants or nicotinic acid produce an insufficient reduction in cholesterol. They also may be used in combination with sequestrants.

FAT CALORIES OF
EATER'S CHOICE RECIPES

| | PER SERVING | | |
RECIPE	TOTAL CALORIES	TOTAL FAT CALORIES	SAT-FAT CALORIES
Soups			
Apple-Squash Soup	148	17	5
Avgolemono Soup	99	6	2
Barley-Vegetable Soup	100	0	0
Bean Soup with Spinach, Squash, and Tomatoes	162	16	2
Blueberry Soup	104	0	0
Broccoli Soup	116	22	4
Cantaloupe Soup	80	4	1
Carrot Soup	76	8	2
Carrot Soup des Basques	96	8	1
Cauliflower Soup	47	7	1
Chilled Strawberry Soup	90	0	0
Cold Ginger-Carrot Soup	60	8	2
Corn Chowder	192	38	8
Cuban Black Bean Soup	215	32	4
Cucumber Soup	78	10	0
Gazpacho I	85	45	6
with croutons	109	47	7
Gazpacho II	83	30	4
with croutons	100	31	5
Ginger Squash Soup	63	11	2
Great Black Bean Soup	233	17	2
Green Pesto Soup	75	33	4
Green Tomato Soup	83	20	4
Hot and Sour Soup	105	22	5
Lentil and Everything but the Kitchen Sink Soup	94	18	2

RECIPE	PER SERVING		
	TOTAL CALORIES	TOTAL FAT CALORIES	SAT-FAT CALORIES
Lentil Soup	146	13	1
with yogurt	153	13	1
Matzo Ball Soup	167	26	6
Mild Fish Chowder	181	20	4
Minestrone	120	18	2
Monhegan Island Fish Chowder	165	21	3
Mulligatawny Soup	121	11	4
Mushroom Soup	95	18	5
Oriental Noodle Soup	64	8	1
Peanut Butter Soup	136	83	13
Potato Soup with Leeks and Broccoli	122	25	3
Sour Cherry Soup	165	0	0
Sweet Cabbage Soup	56	1	0
Tarragon Squash Soup	122	4	2
Tomato-Rice Soup	93	0	0
Tortilla Soup	155	36	4
Vegetable Soup Provençal	74	17	3
Vegetable Soup with Spinach, Potatoes, Rice, and Corn	137	21	3
Watercress Soup	82	12	7
Zucchini Soup	80	2	1

Chicken

RECIPE	TOTAL CALORIES	TOTAL FAT CALORIES	SAT-FAT CALORIES
Alex's Chinese Chicken with Onion, Mushrooms, and Zucchini	232	72	11
Apricot Chicken Divine	215	23	5
Baghdad Chicken	210	48	8
Balsamic Chicken with Potatoes and Onions	203	33	6
Bar-B-Que Chicken			
breast	173	13	4
thigh	126	24	6
Blackened Chicken	154	37	7
Cajun Chicken	204	36	3
Chicken with Apples and Onions	245	48	10
Chicken with Apricots, Sweet Potatoes, and Prunes	301	34	7
Chicken Couscous	291	51	10
Chicken Curry	210	58	13
Chicken with Dried Fruit and Lemon	226	13	4

| RECIPE | PER SERVING | | |
	TOTAL CALORIES	TOTAL FAT CALORIES	SAT-FAT CALORIES
Chicken Fajitas	212	38	6
Chicken Kiev	243	108	23
Chicken Marrakesh	132	13	4
Chicken Nuggets Chez Goor	191	43	5
with honey-mustard sauce	211	43	5
Chicken Paprikash	157	25	5
Chicken with Rice, Tomatoes, and Artichokes	289	28	5
Chicken Smothered in Vegetables	199	44	8
Chicken Verde	217	73	14
Chinese Chicken			
breast	183	13	3
drumstick	130	19	5
thigh	134	24	5
Coq au Vin			
breast	217	97	10
drumstick	162	103	12
thigh	166	108	12
Creamy Chicken Pie	300	114	23
Cuban Chicken	252	35	7
Fifties Chicken	200	33	7
Ginger Chicken with Green Onions	172	51	9
Grilled Apricot-Ginger Chicken	191	29	6
Hunan Chicken with Onions and Red and Green Peppers	192	58	9
Indonesian Chicken with Green Beans	190	69	11
Lower-Fat Approach	175	54	9
Indonesian Peanut Chicken	218	108	18
Keema Matar	279	106	17
Kung Pao Chicken with Broccoli	191	60	10
Lemon Chicken	176	14	4
Lemon-Mustard Chicken	191	73	16
Lime-Peanut-Ginger Chicken	190	79	13
Ma-Po Bean Curd	136	47	10
Mongolian Hot Pot			
sauce	69	0	0
meat and vegetables	199	40	7
broth	184	trace	trace
total	452	40	8
Orange-Soy Chicken	136	29	5
Peppery Chicken	182	23	5

| | PER SERVING | | |
RECIPE	TOTAL CALORIES	TOTAL FAT CALORIES	SAT-FAT CALORIES
Phyllo-Wrapped Chicken with Rice, Artichokes, and Cream Sauce	292	79	18
Pineapple Chicken	210	13	4
Sate Ajam	151	23	5
Sesame Chicken Brochettes	160	20	5
Shepherd's Chicken Chili Pie	218	34	7
Singapore Chicken	176	62	10
Szechuan Chicken with Sweet Red Pepper and Pineapple	203	21	5
Tandoori Chicken	152	13	4
Thai Chicken with Asparagus	201	42	8
Tortillas con Pollo	217	50	4
Vegetables, Chicken, and Cellophane Noodles	111	44	7

Turkey

Basic Turkey Cutlet			
cutlet made with fat	211	60	12
cutlet made without fat	158	8	4
Breaded Turkey Cutlet	273	115	22
Broccoli Baked Turkey	145	32	19
Creamy Turkey Casserole	255	49	22
Turkey with Capers			
cutlets made with fat	237	79	13
cutlets made without fat	184	26	5
Turkey Cutlets with Artichoke-Cream Sauce			
cutlet made with fat	248	85	17
cutlet made without fat	206	43	11
Turkey Mexique	160	30	6
Turkey Niçoise			
cutlets made with fat	219	73	13
cutlets made without fat	184	38	7
Turkey Roll-Ups Firenze	176	32	10
Turkey Sautéed with Onions and Almonds	200	43	8
Turkey Scaloppine Limone			
cutlets made with fat	246	70	14
cutlets made without fat	194	18	6

| RECIPE | PER SERVING | | |
	TOTAL CALORIES	TOTAL FAT CALORIES	SAT-FAT CALORIES
Turkey Scaloppine Marsala			
cutlets made with fat	268	70	14
cutlets made without fat	216	18	6
Turkey with Snow Peas	190	26	9
Turkey with Sweet Red Pepper Sauce			
cutlets made with fat	237	59	11
cutlets made without fat	185	6	2
Turkey Véronique	234	60	12

Fish and Shellfish

RECIPE	TOTAL CALORIES	TOTAL FAT CALORIES	SAT-FAT CALORIES
Broiled Ginger Fish	209	50	6
Broiled Monkfish with Orange Sauce	194	52	13
Cajun Fish	188	58	9
Curry Fish	251	52	12
with teaspoon of each condiment	317	65	18
Dill Fish	115	12	4
Fennel Fish	134	42	4
Fish Baked in Olive, Chili Pepper, and Tomato Sauce	163	34	8
Fish with Mushroom Sauce	302	84	14
Fish with Peppercorns, Thyme, and Mustard	70	23	5
Fish in Wine Sauce	40	1	0
Flounder Fillets Stuffed with Fennel Rice	140	44	10
Honey-Curry Scallops	140	8	4
Marinated Fish Steaks			
monkfish	297	46	16
swordfish	297	90	16
Oriental Fish Kebabs	243	51	10
Phyllo-Wrapped Fish and Mushroom Sauce	431	118	22
without sauce	342	61	10
Salmon with Cucumber-Grape Sauce			
Atlantic	528	82	30
Chinook	540	114	60
pink	330	60	24
sockeye (red)	365	99	42
Salmon Soufflé	149	32	9

RECIPE	PER SERVING		
	TOTAL CALORIES	TOTAL FAT CALORIES	SAT-FAT CALORIES
Scallops Provençal	190	55	8
Scallop or Shrimp Caribbean			
scallops	170	26	3
shrimp	170	35	3
Scallop or Shrimp Creole			
scallops	184	25	7
shrimp	184	35	7
Scallop or Shrimp Curry			
scallops	187	25	7
shrimp	187	36	7
Shangai Fish	117	12	4
Shrimp with Green Peppers	174	36	6
Spicy Shrimp Louisiana	95	35	3

Vegetables

RECIPE	TOTAL CALORIES	TOTAL FAT CALORIES	SAT-FAT CALORIES
Acorn Squash	55	15	3
Afghan Squash	30	10	2
Artichoke	26	0	0
margarine per tablespoon	90	90	18
Bouillon Potatoes	106	0	0
Braised Mushrooms Oriental	83	55	6
Broccoli and Mushrooms	65	21	5
Caraway Carrots	40	10	2
Carrots and Leeks	61	20	3
Cauliflower Sauté	57	30	4
Celery-Mushrooms	44	22	5
Chickpeas with Lemon and Herbs	170	46	5
Curried Beans	155	25	4
Curried Whipped Potatoes	178	20	3
Curried Zucchini	43	22	3
Eggplant with a Greek Influence	51	35	4
Fluffy Sweet Potatoes	133	38	9
Glazed Acorn Squash	58	0	0
Green Beans Basilico	49	21	4
Hot and Garlicky Eggplant	35	15	2
Indian Vegetables	86	10	2
Italian Mixed Vegetables	35	15	2
Keema Eggplant	100	24	4
Lentils and Potatoes	55	23	3
Muriel's Chinese Vegetables	72	27	4
Potato Skins	79	20	3

	PER SERVING		
RECIPE	**TOTAL CALORIES**	**TOTAL FAT CALORIES**	**SAT-FAT CALORIES**
Potatoes Lyonnaise	90	37	7
Ratatouille	36	12	2
Sesame Broccoli	50	20	3
Spaghetti Squash with Tomato Sauce	127	20	3
Spiced Sweet Potatoes	75	0	0
Spinach Oriental	50	30	4
Spinach and Tomatoes	60	29	4
Steamed Zucchini Matchsticks	17	0	0
with margarine	24	7	2
Sweet Potatoes with Oranges, Apples, and Sweet Wine	180	0	0
Sweet Vegetable Mélange	90	15	2
Vegetable Soufflé	75	22	5
Tahini Sauce	20	11	1

Pizza, Chili, Quiche, and Tortillas

Calzone	366	68	11
Chili Non Carne	127	15	3
Focaccia	117	21	3
Pawtucket Chili	110	16	3
Pissaladière	241	77	10
Pizza			
slice	148	36	4
Spinach Quiche	200	70	17
Tomato Quiche	220	108	21
Tomato Tart	173	63	8
Tortillas	90	20	0

Pasta, Rice, and Other Grains

Asparagus Pasta	411	11	2
with chicken	476	18	4
Barley Plus	157	20	4
Basic Tomato Sauce	74	15	2
Bulgur with Tomatoes and Olives	79	23	2
Dan-Dan Noodles	252	32	5
Easy Spaghetti Sauce à la Sicilia	285	24	6
Fried Rice	167	33	6
Indian Rice	97	10	2
Lemon Rice with Spinach and Red Pepper	95	10	1
Olive-Artichoke Rice	105	36	5

	PER SERVING		
RECIPE	TOTAL CALORIES	TOTAL FAT CALORIES	SAT-FAT CALORIES
Pasta Mexicali	168	17	3
Pasta with Pesto	313	80	17
Peasant Pasta	260	68	11
Rice Pilau with Apricots and Raisins	100	15	3
Salmon Pasta Niçoise			
with salmon	408	129	22
with tuna	385	108	18
Spaghetti Touraine	208	89	13
Zesty Fresh Tomato Sauce	64	24	3

Salads

Chicken Salad with Shallots and Mushrooms	140	48	11
Coriander Chicken Salad	90	21	12
Cucumber Salad	20	0	0
Curried Tuna Salad with Pears	220	49	11
Dijon Chicken-Rice Salad	285	71	12
Eastern Spinach Salad	55	20	3
Fruit Salad with Cottage Cheese or Yogurt			
Spring or summer salad			
with cottage cheese	280	10	7
with nonfat yogurt	250	0	0
Fall or winter salad			
with cottage cheese	270	10	7
with nonfat yogurt	245	0	0
Indonesian Vegetable Salad	32	0	0
1 tablespoon dressing	43	30	5
Oriental Chicken Salad	325	145	20
Potato Salad	105	22	5
Salade Niçoise	195	105	11
Tabbouli	135	31	5
Tarragon-Raisin Chicken Salad	180	36	12

Sandwiches, Dips, and Drinks

Baba Ghanoush	12	7	1
Bagel Chips	38	2	0
Chickpea Sandwich or Dip			
sandwich	195	39	4
tablespoon	20	5	1

RECIPE	PER SERVING		
	TOTAL CALORIES	TOTAL FAT CALORIES	SAT-FAT CALORIES
Eggplant Appetizer	46	32	6
Faux Guacamole			
per tablespoon	7	0	0
pita bread, per quarter	33	2	0
Frothy Fruit Shake	105	2	0
Tofu (Mock Egg Salad) Sandwich			
per sandwich	150	54	9
per tablespoon	9	3	1
Vegeburgers	73	N/A	3
Yogurt Cheese			
per tablespoon	7	0	0

Breads

RECIPE	TOTAL CALORIES	TOTAL FAT CALORIES	SAT-FAT CALORIES
Anadama Bread			
loaf	1919	257	42
slice	113	15	2
Apple Oat Bran Muffins	125	32	4
Apricot Oat Muffins	135	32	4
Banana-Carrot Muffins	195	64	11
modified	155	51	8
Bran Muffins	116	23	4
Buttermilk Herb Bread			
loaf	1874	338	75
slice	110	20	4
Buttermilk Pancakes			
total batter	495	90	6
per pancake	31	13	1
Buttermilk Waffles			
total batter	1261	260	40
per waffle	158	32	5
Cardamom Bread			
loaf	1663	255	41
slice	98	15	2
Challah			
loaf	1670	317	47
slice	70	13	2
Cinnamon Applesauce Bread			
loaf	2425	177	24
slice	143	10	1
Cinnamon French Toast	106	29	8

RECIPE	PER SERVING		
	TOTAL CALORIES	TOTAL FAT CALORIES	SAT-FAT CALORIES
Cranberry Bread			
loaf	1899	254	55
slice	112	15	3
Cumin Wheat Bread			
loaf	1814	252	35
slice	107	15	2
Focaccia Genovese	116	13	2
French Bread I			
loaf	874	133	19
slice	87	13	2
French Bread II			
round loaf	942	24	4
slice	94	2	0
baguette	471	12	2
slice	52	1	0
Gingerbread Muffins	177	59	9
Ginger-Orange Bread			
loaf	1678	279	46
slice	99	16	3
Honey Whole-Wheat Bread			
loaf	2222	342	39
slice	130	17	2
Mother's Oat Bran Muffins			
with walnuts	160	49	6
without walnuts	144	36	5
Oatmeal Bread			
loaf	1601	167	33
slice	94	10	2
Onion Flat Bread			
loaf	667	56	7
slice	83	7	1
Orange Oat Muffins	110	34	4
Peanut Butter Bread			
loaf	1358	321	50
slice	78	18	3
Peppery Breadsticks	41	2	0
Pumpernickel Bread			
loaf	2273	301	39
slice	92	12	2
Sesame Breadsticks			
total	1423	196	30
breadstick	41	6	1

RECIPE	PER SERVING		
	TOTAL CALORIES	TOTAL FAT CALORIES	SAT-FAT CALORIES
Shaker Daily Loaf			
loaf	1512	117	28
slice	90	7	2
Whole-Wheat Bagels	115	23	1
Whole-Wheat Banana Raisin Bread			
loaf	2494	195	30
slice	147	11	2
Desserts			
Apple Cake	220	114	13
Apple-Nut Cookies	62	25	4
Apple Pandowdy	243	74	11
Applesauce Cake	250	89	14
Banana Cake	263	110	12
Carrot Cake sans Oeufs	122	40	5
Chocolatey-Chocolate Cocoa Cake	273	71	13
Cinnamon Sugar Coffee Cake	299	98	20
Cinnamon Sweet Cakes	148	61	8
Cocoa Angel Food Cake	119	<1	0
Cocoa Brownies	115	54	9
Deep-Dish Pear Pie	236	61	11
Divine Buttermilk Pound Cake	175	66	13
with Mocha Frosting	225	81	18
with Walnut Glaze	199	71	14
Ginger Cake	183	63	14
with Pear Sauce	194	63	14
Glazed Cinnamon Buns	120	19	3
Honey Graham Crackers	58	12	2
Key Lime Pie (with Graham Cracker Crust)	210	36	8
Lemon Loaf	290	142	21
without walnuts	215	76	15
Mandelbrot	46	18	2
Marble Cake	238	75	15
Marvelous Cookies	80	39	5
Meringue Shells with Fresh Strawberries and Warm Raspberry Sauce	130	0	0
Mocha Cake	140	50	10
with icing	174	61	13
Nutmeg Torte	204	54	11
Oatmeal Cookies	65	25	3

	PER SERVING		
RECIPE	TOTAL CALORIES	TOTAL FAT CALORIES	SAT-FAT CALORIES
Orange Cake	180	74	15
Peach Pound Cake	210	74	16
Pears Hélène	205	23	5
Philip Wagenaar's Raisin-Ginger-Orange Cake	236	43	9
Pineapple Pound Cake	177	47	9
Pumpkin Cake	128	34	7
Spice Cake	238	96	19
with frosting	288	118	24
Strawberry-Rhubarb Pie	240	63	11
Strawberry Tart	215	57	10
Tante Nancy's Apple Crumb Cake	225	66	15
The York Blueberry Cake	141	46	8

GLOSSARY

Aerobic exercise. Steady, repetitive exercise that uses the large muscles and requires a steady supply of oxygen — in contrast to exercise that requires bursts of activity separated by periods of inactivity. Examples of aerobic exercises include walking, swimming, running, and biking. Aerobic exercise burns more fat than active sports, which burn more carbohydrate.

Angina pectoris. An episode of chest pain, often caused by a temporary restriction of oxygenated blood due to narrowing of the coronary arteries supplying the heart muscle. An angina attack is not to be confused with a heart attack, which results from a severe and prolonged lack of oxygenated blood to a part of the heart.

Angiography or angiocardiography. A diagnostic method involving injection of an x-ray dye into the bloodstream. Chest x-rays taken after the injection show the inside dimensions of the heart and blood vessels outlined by the dye.

Aorta. The main trunk artery that carries oxygenated blood from the heart. Lesser arteries branching off from the aorta conduct blood to all parts of the body except the lungs.

Arteriosclerosis. A group of diseases characterized by thickening and loss of elasticity of artery walls. This may be due to an accumulation of fibrous tissue, fatty substances (lipids), and/or minerals.

Artery. A blood vessel that carries blood away from the heart to the various parts of the body. Arteries usually carry oxygenated blood, except for the pulmonary artery, which carries unoxygenated blood from the heart to the lungs for oxygenation.

Atherosclerosis. A type of arteriosclerosis in which the inner layer of the artery wall is made thick and irregular by deposits of a fatty substance. These deposits (called plaques) project above the surface of the inner layer of the artery and thus decrease the diameter of the internal channel of the vessel.

Bile acids. Breakdown products of cholesterol formed in the liver and excreted into the intestine, where they play an important role in the absorption of fats from the foods we eat.

Cholesterol. A fatlike substance found in the cell walls of all animals, including humans. Cholesterol is transported in the bloodstream. Some of it is manufactured by the body and some comes from the foods of animal origin that we eat.

A healthy level of cholesterol is below 200 mg/dL. A higher level is often associated with increased risk of coronary atherosclerosis.

Cholestyramine. A drug used to lower blood levels of cholesterol.

Chylomicrons. Largest of the lipoproteins; produced by the intestine to transport dietary fats to the adipose tissue (fat deposits).

Coronary arteries. Arteries, arising from the base of the aorta, which conduct blood to the heart muscle. These arteries, and the network of vessels branching off from them, come down over the top of the heart like a crown (corona).

Coronary atherosclerosis. Commonly called coronary heart disease. An irregular thickening of the inner layer of the walls of the coronary arteries that conduct blood to the heart muscle. The internal channels of these arteries become narrowed and the blood supply to the heart muscle is reduced.

Coronary bypass surgery. Surgery to improve the blood supply to the heart muscle when narrowed coronary arteries reduce flow of the oxygen-containing blood that is vital to the pumping heart. This reduction in blood flow causes chest pain and leads to increased risk of heart attack. Thus coronary bypass surgery involves constructing detours through which blood can bypass narrowed portions of coronary arteries to keep the heart muscle supplied. Veins or arteries taken from other parts of the body where they are not essential are grafted onto the heart to construct these detours.

Coronary heart disease. Also called coronary artery disease and ischemic heart disease. Heart ailments caused by narrowing of the coronary arteries and therefore a decreased blood supply to the heart.

Electrocardiogram (often referred to as ECG or EKG). A graphic record of the electric currents generated by the heart.

Enzyme. A protein that speeds up specific biochemical processes in the body. Enzymes are universally present in living organisms.

Fats. Also known as lipids. Fats are one of the five major classes of nutrients; the other four are proteins, carbohydrates, minerals, and vitamins. Fats in foods and in the body generally occur as triglycerides.

Heart attack. The death of a portion of heart muscle, which may result in disability or death of the individual, depending on how much of the heart is damaged. A heart attack occurs when a blockage in one of the coronary arteries prevents an adequate oxygen supply to the heart. Symptoms may be none, mild, or severe and may include chest pain (sometimes radiating to the shoulder, arm, neck, or jaw), nausea, cold sweat, and shortness of breath.

Heart disease. A general term applied to ailments of the heart or blood vessels. Some of these are present at birth (congenital) and are either inherited or are the result of environmental influences on the embryo as it develops in the womb. The majority of cases of heart disease, however, are acquired later in life, for example, through the development of atherosclerosis.

High blood cholesterol (hypercholesterolemia). An excess of a fatty substance called cholesterol in the blood, which is often associated with the premature development of atherosclerosis and therefore with increased risk of heart attack and stroke.

High blood pressure (hypertension). An unstable or persistent elevation of blood pressure above the normal range. Uncontrolled, chronic high blood pressure strains the heart, damages arteries, and creates a greater risk of heart attack, stroke, and kidney problems.

High density lipoprotein (HDL). The smallest and most dense lipoprotein, HDL removes cholesterol from LDL and cells and transports it back to the liver, where the cholesterol is broken down into bile acids and excreted into the intestine. HDL is protective against the development of heart disease; high levels of HDL are associated with low risk of heart disease.

Lifestyle. An individual's typical way of life, including diet, kinds of recreation, job, home environment, location, temperament, and smoking, drinking, and sleeping habits.

Lipid. A fatty substance.

Lipoprotein. A complex particle consisting of lipid (fat), protein, and cholesterol molecules bound together to transport lipids through the blood. Lipoproteins are classified according to their density. Four important lipoproteins are Very Low Density Lipoprotein (VLDL), Low Density Lipoprotein (LDL), High Density Lipoprotein (HDL), and chylomicrons.

Liver. A large organ in the upper right side of the abdominal cavity, which is involved in the metabolism of fats, produces bile, and performs various other metabolic functions.

Low Density Lipoprotein (LDL). LDL particles are formed by removal of triglycerides from VLDL. LDL is rich in cholesterol. High levels of LDL in the blood are associated with the premature development of atherosclerosis and an increased risk of heart attack.

Metabolism. A general term designating all chemical changes that occur to substances within the body.

Monocytes. A type of white blood cell that engulfs foreign objects. Monocytes engorged with LDL and chylomicron remnants infiltrate the arterial wall and cause thickening, known as atherosclerosis.

Monounsaturated fat. A fat chemically constituted so that it is capable of absorbing additional hydrogen but not as much hydrogen as polyunsaturated fat. These fats in the diet have recently been shown to lower blood cholesterol levels. One example of a monounsaturated fat is olive oil.

Obesity. An increase in body weight beyond physical and skeletal requirements due to an accumulation of excess fat. This puts a strain on the heart and increases the chance of developing two major heart attack risk factors: high blood pressure and diabetes.

Plaque. Also called atheroma. A deposit of fatty (and other) substances in the inner lining of the artery wall, characteristic of atherosclerosis.

Polyunsaturated fat. A fat chemically constituted so that it is capable of absorbing additional hydrogen. These fats are usually liquid oils of vegetable origin, such as corn oil or safflower oil. A diet with a high polyunsaturated fat content tends to lower the amount of cholesterol in the blood. These fats are sometimes substituted for saturated fat in a diet in an effort to lessen the hazard of fatty deposits in the blood vessels.

Saturated fat. A fat chemically constituted so that it is not capable of absorbing any more hydrogen. These are usually the solid fats of animal origin, such as the fats in milk, butter, meat, etc. A diet high in saturated fat content tends to increase the amount of cholesterol in the blood. These fats are restricted in the diet in an effort to lessen the hazard of fatty deposits in the blood vessels.

Sodium. A mineral essential to life, found in nearly all plant and animal tissue. Table salt (sodium chloride) is nearly half sodium. In some types of heart disease, the body retains an excess of sodium and water, and therefore sodium intake is restricted.

Stroke. A blocked blood supply to some part of the brain.

Triglyceride. The main type of lipid (fatty substance) found in the fat tissue of the body and also the main type of fat found in foods. Triglycerides are composed of three fat molecules attached to an alcohol molecule called glycerol. High levels of triglycerides in the blood may be associated with a greater risk of coronary atherosclerosis.

Unsaturated fat. A fat whose molecules have one or more double bonds, so that it is capable of absorbing more hydrogen. Monounsaturated fats, such as olive oil, have only one double bond (the rest are single), and recent evidence indicates that they may lower blood cholesterol levels. Polyunsaturated fats, such as corn oil and safflower oil, have two or more double bonds per molecule and tend to lower blood cholesterol.

Very low density lipoprotein (VLDL). The lightest and largest of the lipoproteins manufactured by the liver, VLDL particles carry triglycerides from the liver to muscle and fat cells throughout the body. VLDL particles are produced and released in large amounts after meals.

TABLE OF EQUIVALENT MEASURES

Volume Measures

1 gallon	4 quarts
1 quart	4 cups 2 pints
1 pint	2 cups
1 cup	8 fluid ounces 16 tablespoons
½ cup	4 fluid ounces 8 tablespoons
⅓ cup	5 tablespoons + 1 teaspoon
¼ cup	2 fluid ounces 4 tablespoons
1 tablespoon	3 teaspoons ½ fluid ounce

Weight Measures

1 pound	16 ounces 454 grams
3.5 ounces	100 grams
1 ounce	28.35 grams

REFERENCES AND RESOURCES

Chapter 1

American Heart Association. *Heart Facts 1985.*

Assembly of Life Sciences, National Research Council. *Diet, Nutrition, and Cancer Committee Report on Diet, Nutrition, and Cancer.* Washington, D.C.: National Academy Press, 1982.

National Cancer Institute, U.S. Department of Health and Human Services. *Diet, Nutrition & Cancer Prevention: A Guide to Food Choices.* NIH Publication No. 85-2711. Washington, D.C.: Government Printing Office, 1984.

National Institutes of Health. *Heart Attacks.* Medicine for the Layman, NIH Publication No. 80-1803. Washington, D.C.: Government Printing Office, 1980.

Pooling Project Research Group. "Relationship of Blood Pressure, Serum Cholesterol, Smoking Habit, Relative Weight, and ECG Abnormalities to Incidence of Major Coronary Events." *Journal of Chronic Diseases* 31 (1978):201–306.

Chapter 2

Brown, M. S., and J. L. Goldstein. "How LDL Receptors Influence Cholesterol and Atherosclerosis." *Scientific American* 251 (November 1984):58–66.

Department of Health, Education, and Welfare. *A Handbook of Heart Terms.* DHEW Publication No. (NIH) 78-131. Washington, D.C.: Government Printing Office.

Department of Health, Education, and Welfare. *The Human Heart: A Living Pump.* DHEW Publication No. (NIH) 78-1058. Washington, D.C.: Government Printing Office.

Heiss, G., et al. "Lipoprotein-Cholesterol Distributions in Selected North American Populations: The Lipid Research Clinics Prevalence Study." *Circulation* 61 (1980):302.

Lipid Research Clinics Program. *The Lipid Research Clinics Population Studies Data Book, Volume 1. The Prevalence Study.* NIH Publication No. 80-1527. Washington, D.C.: Government Printing Office, 1980.

Inter-Society Commission for Heart Disease Resources. "Optimal Resources for Primary Prevention of Atherosclerotic Diseases." *Circulation* 42 (1970, revised 1972):A55–A95.

Chapter 3

Blackburn, H. "Diet and Mass Hyperlipidemia: A Public Health View." In *Nutrition, Lipids, and Coronary Heart Disease — A Global View,* edited by R. I. Levy, et al., 309–48. New York: Raven Press, 1979.

Blankenhorn, D. H., Nessim, S. A., et al. "Beneficial Effects of Combined Colestipol-Niacin Therapy on Coronary Atherosclerosis and Coronary Venous Bypass Grafts." *Journal of the American Medical Association* 257 (1987):3233.

Blankenhorn, D. H., et al. "The Influence of Diet on the Appearance of New

Lesions in Human Coronary Arteries." *Journal of the American Medical Association* 263 (1990): 1646–52.

Gordon, T., et al. "High Density Lipoprotein As a Protective Factor Against Coronary Heart Disease: The Framingham Study." *American Journal of Medicine* 62 (1977):707.

Kannel, W. B., et al. "Serum Cholesterol, Lipoproteins, and the Risk of Coronary Heart Disease: The Framingham Study." *Annals of Internal Medicine* 74 (1971):1–12.

Kato, H., et al. "Epidemiologic Studies of Coronary Heart Disease and Stroke in Japanese Men Living in Japan, Hawaii, and California. Serum Lipids and Diet." *American Journal of Epidemiology* 97 (1973):372–85.

Keys, A., ed. "Coronary Heart Disease in Seven Countries." *Circulation* 41 (1970):Supplement 1.

LaRosa, J. C., et al. "The Cholesterol Facts. A Summary of the Evidence Relating Dietary Fats, Serum Cholesterol, and Coronary Heart Disease. A Joint Statement by the American Heart Association and the National Heart, Lung, and Blood Institute." *Circulation* 81 (1990):1721.

Lipid Research Clinics Program. "The Lipid Research Clinics Coronary Primary Prevention Trial Results. I: Reduction in Incidence of Coronary Heart Disease." *Journal of the American Medical Association* 251 (1984):351.

Lipid Research Clinics Program. "The Lipid Research Clinics Coronary Primary Prevention Trial Results. II: The Relationship of Reduction in Incidence of Coronary Heart Disease to Cholesterol Lowering." *Journal of the American Medical Association* 251 (1984):365.

McGill, H. C., ed. *The Geographic Pathology of Atherosclerosis.* Baltimore: Williams and Wilkins Co., 1968.

Ornish, D., et al. "Can Lifestyle Changes Reverse Coronary Heart Disease? The Lifestyle Heart Trial." *Lancet* 336 (1990):129–33.

Stamler, J. George Lyman Duff Memorial Lecture. "Lifestyles, Major Risk Factors, Proof, and Public Policy." *Circulation* 58 (1978):3.

Stamler, J. "Population Studies." In *Nutrition, Lipids, and Coronary Heart Disease — A Global View,* edited by R. I. Levy, et al., 25–88. New York: Raven Press, 1979.

Chapter 4

American Heart Association. *Eating for a Healthy Heart. Dietary Treatment of Hyperlipidemia.* AHA Publication No. 50-063-A.

American Heart Association. *Recommendations for Treatment of Hyperlipidemia in Adults.* Joint Statement of the Nutrition Committee and the Council on Arteriosclerosis. AHA Special Report No. 72-204-A, 1985.

Goor, R., et al. "Nutrient Intakes Among Selected North American Populations in the Lipid Research Clinics Prevalence Study: Composition of Fat Intake." *American Journal of Clinical Nutrition* 41 (1985):299.

"Highlights of the Report of the National Cholesterol Education Program Expert Panel on Detection, Evaluation, and Treatment of High Blood Cholesterol in Adults." *Archives of Internal Medicine* 148 (1988):36–69.

Chapter 5

Anderson, J. T., F. Grande, and A. Keys. "Cholesterol-Lowering Diets: Experimental Trials and Literature Review. *Journal of the American Dietary Association* 62 (1973):133.

Dennison, D. *The DINE System: The Nutritional Plan for Better Health.* St. Louis: C. V. Mosby, 1982.

Hegsted, D. M., et al. "Quantitative Effects of Dietary Fat on Serum Cholesterol in Man. *American Journal of Clinical Nutrition* 17 (1965):281.

Keys, A., J. T. Anderson, and F. Grande. "Serum Cholesterol Response to Changes in the Diet. II: The Effect of Cholesterol in the Diet." *Metabolism* 14 (1965):759.

U.S. Department of Agriculture. *Composition of Foods.* Agriculture Handbook No. 8. Washington, D.C.: Government Printing Office, rev. December 1963.

Chapter 6

The fat tables are based on data from the following sources:

Dennison, D. *The DINE System: The Nutritional Plan for Better Health.* St. Louis: C. V. Mosby, 1982.

U.S. Department of Agriculture. *Composition of Foods.* Agriculture Handbook No. 8. Washington, D.C.: Government Printing Office, 1963.

U.S. Department of Agriculture. *Composition of Foods.* Agriculture Handbook No. 8. Washington, D.C.: Government Printing Office, sec. 1–12 rev. 1976–84.

U.S. Department of Agriculture. *Nutritive Value of Foods.* Home and Garden Bulletin No. 72. Washington, D.C.: Government Printing Office, rev. 1981.

U.S. Department of Agriculture. *Nutritive Value of American Foods in Common Units.* Agriculture Handbook No. 456. Washington, D.C.: Government Printing Office, November 1975.

Chapter 7

Block, G., et al. "Nutrient Sources in the American Diet: Quantitative Data from the NHANES II Survey. II: Macronutrients and Fats." *American Journal of Epidemiology* 122 (1985):27–40.

Chapter 8

American Heart Association. *Diet in the Healthy Child.* AHA Publication No. 72-203-A; also in *Circulation* 67 (1983):1411A.

Anderson, J. W., et al. "Hypocholesterolemic Effects of Oat Bran or Bean Intake for Hypercholesterolemic Men." *American Journal of Clinical Nutrition* 40 (1984):1146–55.

Kirby, R. W., et al. "Oat Bran Intake Selectively Lowers Serum Low-Density Lipoprotein Cholesterol Concentrations of Hypercholesterolemic Men." *American Journal of Clinical Nutrition* 34 (1981):824–29.

Liebman, B. "What Is This Thing Called Oat Bran?" and "Hot Cereals." *Nutrition Action Health Letter* 12, No. 9 (December 1985):7–11. Center for Science in the Public Interest, 1501 16th Street N.W., Washington, D.C. 20036.

Chapter 9

American Diabetes Association. "Glycemic Effects of Carbohydrates. A Policy Statement of the American Diabetes Association." *Diabetes Forecast* (May/June 1985):20–21; also in *Diabetes Care* (November/December 1984).

Case, R. B., et al. "Type A Behavior and Survival After Acute Myocardial Infarction." *New England Journal of Medicine* 312 (1985):737–41.

Food and Nutrition Board, National Research Council, National Academy of Sciences. *Recommended Dietary Allowances.* 9th edition. Washington, D.C., 1980.

Friedman, M., and R. Rosenman. *Type A Behavior and Your Heart.* New York: Alfred A. Knopf, 1974.

National Institutes of Health. *Exercise and Your Heart.* NIH Publication No. 81-1677, 1981. Available from the National Heart, Lung, and Blood Institute, Bethesda, MD 20205.

Ruberman, W., et al. "Psychosocial Influences on Mortality After Myocardial Infarction." *New England Journal of Medicine* 311 (1984):552–59.

The Sodium Content of Popular Prepared Food Items. Available from Consumer Affairs, Morton Salt Division, Morton Norwich Products, 110 Wacker Drive, Chicago, IL 60606

U.S. Department of Agriculture. *The Sodium Content of Your Food.* Home and Garden Bulletin No. 233. Washington, D.C.: Government Printing Office.

U.S. Department of Health and Human Services. "Health Implications of Obesity." *National Institutes of Health Consensus Development Conference Statement* 5, No. 9 (1985). National Institutes of Health, Office of Medical Applications of Research, Building 1, Room 216, Bethesda, MD 20205.

U.S. Department of Health and Human Services. *Sodium: Facts for Older Citizens.* HHS Publication No. 83-2169. Available from the U.S. Food and Drug Administration, 5600 Fishers Lane, Rockville, MD 20857

U.S. Department of Health and Human Services. "Treatment of Hypertriglyceridemia." *National Institutes of Health Consensus Development Conference Statement* 4, No. 8 (1983). National Institutes of Health, Office of Medical Applications of Research, Building 1, Room 216, Bethesda, MD 20205.

U.S. Department of Health and Human Services, Public Health Service, National Institutes of Health. *The 1984 Report of the Joint National Committee on Detection, Evaluation, and Treatment of High Blood Pressure.* NIH Publication No. 84-1088; also in *Archives of Internal Medicine* 144 (1984):1045–57.

U.S. Surgeon General. *The Health Consequences of Smoking: Cardiovascular Disease.* A Report of the Surgeon General, November 1983. Available from the Office on Smoking and Health, 5600 Fishers Lane, Parklawn Building, Room 110, Rockville, MD 20857.

Chapter 12

National Cholesterol Education Program. "Report of the Expert Panel on Blood Cholesterol Levels in Children and Adolescents."

INDEX